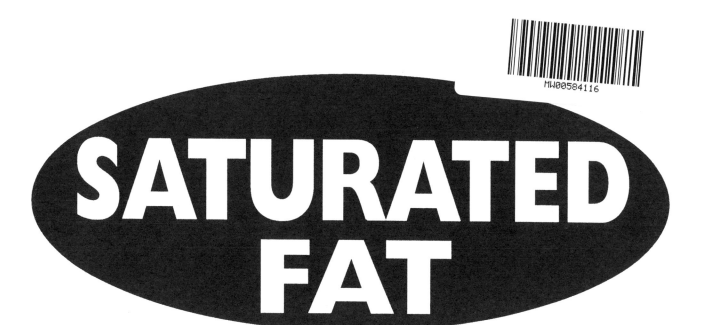

SATURATED FAT

MAY
SAVE
YOUR
LIFE

by
Bruce Fife
N.D.

Foreword by Charles T. McGee, M.D.

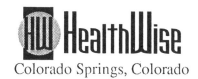

HealthWise
Colorado Springs, Colorado

Acknowledgments:
Grateful acknowledge is given to Charles T. McGee, M.D., and Maria
Miles, M.S., C.N., for their help and encouragement in preparing this
work.

Cover design by Michael Donahue

Published by **HealthWise Publications** an imprint of:
Piccadilly Books, Ltd.
P.O. Box 25203
Colorado Springs, CO 80936, USA

International sales and inquires contact:
 EPS
 20 Park Drive
 Romford Essex RM1 4LH, UK
or
 EPS
 P.O. Box 1344
 Studio City, CA 91614, USA

Library of Congress Cataloging-in-Publication Data

Fife, Bruce, 1952-
        Saturated fat may save your life / Bruce Fife.
            p.   cm.
        Includes bibliographical references and index.
        ISBN 0-941599-49-3 (pbk.)
        1. Saturated fatty acids in human nutrition. 2. Unsaturated fatty acids
    in human nutrition. 3. Antioxidants--Physiological effect.
    I. Title.
    QP752.S37F53   1999
    613.2'84--dc21   99-37568

Simultaneously Published in Australia, UK, and USA
Printed in Canada

TABLE OF CONTENTS

FOREWORD

In 1976 I attended a most unusual alternative medicine meeting. One presenter, Alsoph Corwin, Ph.D., professor of chemistry emeritus of Johns Hopkins University, appeared on stage dressed in full chef's uniform complete with a tall white hat topped with ruffles. He explained that in place of a lecture he was giving us a cooking lesson.

First, he filled a laboratory beaker with cold pressed vegetable oil. With the lights off he passed what I remember as an ultraviolet light through the oil onto a white screen. The screen remained white. After bringing the oil to a boil he again passed light through the oil. This time the screen filled with a pink color.

Dr. Corwin explained this change occurred because the shape of fatty acid molecules in the oil had been altered by heating, and this changed optical properties of the oil. Angled *cis* bonds between carbons had been straightened out to form abnormal *trans* bonds. He went on to elaborate how pervasive trans fatty acids were in the modern diet as well as suspected health risks that may follow their consumption.

This served as my introduction to lipids (fats). My readings in nutrition to that point extended into vitamins, minerals, high- and low-fat diets, vegetarianism, and such, but the dark and ominous area of lipids I intentionally postponed repeatedly. Suddenly oils, butter, and lard expanded into terms such as saturated, unsaturated, monounsaturated, polyunsaturated, hydrogenated, cis, trans, cholesterol, cholesterol esters, monoglycerides, diglycerides, triglycerides, EPA, GLA, HDL, HDL-1, HDL-2, HDL-3, native LDL, oxidized LDL, phospholipids, and on and on. What a headache to decipher. But there is a purpose involved in understanding fats and it involves most of the common modern diseases that kill us.

As our population ages we are becoming more aware of the preponderance of degenerative diseases such as heart attack, diabetes, cancer, arthritis, allergies, osteoporosis, and a long list of others. Oddly, people in primitive lifestyle cultures seldom suffer degenerative diseases, which led Europeans to call them "diseases of civilization." But when exposed to the diets and ways of modern civilization these same people develop degenerative diseases the same as we. Obviously this can not be explained by some temporary genetic protection.

Two pioneers stand out as making great strides in explaining why we suffer from these "diseases of civilization." American dentist Weston Price studied oral health patterns in primitive people around the world from 1930 to 1940. British epidemiologist T.L. Cleave, M.D., studied the onset of degenerative diseases in developing areas of the world from about 1940 to 1970. Both discovered a similar pattern. People remained free of degenerative diseases as long as they continued to eat only the fresh unprocessed foods of their region, regardless of the mix of foods available or fat content. All other variables pale by comparison.

As soon as a store opened selling what is commonly called "junk" food (candy, white flour crackers, soda pop, jam, jellies, etc.) the oral health of unborn children and those born afterward quickly degenerated. Tooth decay became rampant and crooked teeth were seen for the first time. Exceptions occurred only when a mother rejected the modern foods and remained on the traditional diet. Other forms of physical degeneration followed down the road. Cleave found diseases such as diabetes, high blood pressure, and heart attacks began to be seen about 20 to 30 years after the introduction of refined carbohydrates into the diet. This lag made the connection very abstract and difficult to piece together. I have been unable to find records of any exception to this general pattern.

The dietary changes involved were numerous and involved the introduction of previously absent white flour, white rice, refined sugar, heat treated oils, and other refined foods. It is easy to show these changes decrease intake of vitamins, minerals, and antioxidants. There may be more subtle changes as well. I believe we are naive to conclude other, yet undiscovered changes may not be going on, possibly in the area of electromagnetic properties of foods as believed in Chinese medicine. At the same time, pollutants are entering the environment increasing the need for micronutrients and antioxidants. These changes in diet and health occurred worldwide over the past century and have made healthy primitive people a thing of the past.

All is not lost. Some good things have happened giving us ways to fight back and protect our own personal health. First of all, it is easier to return to a healthy diet than it was 25 or 30 years ago. With improvements in transportation, fresh fruits and vegetables are available throughout the year, not only in season, and sales of fresh produce have risen sharply. Whole grain products also are more widely available and gaining in market share.

Also important are the increasing numbers of people taking supplements of vitamins, minerals, and antioxidants. It is hard to find a closer association than the 50% decline in deaths from heart attacks since 1968 and the increase in consumption of vitamins, especially the antioxidant vitamin E, as well as vitamin B-6, and folic acid both of which help keep down blood levels of homocysteine. It has even become commonplace for cardiology offices to recommend vitamin E supplements to their patients. A mere 10 years ago TV evening news programs condemned vitamin supplements as a waste of money and implied those who took them were not functioning with a full deck (even though surveys found vitamin users had above average educational levels).

The message is clear. You can prevent or ameliorate most degenerative diseases, but you will need to make the effort yourself. If you go along with what everyone else is doing you will become another degenerative disease statistic. This book provides many avenues to aid you in this direction as Dr. Fife takes aim at the role of lipids in health and disease. But remember, the playing field is not level and the water has been muddied intentionally by vested interests with huge financial stakes at risk.

Lurking behind the scenes are powerful multinational corporations that have products to protect and make sales directly related to your buying habits and lack of reliable information. These interests have long tentacles of influence that reach into nutrition education in schools and universities, media advertising, and on to governmental agencies that determine public health policy and what research ideas get funded or not. Food processing giants promote the cholesterol theory and the saturated fat phobia that leads people to buy trans fat containing oils and margarine. Drug companies are happy to support the cholesterol hypothesis as it leads to the sale of expensive cholesterol-lowering drugs. The fat theory had been good for both industries enriching their bottom lines by the billions.

Fortunately you have the option of going down another path to seek answers elsewhere. If you use your head, you may be able to die young at a ripe old age.

Charles T. McGee, M.D.

Introduction

A NEW LOOK AT DIET AND HEALTH

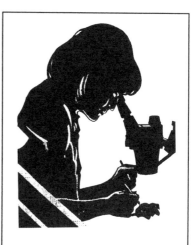

Carmen, a 62-year-old patient, was surprised when her doctor told her that X-rays showed several small tumors in her breast. "I've been very careful about what I eat," she told him. "I watch my weight, don't eat much red meat, sweets, or other bad foods. I can't understand why I should have this problem."

"How much fat and oil do you eat," the doctor asked?

"I avoid most foods high in saturated fat and cholesterol. I eat chicken and fish occasionally. The only oil I use is the healthy kind—polyunsaturated like safflower and margarine made from soybean oil."

"I'm going to put you on a *saturated fat* diet," he said deliberately waiting for her reaction.

"What!" she questioned? "I've tried to avoid saturated fat. Isn't it unhealthy?"

"That all depends. Some fats can increase the risk of certain disease, but not all fats are the same. Fat is essential to good health and some saturated fats actually promote improvement in circulation and boost the immune system. This may be what you need to rid yourself of these lumps. It's either this or surgery or drug therapy. You make the choice."

"It sounds too simple."

"I believe the less dramatic treatments, like dietary changes, should be a patient's first step at correcting degenerative problems like cancer that have taken years to develop. If that doesn't work we can always try another route."

The doctor had Carmen eliminate all vegetable oils including margarine and shortening from her diet. These were to be replaced with butter (high in saturated fat and cholesterol) and coconut oil (one of the richest sources of dietary saturated fat). He also had her take a daily vitamin supplement. Eggs were allowed as were moderate amounts of meat, chicken, and fish. But under no circumstances was she to have vegetable oils or foods containing them.

It was easy to replace vegetable oil with butter and coconut oil. She enjoyed the rich flavor they gave her foods. The hard part was avoiding packaged foods prepared with vegetable oils. Most frozen and packaged foods use vegetable oil in one form or another. But she soon found which brands didn't and began cooking more foods from scratch. Besides, she said, "They tasted better now that I could use the more flavorful saturated oils."

"At first I was concerned about adding saturated fat to my diet. I thought it would clog up my arteries and perhaps lead to heart disease. My doctor reassured me that this wouldn't happen."

After three months Carmen returned to the doctor for a follow-up examination. "I was surprised when the mammograms revealed absolutely no signs of the

"A wise man ought to realize that health is his most valuable possession."

—Hippocrates

"To a greater extent than most of us are willing to accept, today's disorders of overweight, heart disease, cancer, blood pressure, and diabetes are by and large preventable. In this light, true health insurance is not what one carries on a plastic card, but what one does for oneself."

—Lawrence Power, M.D.

tumorous lumps which I had previously. This 'saturated fat diet' really worked."

THE SATURATED FAT MYTH

If you want to reduce body fat as well as reduce your risk for stroke, heart disease, atherosclerosis, cancer and many other degenerative diseases you should eat *more* saturated fat and *less* polyunsaturated fat. In fact, using saturated fat in your diet may be one of the healthiest decisions you can make—*if* it is the right kind. Sound farfetched? It's not.

It comes as a surprise to most people to learn that there are many different types of saturated fat. Each of these fats affect our bodies in different ways. For decades scientific studies on dietary fats falsely accused *all* saturated fats of raising blood cholesterol levels and contributing to cardiovascular disease. While excess consumption of saturated fats in general may contribute to some health problems, not all saturated fats are the same. Tropical oils (coconut, palm, and palm kernel oils) are especially high in saturated fat, yet provide many health benefits.

It's been noted that Polynesians and the Bicolanos of the Philippines, whose daily diet consists of a great deal of saturated fat from coconut oil, have low blood cholesterol levels and little coronary heart disease. This has been an enigma. These observations conflict with the current belief that saturated fat contributes to heart disease. According to the prevailing theories, these island people should have a high incidence of cardiovascular disease. But they don't.

Most of our lives we've been told that unsaturated oils are good and saturated oils are bad. Many of you reading this now may have doubts that some saturated oils are not as bad as what you've been told and that they may even be beneficial. Although saturated fat has been labeled a major player in the development of heart disease and cardiovascular degeneration, recent research proves otherwise. In fact, some types of saturated fats have the opposite effect, reducing risk of cardiovascular disease and lowering total blood fat content, making them far more healthy than even most unsaturated oils—including the highly regarded olive oil.

Because saturated fat has been labeled as the bad guy among oils, presumably less harmful ones have replaced them in much of our foods. These presumably less harmful oils are the polyunsaturated fats. You see the word "polyunsaturated" proudly displayed on foods as if it had some healthful benefit. We have tended to believe these marketing gimmicks as honest concerns for consumers' health.

Some research suggests that polyunsaturated oils may reduce the risk of cardiovascular disease by lowering blood cholesterol. Although they may reduce cholesterol levels, they do not remove plaque deposits or heal damaged arteries.

Some of polyunsaturated oils may reduce the risk of heart and circulatory disease by thinning the blood. That is, some oils lower the blood's ability to form clots, thus reducing the chance of having a clot plug up an artery to a vital organ causing serious or even fatal consequences. But other types of polyunsaturated oils have just the opposite effect—they increase the blood's tendency to clot, thus increasing risk of heart attack and stroke. Unfortunately, the vast majority of the polyunsaturated oils in our foods are the wrong kind.

Recent research has demonstrated that all polyunsaturated oils stimulate growth of tumors and can cause cancer. Because they have been linked to cancer, diabetes, obesity, and other health problems, many researchers now consider them more dangerous than saturated fat.

It appears that saturated fats, particularly certain types of saturated fat, are actually beneficial and that polyunsaturated fats are the ones that are truly hazardous to your health. This new view on health opens many exciting possibilities and solves the riddle to many enigmas in medicine that have baffled researchers and health care professionals for years.

A BIG FAT LIE

The warning to reduce consumption of fat, specifically saturated fat and cholesterol, is found everywhere we look. Many doctors are now advocating very low-fat diets to help fight heart disease and other degenerative conditions. Over the past few decades fat has emerged as the biggest threat to health that mankind has ever faced. Everybody blames their health problems on excess fat. It has become a convenient battle cry. But how bad is it really? After all, people have been eating saturated fat and cholesterol for thousands of years. Why, suddenly, is it now considered a health problem when it wasn't before? Much of what we hear is nothing more than a big fat lie. Fat is actually a necessary part of our diet and a vital component of our bodies.

We often think that the less fat we have on our bodies and the less we eat, the better. If you weigh 150 pounds, but are not overweight, your body would contain 30 pounds of fat. This fat serves an important purpose. We need it to be healthy. In fact, without it we would be dead. Fat provides a protective cushion for delicate organs, helps regulate body temperature by insulating us against environmental extremes, is involved in the production of vital hormones, and provides a readily accessible source of energy when food is restricted or physical activity is increased. Vitamins A, D, E, and K, as well as beta-carotene, all of which are essential to good health and the maintenance of life, are found in the lipid (fat) component of vegetable and animal foods. Fats, or lipids form a major part of the structure in all of our cells, particularly the cell membrane.

Every cell in our bodies must have a continual source of energy to keep it functional and living. This need for energy is so vital to the life of the cell that interruption even for a moment would bring death. This need for a continual supply of energy is satisfied primarily by the fat stored in our bodies. Fat provides the calories we need between meals and during times of prolonged fasting. Stored fat supplies about 60 percent of the body's ongoing energy needs when we are at rest. When exercising or during prolonged periods without food, fat stores make an even greater contribution to our energy needs.

One of the most important fats in our bodies is cholesterol—yes, cholesterol, the so-called evil villain of the dinner plate. Cholesterol is so important to the basic operations of life that without it, every cell in our body would become dead masses of fat and protein. Cholesterol is found in all body tissues and comprises an integral part of the cell membrane. Nine-tenths of all the body's cholesterol is located in the external and internal membranes of cells. It is essential in the production of nerve tissues. It is used by the body to make bile acids necessary for digestion of fats and fat-soluble vitamins. We get most of our vitamin D from cholesterol. Our bodies transform cholesterol into a variety of important hormones such as estrogen, progesterone, testosterone, DHEA, cortisol, and others. If we had no cholesterol we would be sexless. That is, there would be no male or female differentiation and reproduction would be impossible.

Cholesterol deficiency, however, is usually not a problem. Its presence is so vital to health that if we don't get it in our diet, the body will synthesize it in the liver from other nutrients. Your liver is manufacturing cholesterol right now at the rate of about 50,000,000,000,000,000 molecules per second. The raw materials that the liver uses to make cholesterol can be derived from carbohydrate, protein, or fat (both saturated or unsaturated).

The body tries to maintain a balance between the amount we eat and the amount manufactured in the liver. If we eat little then the liver will produce more. If we eat more

the liver produces less. This is why even drastic decreases in dietary cholesterol intake often produce only small drops in blood cholesterol levels.[1] Often we eat too much and the body has an excess. The excess is then broken down by the liver and converted into triglycerides (fat molecules) to be stored as body fat.

Fat is not the villain it is often made out to be; however, not all fats are alike. Some dietary fats are good for us, some are not so good, and others are downright dangerous. The problem is that many of the good fats are condemned as bad and the truly bad ones are praised as good. Even many health professionals are confused and lead people astray with erroneous dietary advice. Many people right now are consuming oils they think are good for them or at least not harmful, but in actuality they are destroying their health. Are you one of these people?

A PARADIGM SHIFT

In science you'll find that every significant breakthrough required a break with, or a breakaway from, old ways of thinking. If ideas don't change there is no progress, no improvement. We become stagnant. The way we see and interpret the world is called a paradigm. It's the philosophy upon which we base our decisions and govern our life. All great breakthroughs in science involved paradigmatic shifts in thinking or in the accepted ideas of the time. By looking at things differently, from a totally different perspective, revolutionary changes can occur.

When the germ theory was first proposed in the late 19th century it was a paradigmatic shift in thinking. Before that time sanitary conditions were appalling. Hospitals were often breeding grounds for disease. Soldiers in war died more from infections than they did in battle. A minor injury could be just as deadly as a serious battle wound. Operating tables were simply doused with a bucket of water to "clean" them for the next patient. Childbed fever, a mysterious disease, which killed women and their newborn infants, rose to epidemic proportions, claiming the lives of up to 50 percent of the women in certain hospitals. Its cause was finally shown to be a result of physicians simply not washing their hands between patients or even after performing autopsies. No wonder so many relatively healthy people died when they went to the hospital!

When Louis Pasteur introduced the germ theory an entirely new understanding of disease was discovered. With the germ theory, childbed fever and many other illnesses were finally understood. Measures could be taken to prevent the spread of infectious disease. Attention to hygiene and sanitation over the past century and a half has done more to improve health and lengthen life expectancy than any

---

Saturated Fat and Cholesterol

- Dietary fat supplies fat-soluble vitamins A, D, E, K, and beta-carotene.
- Cholesterol is necessary in making estrogen, progesterone, testosterone, and DHEA.
- Saturated fat and cholesterol are vitally important structural components of every cell in our bodies.
- Fat is necessary for proper digestion and absorption of dietary nutrients.

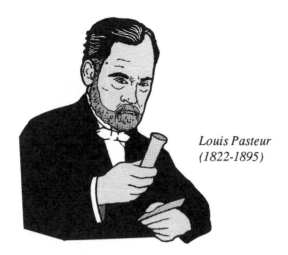

Louis Pasteur
(1822-1895)

other advancement in medical science. With this paradigmatic shift in thinking new, more effective, medical procedures and treatments were developed. Medical science took a giant leap forward.

History is full of examples of how a paradigm shift has revolutionized science. But changes in thinking aren't always welcomed with open arms, in fact, they usually encounter stiff opposition for many years. Often, a generation must pass before a new paradigm is fully accepted.

At one time, bloodletting was an accepted, time-honored treatment for most every illness from scurvy to pneumonia. The theory was that the removal of diseased blood or fluid from the body would facilitate healing. If one bleeding wasn't enough, it was performed again and again, if necessary, until the patient improved—or died. The latter was often the case. Bloodletting was a standard medical procedure for hundreds of years. If you were a doctor back then and refused to use this method of treatment, saying it was useless and perhaps even harmful, you would be branded a quack and ridiculed as incompetent or even dangerous. In retrospect, we can see it was really the other way around. Since that time, medical science has gone through a paradigm shift in regard to bloodletting.

Those insightful pioneers who propose changes in the established way of thinking are often persecuted. The classic example of this is Galileo. During his day it was believed that the earth was the center of the universe and the sun, moon, and planets revolved around it. This idea had prevailed for well over a thousand years. Anyone could plainly see that the sun, moon, and stars, *moved* overhead. The concept was endorsed by the Church because the Bible stated that the sun "moved" in the heavens. All the respected authorities both ancient and modern accepted this belief.

With the invention of the telescope, Galileo observed the heavens and made astonishing discoveries that revealed that the earth was not the center of the universe and that it moved around the sun along with the other planets. This aroused severe antagonism from traditionalist professors of science and also from Church authorities. In 1616 the Church declared these new ideas contrary to Holy Scriptures and any book teaching it was prohibited—this prohibition was not lifted until 1757—141 years later. Despite the scientific evidence presented by Galileo, he was forbidden to teach his new theory. Eventually he was forced to recant his observations and sentenced to life in prison. His sentence was served in the solitude of his home where he was confined until the day he died.

When people heard Galileo's theories they scoffed. It's impossible. He's eccentric. A troublemaker they thought. They must have reasoned, "We can see the sun, moon, and stars and they all move around the earth, not the sun. If the earth moved, we would be sure to feel it, but we don't." To the people of his day Galileo's ideas made no sense. It was only later through the works of Kepler and Newton that his observations and ideas were proven correct.

Today, we need another paradigmatic shift in thinking. The current paradigm involving the treatment of degenerative disease hasn't worked. In 1971 President Richard Nixon declared "War on Cancer." Millions of dollars poured into funding cancer research in an all out attack. The fight against cancer was on and researchers worked at a frantic pace. People fully expected this enormous effort would soon end in the discovery of the long awaited cure. It's been nearly 30 years since the "war" was declared and we are still no closer to a cure now than we were then. The number of new cancers is higher now than it has ever been. Dr. Samuel Epstein, professor of environmental medicine at the University of Illinois stated: "Our ability to cure most advanced cancers scarcely has improved since 1971. For example, the five-year survival rate for non-localized breast cancer remains a static 18%. Cancers of the breast, of prostate and colon in men have escalated 60%; cancers in children 30%." It seems we have lost the war against cancer.

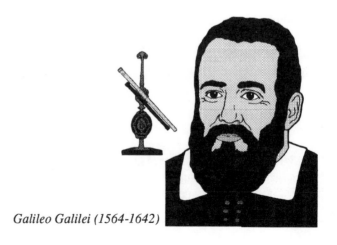

Galileo Galilei (1564-1642)

Heart disease has been our biggest cause of death since the 1950s. Despite the fact that low-fat foods are readily available and we all make efforts to limit consumption of saturated fat and cholesterol, heart disease still remains our number one killer. With the development of new technology, new drugs, and increasing medical knowledge, the occurrence of degenerative disease continues to rise. What we are doing now—our present paradigm—obviously isn't working. We need a paradigmatic shift in thinking in regard to preventing and curing degenerative disease.

Current methods of preventing and treating disease focus primarily on removing or masking the symptoms without solving the underlying problem. Once a person gets cancer, for example, the chances that cancer will return are very high. Some doctors have reported that all of their cancer patients who have been successfully treated with conventional methods eventually get cancer again.

It's time to take a new look at health and disease. If you can change your paradigm, your way of thinking about health, and view food in a new light, you can have better health—much better. Many people have made the shift in thinking and now realize that diet does profoundly affect health. But you need to go even farther and shift from the generally accepted idea that saturated fat and cholesterol are bad and focus on the real threat to health—polyunsaturated oils. This is a hard concept for some of us to accept because we have heard all our lives that saturated fat and cholesterol were bad for us and that vegetable oil was better, or even good for us. We even take vegetable oil supplements (i.e., flaxseed oil, evening primrose oil, etc.) in hopes of improving health. It hasn't helped.

Health conscious people who view eating too much meat and saturated fat as bad and eating vegetables as good often have a hard time accepting the fact that oils from healthy vegetables are bad for us. If vegetables are good for us how can the oil in these healthy foods be bad? The answer is that refined vegetable oils are fractionated foods, not whole foods. Fractionated foods are refined or highly processed foods in which certain chemical constituents become concentrated while, others (such as vitamins and minerals) become depleted. Sugar is a fractionated food. It comes from beets—healthy vegetables. When we eat sugar we aren't eating the beets, we are only eating one highly concentrated part of the plant, the sucrose, and it can have dramatic effects on our bodies. White flour is another fractionated food. In removing the bran, some 20 nutrients are seriously depleted. Only four or five are added back in the "enrichment" process. White rice is another fractionated food. The vitamin- and mineral-rich outer layer is removed in the

"polishing" process. Eating a diet composed predominately of products made of white flour, white rice, and other fractionated food has led to nutrient deficiency disease.

You can achieve better health by not worrying about saturated fat and cholesterol which are found naturally in our foods and start limiting refined polyunsaturated oils and other fractionated foods in your diet. When you can make this paradigm shift you will be on the road to better health.

WHAT THIS BOOK CAN DO FOR YOU

In this book you will learn many facts that will be completely new to you. You will find the answers to many questions and the solution to enigmas on health that have stumped medical professionals for years. You will discover why health in modern industrialized countries is failing despite rapid advances in medical technology.

Some of the material in this book may shock you. Information we have been led to believe for years is grossly misleading and in some cases dangerously false, but continues to be propagated by those who have a financial interest at stake. All of the facts presented in this book are documented by scientific studies and historical accounts.

Simply reducing fat intake has not proven to be effective in preventing disease. There are more factors involved. In this book you will learn how to recognize and avoid those things that can destroy your health. You will learn why the incidence of asthma, diabetes, and cancer are on the rise, why heart disease is our number one killer, but most of all, you will learn how to prevent these conditions from happening to you.

When reading this book I recommend that you cover each chapter in order to gain the most out of the material. Concepts presented build from one chapter to the next. Chapter 1 provides a brief overview of dietary oils. Chapter 2, which discusses the concept of free radicals, aging, and disease, is especially important because it lays the foundation for understanding the concepts presented throughout this book. Most of the following chapters present the facts on oils and how they relate to health and disease. Much of this is new information for most people and will cause you to think differently about diet and health.

In the final chapter of this book I describe the Antioxidant Health Plan, also referred to as the saturated fat diet described earlier in this chapter. This remarkable health plan can make a dramatic difference in your health and well-being. It has been the means by which many people have overcome degenerative health problems and put them on a road to a new and better life.

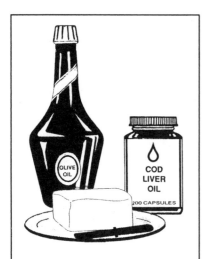

Chapter 1

DIETARY FATS AND OILS

"Many of us have a 'fat tooth' in addition to a sweet tooth."

— Andrew Weil, M.D.

Fat—the word conjures up images of grotesque, greasy tissue hanging off of a slab of meat. Meat isn't the only place we find fat. All living organisms have it. Animals have it, people have it, plants have it, even the tiniest organisms like protozoa and bacteria have it. Fat is an essential tissue to life. For this reason, fat in one form or another is found in all of our foods. And although we like to eliminate it as much as possible, it constitutes an important part of our diet.

Except for some highly processed and refined foods, such a sugar, everything we eat contains some fat or oil. Those foods which are particularly rich in fat are red meat, chicken, fish, dairy, eggs, nuts, and seeds. Fruits and vegetables also supply some fat. Nuts, seeds, and grains are the richest plant sources for oil and it is from these sources we get most of our vegetable oils.

The terms fat and oil are often used interchangeably. Generally speaking, fats are considered solid at room temperature while oils remain liquid. Lard, for example, would be referred to as a fat.

Doctors often use the term "lipid" in referring to fat. Lipid is a general term that includes several fat-like compounds in the body. By far the most abundant and the most important of the lipids are the triglycerides. When we speak of fats and oils we are usually referring to triglycerides. Two other lipids—phospholipids and sterols (which includes cholesterol)—technically are not fats because they are not triglycerides. But they have similar characteristics and are often referred to as fats.

About 95 percent of the lipids in our diet from both plant and animal sources are triglycerides. Our body fat is predominately composed of triglycerides. Triglycerides are comprised of molecules known as fatty acids. In this book I make frequent reference to the *fatty acids*. The three general categories of fatty acids are saturated, monounsaturated, and polyunsaturated.

All oils and animal fats consist of a mixture of these three fatty acids as well as other dietary fats. To say an oil is saturated or monounsaturated is grossly oversimplifying. No oil is purely saturated or polyunsaturated. Olive oil is often called "monounsaturated" because it is predominately monounsaturated, but like all vegetable oils, it also contains some polyunsaturated and saturated fat as well.

Animal fats are generally the highest in saturated fat and cholesterol. Vegetable oils contain virtually no cholesterol, but do have saturated fat as well as monounsaturated and polyunsaturated fat. Most vegetable oils are high in polyunsaturated fats, the exception being palm and coconut oils which are very high in saturated fat.

Some fatty acids are considered essential in our diet to achieve and maintain optimal health. Others, although perhaps not classified as essential, do promote good

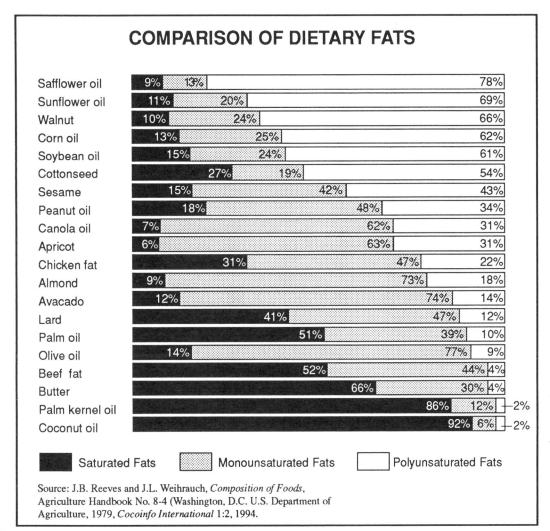

COMPARISON OF DIETARY FATS

	Saturated	Monounsaturated	Polyunsaturated
Safflower oil	9%	13%	78%
Sunflower oil	11%	20%	69%
Walnut	10%	24%	66%
Corn oil	13%	25%	62%
Soybean oil	15%	24%	61%
Cottonseed	27%	19%	54%
Sesame	15%	42%	43%
Peanut oil	18%	48%	34%
Canola oil	7%	62%	31%
Apricot	6%	63%	31%
Chicken fat	31%	47%	22%
Almond	9%	73%	18%
Avacado	12%	74%	14%
Lard	41%	47%	12%
Palm oil	51%	39%	10%
Olive oil	14%	77%	9%
Beef fat	52%	44%	4%
Butter	66%	30%	4%
Palm kernel oil	86%	12%	2%
Coconut oil	92%	6%	2%

◼ Saturated Fats ▦ Monounsaturated Fats ☐ Polyunsaturated Fats

Source: J.B. Reeves and J.L. Weihrauch, *Composition of Foods*, Agriculture Handbook No. 8-4 (Washington, D.C. U.S. Department of Agriculture, 1979, *Cocoinfo International* 1:2, 1994.

Fats and oils contain a mixture of saturated, monounsaturated, and polyunsaturated fatty acids. All vegetable oils contain saturated fat to one degree or another. Likewise, animal fats which are commonly considered saturated, are really a mixture of all three.

health and combat disease if eaten in moderation. Unfortunately, along with the "good" fats almost always come the "bad," so all sources of fat should be eaten in moderation. The best sources of essential fatty acids in our diet are whole foods such as fish, fresh vegetables, fruits, nuts, and seeds—not refined oils.

TRIGLYCERIDES

When you cut into a beef steak, the white fatty tissue you see is composed of triglycerides. Cholesterol is also present but it is intermingled within the meat fibers and undetectable with the naked eye. The fat that is a nuisance to us, the type that hangs on our arms, looks like jelly on our thighs, and makes our stomach look like a spare tire, is composed of triglycerides. It is the triglycerides that make up our body fat and the fat we see and eat in animal foods.

The fat most people talk about in terms of diet and health is cholesterol. Cholesterol, however, is not the major fat of dietary concern. Triglycerides are the ones we need to be most concerned about when it comes to diet and health.

Saturated fat is a triglyceride; so is polyunsaturated fat. Triglycerides are composed of individual fat molecules known as fatty acids. It takes three fatty acid molecules to make a single triglyceride molecule. The fatty acids are attached to a glycerol molecule which acts as a backbone so-to-speak for the triglyceride. All glycerol molecules look exactly alike, but the fatty acids may vary in size and degree of saturation.

Fatty acids are classified by their degree of saturation. The three classifications are saturated, monounsaturated, and polyunsaturated. We hear these terms used all the time, but what do they mean? All fatty acids consist primarily of a chain of carbon atoms with varying amounts of hydrogen

```
    H  H  H  H  H  H  H  O
    |  |  |  |  |  |  |  ||
H — C — C — C — C — C — C — C — O-H
    |  |  |  |  |  |  |
    H  H  H  H  H  H  H
```

Diagram of an 8-carbon chain fatty acid.

atoms attached to them. A molecule that has two hydrogen atoms attached to each carbon is said to be "saturated" with hydrogen because it is holding all the hydrogen atoms it possibly can. This type of fatty acid is called a saturated fat. A fatty acid that is missing a pair of hydrogen atoms on one of its carbons is called a monounsaturated fat. If more than two hydrogen atoms are missing, it's called a polyunsaturated fat.

The concept of saturation can be described using an analogy with a school bus full of kids. The bus could represent the carbon chain and the students the hydrogen atoms. Each seat on the bus can hold two students. A bus that filled to capacity so there are no empty seats would be analogous to a saturated fat. No more students can fit on the bus. If two students get off the bus and leave one seat vacant, that would be analogous to a monounsaturated fat. If four or more students get off the bus leaving two or more empty seats that would be like a polyunsaturated fat. A school bus that is only half filled would be like a fatty acid that is very polyunsaturated.

```
  H  H  H  H  H  H  H  H  H  H  H  H  H  H  H  H  H  O
  |  |  |  |  |  |  |  |  |  |  |  |  |  |  |  |  |  ||
H-C—C—C—C—C—C—C—C—C—C—C—C—C—C—C—C—C—C—O-H
  |  |  |  |  |  |  |  |  |  |  |  |  |  |  |  |  |
  H  H  H  H  H  H  H  H  H  H  H  H  H  H  H  H  H
```

Saturated Fatty Acid

```
  H  H  H  H  H  H  H  H        H  H  H  H  H  H  H  O
  |  |  |  |  |  |  |  |        |  |  |  |  |  |  |  ||
H-C—C—C—C—C—C—C—C—C = C—C—C—C—C—C—C—C—C—O-H
  |  |  |  |  |  |  |  |        |  |  |  |  |  |  |
  H  H  H  H  H  H  H  H        H  H  H  H  H  H  H
```

Monounsaturated Fatty Acid

```
  H  H  H  H  H        H        H  H  H  H  H  H  H  O
  |  |  |  |  |        |        |  |  |  |  |  |  |  ||
H-C—C—C—C—C—C = C—C—C = C—C—C—C—C—C—C—C—C—O-H
  |  |  |  |  |  |  |  |  |  |  |  |  |  |  |  |  |
  H  H  H  H  H  H  H  H  H  H  H  H  H  H  H  H  H
```

Polyunsaturated Fatty Acid

Above are simplified diagrams of 18-carbon chain fatty acids illustrating the difference in the molecular structure between saturated and unsaturead fats.

The length of the fatty acid chain, or size of the school bus, is also important. Some fatty acids contain only two carbon atoms while others have as many as 24. The two carbon fatty acid would be like a bus that has only two seats, so that it can carry a maximum of four students—two in each seat. A fatty acid with 24 carbons would be like a long bus with 24 seats, allowing room 48 students. Long-chain fatty acids (LCFA) are those which have chains 14 or more carbons long. Medium-chain fatty acids (MCFA) are those which have chains between 8 and 12 carbons long. Short-chain fatty acids (SCFA) are those that have chains only 2 to 8 carbons long.*

The degree of saturation and length of the carbon chain of the fatty acids determines their chemical properties and their effects on our health. The more saturated the fat and the longer the chain the harder the fat and the higher the melting point. Saturated fat, like that found in lard, is solid at room temperature. Polyunsaturated fat, like corn oil, is liquid at room temperature. Monounsaturated fat is liquid at room temperature, but in the refrigerator it begins to solidify slightly and becomes cloudy or semi-solid. Short-chain fatty acids (SCFA) are soft and fluid while long-chain fatty acids (LCFA) become thick or waxy. Butter, which is made of many short-chain saturated fatty acids, is very soft when not refrigerated and easily melts when room temperature rises on warm days. Most vegetable oils have very low melting points and, therefore, are liquid. It is the higher melting point and creamy texture of butter and butter substitutes such as margarine and shortening that give many foods their desirable qualities.

Lard and butter have generally been replaced by hydrogenated vegetables oils such as margarine and shortening. This is good for food manufacturers, because hydrogenated oils are cheaper, but it is bad for the consumer because of the health consequences. The degree of saturation and length of the carbon chain of the fatty acids is extremely important in terms of health and we will return to this topic in a later chapter. For more details on the chemical aspects of fatty acids see the appendix.

REFINED OILS

Traditionally, most oils used throughout the world come from animal fat and butter. A couple of generations ago people cooked almost all of their food using oils high in saturated fat and cholesterol.

Some peoples in certain areas of the world developed processes to extract oil from plants. One of the most popu-

---

*Long-, medium-, and short-chain fatty acids that make up a triglyceride molecule are referred to as long-, medium-, and short-chain triglycerides.

lar vegetable oils was derived from the fruit of the olive tree. Olive oil has been an important commodity since biblical times. Oil was squeezed out of the tiny fruit by screw-type presses or pounded out using a wooden funnel and hammer. The oil derived from this process also contained other substances such as water and phytochemicals (plant chemicals including vitamins and minerals). This made the oil dark in color and highly flavored which imparted the aroma and taste that made it popular. Olive oil is often extracted in a similar manner today, although much is also produced using more modern methods.

Modern processing removes all of the nonoil components of the plant, making it essentially colorless, tasteless, odorless and lacking in important nutrients. Tasteless oil is desirable if you don't like the flavor of the natural oil or desire not to have the taste of your foods affected by the oil.

The majority of vegetable oils today are highly processed and refined. In the refining process, the oil is separated from its food source with petroleum solvents and then boiled to evaporate the solvents. The oil is refined, bleached, and deodorized which involves heating to temperatures of about 400° F (200° C). Chemical preservatives are frequently added to retard oxidation.

The less processing an oil undergoes, the less damaging it is on health. The most natural oils are extracted from seeds by mechanical pressure and low temperatures, and without the use of chemicals. Oils derived by this process are referred to a "expeller pressed" or "cold pressed." These oils contain no colorings, preservatives, or chemical additives. The term "cold pressed" is not really accurate. In reality all oils are subjected to some heat in processing. Expeller pressed oils are processed at lower temperatures than refined oils—160° F (70° C) as opposed to temperatures up to 400° F (200° C).

All oils, whether cold pressed, saturated, or unsaturated are degraded or oxidized when heated. High temperatures, such as in deep frying, destroys the nutritive value of oil and alters its chemical structure. Deep-frying oxidizes all types of fats including monounsaturated and polyunsaturated vegetable oils. In fact, unsaturated vegetable oils are less stable than saturated fat and, therefore, degrade more quickly. Oxidized oils have been found to induce damage to interstitial tissues and blood vessel walls and cause numerous organ lesions in animals. Some experts believe they, even more than cholesterol or saturated fat, contribute to the development of atherosclerosis or hardening of the arteries.[1,2] The logical conclusion is to avoid using oils that have been heat processed and to not cook foods in oils at high temperatures.

The less saturated a fat is the more easily it is destroyed by heat and the more quickly it oxidizes and becomes rancid. Using high heat in the processing of polyunsaturated oils chemically alters them and they become dangerous to health. Vegetable oils should never be heated above about 325° F (160° C). Saturated fats are more tolerant to heat and make better cooking oils. Coconut, palm, and palm kernel oils, and even butter would be better for cooking.

By far the best cooking oil you can use and one of the best all round oils is coconut oil. Coconut oil has a high saturated fat content, more than lard or butter, making it a good cooking oil. Non-hydrogenated, cold processed coconut oil is perhaps the healthiest all-purpose oil you can use.

When you see oils in the store, if they are colorless, tasteless, and odorless, you know they have been highly refined and processed and contain chemical preservatives. Even if the label says "cold pressed" it could have gone through many additional stages of processing to remove all nutrients thus making it a "dead" oil. A lot of the vegetable oils in health food stores are of this type.

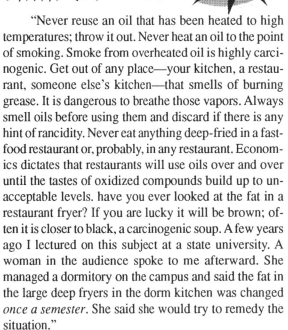

HEAT DAMAGED OILS

"Never reuse an oil that has been heated to high temperatures; throw it out. Never heat an oil to the point of smoking. Smoke from overheated oil is highly carcinogenic. Get out of any place—your kitchen, a restaurant, someone else's kitchen—that smells of burning grease. It is dangerous to breathe those vapors. Always smell oils before using them and discard if there is any hint of rancidity. Never eat anything deep-fried in a fastfood restaurant or, probably, in any restaurant. Economics dictates that restaurants will use oils over and over until the tastes of oxidized compounds build up to unacceptable levels. have you ever looked at the fat in a restaurant fryer? If you are lucky it will be brown; often it is closer to black, a carcinogenic soup. A few years ago I lectured on this subject at a state university. A woman in the audience spoke to me afterward. She managed a dormitory on the campus and said the fat in the large deep fryers in the dorm kitchen was changed *once a semester*. She said she would try to remedy the situation."

— Andrew Weil, M.D,
Natural Health, Natural Medicine

Extra virgin olive oil found in almost any grocery store is one of the least processed. It retains its aroma and flavor which enhances many dishes. It spoils quickly so must be refrigerated after opening and used within a reasonable amount of time. For this reason, it is best to purchase small quantities at a time. Virgin olive oil and especially the so-called "light" olive oil are much too refined. The best olive oil is the *extra* virgin.

HYDROGENATION

The hydrogenation of vegetable oils is done to create an artificial saturated fat. Throughout history fats used in most cultures for all cooking and baking needs were saturated like lard, beef fat, and butter. When vegetable oils came on the scene in the early 20th century they didn't produce the same desirable qualities in foods that saturated fats did. Chemists then set out to make an inexpensive saturated fat out of relatively cheap unsaturated vegetable oils.

The process, which is still used today, begins with refined vegetable oils which have already become rancid as a result of the extraction process. The oil is mixed with tiny metal particles—usually nickel oxide, which is very toxic and impossible to completely remove—to act as a chemical catalyst. Under high pressures and temperatures hydrogen gas is squeezed into the oil and chemically bonded to the fat molecules. Emulsifiers and starch are then forced into the mixture to give it a better consistency. The mixture is again subjected to high temperatures in a steam-cleaning process to remove its horrible odor. The hydrogenation process is now complete, but the resulting oil is a disgusting gray color, more like what you would expect to see in a jar of axle grease, so it is bleached to give it a more appetizing white appearance. The final result is hydrogenated vegetable oil or, as we see it on the store shelves, shortening.

Food producers saw that they could use this same process to make a cheap butter substitute. This process involves taking the shortening and adding coal-tar dyes and chemical flavorings to make it resemble butter and, as a result, margarine was born. This mixture is compressed and packaged in blocks or tubs, ready to be enjoyed on a slice of bread. Just knowing how margarine and shortening are made is enough to keep me from eating it.

In the process of hydrogenation, liquid vegetable oils become solid fats. Another thing happens that has significant health implications. A new fatty acid, unlike those normally found in nature, is created. This is called the *trans* fatty acid. This toxic fatty acid is foreign to our bodies and can create all sorts of trouble.*

"These are probably the most toxic fats ever known," says Walter Willett, M.D., professor of epidemiology and nutrition at Harvard School of Public Health. Willett, who has researched the effects of trans fats on the body, disagrees with those who say that the hydrogenated fats found in margarine or shortening are less likely to raise cholesterol than the saturated fats found in butter: "It looks like trans fatty acids are two to three times as bad as saturated fats in terms of what they do to blood lipids."[3]

Studies now clearly show that trans fatty acids can contribute to atherosclerosis and heart disease. For example, swine fed a diet containing trans fatty acids developed more extensive atherosclerotic damage than those fed other types of fats. [4]

In one study, humans consumed known amounts of trans fatty acids. This dietary change increased blood LDL (bad cholesterol) and lowered the HDL (good cholesterol), both regarded to be undesirable changes.[5] Trans fatty acids have been shown to raise blood cholesterol levels even more than saturated fat.[6] Since it also lowers the good HDL cholesterol, unlike saturated fat, many researchers now believe it has a greater influence on the development of cardiovascular disease than any other dietary fat.[7]

This observation appears to be valid. The *New England Journal of Medicine* reported the results of a 14-year study of more than 80,000 nurses (*New England Journal of Medicine* November 20, 1997). The research documented 939 heart attacks among the participants. Among the women who consume the largest amounts of trans fats, the chance of suffering a heart attack was 53 percent higher than among those at the low end of trans fat consumption.

Another interesting fact uncovered by this study was that total fat intake had little effect on the rate of heart attack. Women in the group with the largest consumption of total fat (46 percent of calories) had no greater risk of heart attack than those in the group with the lowest consumption of total fat (29 percent of calories).

The researchers, from the Harvard School of Public Health and Brigham and Women's Hospital in Boston who

---

*Trans fatty acids are formed as a result of the heat treatment of oils. The more heat applied for a longer time the more cis double bonds are converted to trans bonds. According to Russ Hume Hall, Ph.D., in his book *Food For Nought,* page 245, vegetable oils are subjected to a deodorizing process (nothing to do with hydrogenation) in which they are heated to 330° to 380° F (165° to 193° C) in a partial vacuum for 12 hours. This converts between 15-19% of the fatty acid molecules in liquid vegetable oils to trans fatty acids. Hydrogenation of oils is a separate process that is used to make oils more solid and also requires high temperatures which increases the incidence of trans bonds to the 40-48% range as in margarine. Therefore, any vegetable oil that has been subjected to high temperatures contains trans bonds. Most liquid vegetable oils sold in stores have undergone heat treatment and contain trans fatty acids.

conducted the study, said this suggested that limiting consumption of trans fats would be more effective in avoiding heart attacks than reducing overall fat intake. About 10 percent of the fat in the typical Western diet is trans fat.

Trans fatty acids affect more than just our cardiovascular health. According to Mary Enig, Ph.D., when monkeys were fed trans fat-containing margarine in their diets, their red blood cells did not bind insulin as well as when they were not fed trans.[8] This suggests a link with diabetes. Trans fatty acids have been linked with a variety of adverse health effects which include: cancer, ischemic heart disease, MS, diverticulitis, complications of diabetes, and other degenerative diseases.[9]

Hydrogenated oil is a product of technology and may be the most destructive food additive currently in common use. If you eat margarine, shortening, hydrogenated or partially hydrogenated oils (common food additives), then you are consuming trans fatty acids.

Many of the foods you buy in the store and in restaurants are prepared with or cooked in hydrogenated oil. Fried foods sold in grocery stores and restaurants are usually cooked in hydrogenated oil because it makes foods more crispy and is more resistant to spoilage than other oils. Many frozen, processed foods are cooked or prepared in hydrogenated oils. Hydrogenated oils are used in making French fries, biscuits, cookies, crackers, chips, frozen pies, pizzas, peanut butter, cake frosting, and ice cream substitutes such as mellorine.

The liquid vegetable oils you buy in the store aren't much better. The heat used in the extraction and refining process also creates trans fatty acids. So that bottle of corn or safflower oil you have on the kitchen shelf contains trans fatty acids even though it has not been hydrogenated. Unless the vegetable oil has been "cold pressed" or "expeller pressed," it contains trans fatty acids. Most all of the common brands of vegetable oil and salad dressings contain trans fatty acids.

Liquid vegetable oils contain an average of 15 percent trans fatty acids. In comparison, margarine and shortening average about 35 percent, but some brands may run as high as 48 percent.

> "When I was discussing fats with a group of medical students and mentioned solid vegetable shortenings, one student asked, 'Why do they call it shortening? What does it shorten?' Before I could respond, another student answered, 'Your life.'"
> — Andrew Weil, M.D.,
> *Natural Health, Natural Medicine*

When monounsaturated and polyunsaturated oils are used in cooking, especially at high temperatures, trans fatty acids are formed. So even if you use cold pressed oil from the health food store or olive oil, if you use it in your cooking, you are creating unhealthy trans fatty acids. The purpose of buying the "healthy" oil is defeated if you cook it.

You might ask: does the amount of trans fatty acids that are produced when you heat oils at home pose any real danger? Studies show diets containing heat-treated liquid corn oil were found to produce more atherosclerosis than those containing unheated corn oil.[10] So, *yes any unsaturated vegetable oil becomes toxic when heated.* And even a small amount, especially if eaten frequently over time, will affect your health.

Saturated fats, from any source, are much more tolerant to temperatures used in cooking and do not form trans fatty acids, and therefore, make much better cooking oils. Saturated fats are the only oils that should be used in cooking, just as they were in our grandparents' day and throughout all of history. Modern technology in an effort to create a cheap source of oil from polyunsaturated vegetable sources has created a major health problem. This will be discussed further in later chapters.

FAKE FATS

Turning on the evening news, Jean, a 49-year-old, sat down to enjoy a bag of potato chips before going to bed. These chips weren't the ordinary type she'd eaten before, but a new brand made with the fat substitute olestra. At the time, this product was recently introduced on the market and heavily promoted as a "healthy" alternative to those made with ordinary fat. It was touted as a way to help reduce fat calories and cut risk of heart disease.

"Normally I can eat anything without becoming sick," she says. An hour after going to bed she suffered gas pains "so sharp and of such a magnitude that I would say it was almost like the beginning of labor."

As the pains began to subside she was hit with repeated waves of diarrhea. The rest of the night was spent in torment. Jean is just one of thousands who have had messy runins with olestra.

Olestra (also known by the trade name Olean) is a fat substitute made from sugar and soybean oil. It is designed to have the taste and texture of fat, but because its molecules are too large for the body to digest, it generally passes through the digestive tract unabsorbed. The advantage to a fat that passes through the body without being digested is obvious—no calories! The makers of olestra have promoted products made with this new fat as safe and healthy, cheerfully trumpeting that you can "eat like a kid again," snacking on junk foods without guilt. Olestra was created for use in snack foods and Frito-Lay has developed an entire line of WOW! potato and corn chips made with the artificial fat.

Regular chips deliver 150 calories and 10 grams of fat per serving, while the new WOW! chips deliver only 75 calories and 0 grams of fat. It sounds like a junk food junkie's dream, but watch out. This fake fat can have serious health consequences. Because it is not digested well, it can have a laxative effect, especially if eaten in large quantities. This is what Jean discovered after her late evening snack. Olean's manufacturer, Procter & Gamble, received more than 13,000 reports of adverse reactions from customers when Frito-Lay started test-marketing olestra-containing chips in select cities. Complaints ranged from mild stomach upset to cramps so severe that, in scores of cases, the victims needed to be hospitalized. While most people may not experience any immediate problems, especially if they only eat the chips occasionally, repeated use may cause some serious problems down the line.

An even bigger danger than abdominal cramping and loose stools is the fact that olestra inhibits the absorption of important fat-soluble vitamins (A, D, E, and K). Each of these vitamins are essential to health. Since olestra is pushed through the digestive tract without being absorbed, it pulls these vitamins out along with it. So even if you eat vegetables containing these vitamins with an olestra-containing food, these vitamins will not do you any good. Also, eating foods containing olestra means that other foods containing vitamins are eaten less. All of this combined can lead to serious vitamin deficiencies. Because of these potential health problems, the FDA has required all products made with this artificial fat to carry warning labels which read: "This Product Contains Olestra. Olestra may cause abdominal cramping and loose stools. Olestra inhibits the absorption of some vitamins and other nutrients."

To compensate for the loss of these nutrients, products containing olestra are required to add the four fat-soluble vitamins. However, manufacturers are not required to add beta-carotene or other carotenoids—another group of fat-soluble nutrients. The carotenoids are potent antioxidants have been shown to offer significant protection against cancer, heart disease, and macular degeneration—the leading cause of blindness in the elderly.

While portrayed as a natural product, because it is made from sugar and soybean oil, it is as synthetic as rubber and even more unnatural than the trans fatty acids found in hydrogenated oils. Olestra is completely unlike any substance found in nature and our bodies have no way of handling it. Because of this, the National Advertising Division of the Council of Better Business Bureaus ruled the Procter & Gamble's ads were inaccurate when they portrayed olestra as a natural product that looks like vegetable oil.

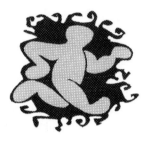

Fake fats are creeping into our foods.

Olestra is only the first of many artificial fats that are now beginning to come onto the market and are finding their way into a variety of foods. Foods you're eating now may be made with one of these synthetic substitutes. Salatrim (also called Benefat) is Nabisco's answer to olestra. Salatrim is used in "Fat-Free" cookies, chocolate chips, and other foods. Like olestra, products containing salatrim can also cause nausea and cramps. But, unlike olestra, products with salatrim are not required to carry warning labels, so you have to carefully read the ingredients label.

Other fake fats to hit the grocery shelves include Oatrim, Z-Trim, and Nu-Trim. These fat substitutes are finding their way into cookies, cakes, brownies, ice cream, pie and all sorts of baked goods and desserts. Because these products are low in absorbable fat and low in calories, products made with them are touted as "Low-Fat," "Non-Fat," or "Heart-Healthy." Watch out for any product with these labels. Since artificial fats are relatively new, their effect on health is still under question.

Food is supposed to nourish us. Products containing these fake fats are only providing empty calories that rob us of the nutrients we need to fight disease and slow down the effects of aging. It's amazing that some people will choose to eat foods simply because they are indigestible.

ANIMAL FATS

For thousands of years the primary type of oil used by man was derived from animals. It wasn't until the early 20th century that technology developed to the point where vegetable oils became readily available. Beginning in the 1950s scientific studies seemed to implicate saturated fat and cholesterol as primary suspects in a number of diseases, most notably heart disease, which by this time had become the number one killer in most industrialized nations. The people living in less affluent countries were not affected by heart disease or other degenerative conditions. Since the people in these poorer countries usually ate less meat and dairy products, this suggested that the cause for our skyrocketing disease rate was connected with animal foods. Fat was considered the primary culprit.

Since then we have been on an anti-fat campaign, especially when it comes to saturated fat and cholesterol, both of which are derived primarily from animals. Many studies seem to verify this hypothesis. But there are some problems with this theory. Some less developed cultures, however, that eat foods high in animal fat, have virtually no heart disease or other related problems. It has also been noted that before vegetable oils were readily available, most people ate oils high in saturated fat and cholesterol, and heart disease, cancer, and other "modern" illnesses were not the problem as they are today.

Just eating foods rich in saturated fat and cholesterol is not the problem—doing so may increase risk—but there are other important factors that also play a part. These factors may be more important than the amount of saturated fat and cholesterol in our diets.

One of the changes that has occurred over the past several decades is the increasing use of chemicals in our environment. This may be one key ingredient in the increased incidence of degenerative disease in industrialized countries.

Because of the pervasiveness of chemicals used in the environment and in raising animals, tallow (fat from beef, lamb, and other animals), lard (pig fat), dairy (butter, milk, cheese, etc.) and other animal products that contain fat are now dangerously toxic. They're toxic not because of the saturated fat, but because of the contaminants they contain. Insecticides, hormones, antibiotics, etc., that are fat-soluble collect in the fatty tissues of animals. When we eat animal products we are eating their lifetime accumulation of toxins.

Cattle are routinely fed hormones to stimulate growth and antibiotics to reduce chance of infection. Synthetic hormones increase milk production of dairy cows. Some of these hormones were originally used by humans but discontinued because they caused cancer and other health problems.[11] In chickens, poisons such as arsenic are added to feed to make egg shells harder and less susceptible to breakage. Corn, soybeans, hay and other crops grown for animal feed are sprayed heavily with pesticides, herbicides, and fungi-

cides, even more so than those for human consumption. All these toxins collect in the fatty tissues of the animals and, when we eat meat or dairy, we are consuming a toxic cocktail.

Farmers have a high incidence of cancer and other diseases as a result of their use and exposure to pesticides. Israel had the world's highest incidence of breast cancer when they allowed the insecticide lindane to be used in dairies, and the cancer rate decreased immediately after the government prohibited its use. *Science News* reported in 1992 and again in 1994 that women with breast cancer have very high levels of agricultural pesticides in their breasts. Crops fed to animals are sprayed heavily with insecticides. Residues from spraying is always present in the produce. Approximately ninety-five percent of the pesticide residue we are exposed to in our food comes not from fruits or vegetables, as you might expect, but from eating meat and dairy products.[12]

Meat contains approximately 14 times more pesticides than do plant foods; dairy products 5.5 times more. By eating foods of animal origin, we ingest greatly concentrated amounts of hazardous chemicals.[13]

Studies have shown that the greatest amount of pesticide residue in foods is found in meat, fish and poultry. The next greatest amount is found in dairy products followed by vegetable oils, leafy vegetables, fruits, legumes, grains, and root vegetables in that order.[14] Note that after animal products, vegetable oil has the highest degree of contamination. This makes sense, since fat-soluble toxins accumulate in the fatty tissues of both animals and plants. When oils are extracted from plants so are the pesticides they have absorbed.

Tons of pesticides are sprayed on corn, soybeans, cotton, sunflowers, and safflower crops which are used to make vegetable oil and to feed livestock. As a result, the fats and oils we eat, particularly from animal products, may be dreadfully contaminated.

Chapter 2

OXIDATION AND FREE RADICALS

THE FREE RADICAL

What do all the following conditions have in common: heart disease, atherosclerosis, stroke, cancer, varicose veins, hemorrhoids, hypertension, wrinkled skin, dermatitis, aging spots, arthritis, digestive problems, reproductive problems, cataracts, loss of energy, diabetes, and failing memory? You might say that all of these conditions are associated with aging, but age is *not* the cause. Indeed, even young people suffer from many of these ills. The one thing that ties all these conditions together, as well as most other degenerative diseases, is *free radicals*. Free radicals, also known simply as *radicals,* are renegade molecules that attack and destroy other molecules. Any tissue in our body can be damaged by free-radical reactions. It is the accumulation of this damage over many years that results in degeneration of body tissues and loss of function that typifies the symptoms of old age.

Of all the factors that affect human health, the free radical is the most insidious. It doesn't attack suddenly like food poisoning or eboli, but is equally as dangerous. A single free radical can do little damage, but the cumulative effect of millions over many years has the power of a stick of dynamite. Like an underwater demolition team, they creep upon us unnoticed, slowly sabotaging our health year after year. Health declines slowly and disease develops ever so gradually that we take little notice. In the meantime, free radicals are also forming alliances with other health-destroying factors such as viruses and toxins to increase the pain and suffering we endure. In one way or another, free radicals are involved in all major diseases that afflict mankind. They are not necessarily the cause of all disease, but they are accomplices. Understanding what free radicals are and where they come from will arm you with knowledge to defend yourself against much of the destruction they can cause to your health.

As you remember from your high school science class, atoms are composed of negatively charged electrons orbiting a positively charged nucleus. Electrons travel around the nucleus within certain limits called orbitals. Each orbital can hold two electrons. Orbitals are arranged into energy levels or shells, depending on their distance from the nucleus. In order to satisfy bonding requirements and maintain a state of equilibrium, electrons tend to associate in pairs within the orbitals. A molecule consists of two or more atoms.

A free radical can be defined as an atom capable of independent existence that contains an unpaired electron in its outer shell. Molecules can be free radicals if one or more of the atoms present has unpaired electrons. An unpaired electron is one that is alone in an orbital.

20

Free radicals of different types vary widely in their chemical reactivity, but in general they are more reactive than nonradicals. The oxygen molecule (O_2) qualifies as a free radical because it contains two unpaired electrons. Fortunately, however, oxygen is not a particularly reactive free radical.[1]

Most biological molecules are nonradicals, containing only paired electrons. An electron occupying an orbital by itself is unstable and, therefore, generally more reactive than nonradicals. Some radicals are very highly reactive and destructive. These radicals will quickly attack and steal an electron from a neighboring atom. The second atom, now with one less electron, becomes a highly reactive free radical itself and pulls an electron off yet another nearby molecule. This process continues in a destructive chain reaction that may affect hundreds and even thousands of molecules.

Once a molecule becomes a radical, its physical and chemical properties change. The normal function of such molecules is permanently disrupted, affecting the entire cell of which they are a part. A living cell attacked by free radicals degenerates and becomes dysfunctional. Free radicals can attack our cells literally ripping their protective membranes apart. Sensitive cellular components like the nucleus and DNA, which carries the genetic blueprint of the cell, can be damaged, leading to cellular mutations and death.

As an analogy, think of your car as one of your body's cells. It serves a useful purpose taking you to and from work so you can provide a living for yourself and family. Your car is very important to your life just as the cells in your heart or brain, or any number of organs, are essential to life. Free radicals can be equated to vandals who strike randomly. When they see your car they may break off a side mirror. You could still get to work and back without it, but the car would not provide optimal function. These radical vandals may attack your tire the next time, making it go flat. This could seriously hamper the car's ability to function. You could still drive it somewhat, but it is far less functional and less effective. If the vandals keep destroying parts of the car or if they just happen to remove a vital component like a battery cable, the entire car becomes useless. Our cells, like this car, are attacked by destructive free-radical vandals that do a little damage here and a little damage there. Some injuries may be relatively minor, others fatal.

The more free radicals that attack our cells, the greater the damage and the greater the potential for serious destruction. If the cells that are damaged are in our heart or arteries, what happens? If they are in the brain, what happens? If they are in our joints, pancreas, intestines, liver, or kidneys, what happens? Think about it. If the cells become damaged, dysfunctional, or die, can these organs fulfill their intended purpose at optimal levels, or do they degenerate?

Free-radical damage has been linked to the loss of tissue integrity and to physical degeneration. As cells are bombarded by free radicals the tissues become progressively impaired. Some researchers believe that free-radical destruction is the actual cause of aging.[2] The older the body gets, the more damage it sustains from a lifetime accumulation of attack from free radicals.

Differences in lifestyle, diet, activity level, and genetics all play a part in how free radicals affect our health. Today some sixty or so degenerative diseases are recognized as having free radicals involved in their cause or manifestation.[3] Additional diseases are regularly being added to this list. The research that linked the major killer diseases such as heart disease and cancer to free radicals has expanded to include most every other degenerative disease.

Free radicals don't necessarily cause all of these diseases, but they are involved as accomplices. In fact, it has been suggested that most of the damage caused by disease is actually the result of the accompanying free-radical destruction and not from the disease process itself.

If you can prevent cellular destruction from free radicals, then tissue degeneration and "aging" slow down. Without the bombardment from free radicals, damaged cells are eventually replaced by newer, healthier cells. Tissues built with these new cells become more functional. Degeneration

Disease and Free Radicals

Some of the most common conditions involving free-radical degeneration

heart disease	asthma
atherosclerosis	hay fever
cancer	food allergies
stroke	phlebitis
diabetes	ulcers
psoriasis	cataract
eczema	colitis
acne	constipation
arthritis	fibrocystic breast
edema	disease
chronic fatigue	Alzheimer's disease
varicose veins	Parkinson's disease
hemorrhoids	failing memory
seizures	senility
prostitis	kidney stones
prostate hypertrophy	gout
multiple sclerosis	depression
PMS	insomnia
dysmenorrhea	lupus

stops. Healing occurs. Organs and tissues are revived. If you junk the car in our example above that has been crippled by free-radical vandals and buy a new one, and vandals never touch your new car and no other damage occurs to it, this car will last the full length of its designed lifetime, providing many years of trouble-free use. Likewise, our cells will live to their full potential, allowing for a long vital life free from the aches and pains caused by free-radical degeneration.

This can happen if you could stop the destructive effects of free-radical chain reactions. That's the problem. Stopping all free-radical reactions is not really possible, nor entirely desirable as some of the natural processes in our bodies generate free radicals.

Free-radical reactions occur in our bodies all the time. They are a necessary part of life and you can never be free from them. Every breath of air we take creates free radicals (especially if the air is polluted by smog or tobacco smoke). Normal metabolic processes in our cells creates free radicals. Chemical reactions with the food we eat (particularly from oils and chemical contaminantes) create free radicals. Because free-radical reactions are a part of life, we can not eliminate them entirely, but we can greatly reduce them by eliminating those which are caused by our food and environment.

Most of the destruction our bodies encounter with free radicals comes from our environment. Eliminate them and the body will respond. Healing and rejuvenation occur. Aging still progresses because we cannot eliminate all free-radical reactions, but by cutting down our exposure to those in our environment we can retard degeneration and perhaps overcome many degenerative conditions.

Oxidation

When you cut an apple open and expose the cut surface to air for any length of time, it turns brown due to oxidizing reactions. When iron oxidizes it rusts. Silver tarnishes. Oxidized fats become rancid. Much of the chemical deterioration that occurs in the world is a result of oxidation. Basically, oxidation is a process in which substances combine with oxygen or other nonmetallic elements.*

Like a Dr. Jekyll and a Mr. Hyde, oxygen has two faces with characteristics that are both good and bad. On the one hand, oxygen is necessary for life. Every cell needs oxygen in order to produce ATP—the energy that fuels metabolism. On the other hand, it generates destructive chemical reactions that cause deterioration and leads to death. It seems that we can't live with it and we can't live without it. To

most microorganisms oxygen is deadly and exposure to this gas readily kills them. For this reason, oxygen in one of its many forms (e.g. hydrogen peroxide and ozone) is used as a disinfectant. Even animals and humans can be seriously injured by breathing too much oxygen-enriched air.[4]

Oxidation can occur with many substances. Common byproducts of oxidation are free radicals. Many different types of free radicals exist with varying levels of reactivity. I will mention just a few of the most notable oxygen species.

The oxygen in the air we breath consists of two oxygen atoms (O_2). Although this oxygen has two unpaired electrons and is therefore classified as a free radical, the electrons are arranged in such a way that it oxidizes most things very slowly at room temperature. The rate of oxidation can be speeded up by the addition of heat or radiation. Also, some molecules are more susceptible to oxidation than others. For example, iron easily oxidizes to form rust, whereas gold is very resistant.

Other forms of oxygen are much more reactive. Singlet oxygen (O) is a powerful oxidizing agent. Oxygen (O_2) can be split by light energy into two singlet oxygen radicals which readily attack body tissues.

If oxygen (O_2) picks up one additional electron it is known as a superoxide radical and inside the body can become an active and potent oxidizing agent and can do considerable damage.

Water (H_2O) can be split to form two free radicals—a hydrogen radical (H) and a hydroxyl radical (OH).** The hydroxyl radical is the most reactive oxygen radical known to chemistry. It has tremendous potential for causing biological damage. It can react with any cell or tissue it comes in contact with, usually setting off free-radical chain reactions.

Radiation

Most of our knowledge about the chemistry of the hydroxyl radical has been provided by radiation chemists, since exposing water to ionizing radiation such as X-rays and gamma rays generates this highly reactive radical.

You may be surprised to learn that most of the damage done to living organisms exposed to excess ionizing radiation is not caused by cellular disruption from the radiation, but by the consequence of the hydroxyl radicals which

---

*Chemically the process of oxidation is much more complex, but this definition is suitable for the purposes of this text.

**The hydrogen radical is not the same as a hydrogen ion. The hydrogen ion has one proton and no electrons and possesses a positive charge. The hydrogen radical has one proton and one electron so possesses no charge. Likewise, the hydroxyl ion has 9 protons and 10 electrons giving it a negative charge, but the hydroxyl radical has 9 protons and 9 electrons so it has no charge but is highly reactive.

are formed by it.[5] While high doses of radiation can cause severe burning and death, most of the biological consequences of excess low-radiation exposure are due to free-radical damage to proteins, DNA, and fats and not by the radiation itself.[6]

When body tissues are exposed to ionizing radiation, most of the energy they take up is absorbed by the water in our tissues. This happens because there is more water available than any other compound. Our body consists of about 60 percent water. The radiation causes one of the bonds in the water molecule to split, producing a hydrogen radical and a hydroxyl radical. The latter species is the most reactive radical known and can attack and damage almost every molecule found in living tissue. Because it is so reactive, the hydroxyl radical does not exist for even a microsecond before combining with a molecule in its immediate vicinity. This event sets off a destructive chain reaction of free radicals. So, if a hydroxyl radical, or one of its offspring, attacks the DNA in our cells, free-radical chain reactions can occur within the DNA which can lead to serious alterations resulting in mutations and the development of cancer.[7]

DNA is our genetic blueprint. If that is altered in any way, new cells that may develop can be mutated. This can give rise to abnormal growths and deformities. If the affected DNA were among the reproductive organs, it may also affect our offspring, giving rise to children with birth defects. Ionizing radiation can easily penetrate our cells and tissues to attack water molecules anywhere in our bodies. So the DNA within our cells is very vulnerable to radiation and injury by the hydroxyl radical.

After the development of the Atomic Bomb during World War II, people became acutely aware of the potential danger of radiation. Fallout from nuclear testing and exposure to toxic waste lead to many health problems. Close proximity to high doses of ionizing radiation causes massive cellular injury and death. As distance between a person and the source increases or as intensity of the radiation declines, the effects of exposure are delayed and often hidden.

Genetically mutated animals and insects that grew to enormous proportions and terrorized unsuspecting humans was the plot for numerous science fiction films in the 1950s and 1960s. This theme with various twists is often used even today. While these mutant monsters are purely the imaginations of science fiction writers, large doses of nonlethal radiation can affect the DNA and cause mutations and cancer. Contrary to what many movies and books depict, those who are adversely affected by harmful doses of radiation do not become radioactive. But they do suffer from heavy free-radical damage.

Ironically, while radiation can cause cancer, it is also used to treat it. Low doses of radiation are beamed directly at cancerous growths or radioactive material may be directly placed within affected tissues. This causes the formation of hydroxyl radicals that destroy the cancer cells. In the process, some healthy cells are also unavoidably sacrificed. It is believed that the overall benefits of radiation treatment outweigh the negative consequences.

Survivors Face Risk of Cancer from Radiation Therapy

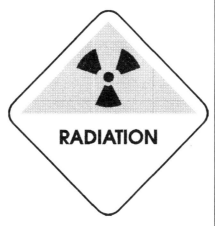

RADIATION

Girls treated for childhood cancer with chest radiation are 20 times more likely to develop breast cancer later in life than other women, and run an extremely high risk of getting it by their early 20s, a study suggests. The researchers proposed that these women get their first mammogram at age 25—15 years earlier than recommended for most women.

Doctors have long wondered whether childhood cancer survivors needed special screening because of growing evidence that they face a higher risk of cancer later on than other people. Radiation kills cancer cells, but it is also known to damage other cells, which can, in turn, become cancerous.

In a study reported in the journal *Cancer* (February 12, 1998 issue) researchers at St. Jude Children's Research Hospital in Memphis Tenn., traced medical records of 3,436 girls treated for cancer at the institution between 1962 and 1995. Some had been diagnosed before age 10.

They found that 12 of these girls later developed breast cancer, about 20 times the rate of the general female population. Four of them or one-third, developed breast cancer before age 25—one at the age of 12. Normally, only 0.2 percent of breast cancers occur before age 25.

"That's a phenomenal finding" said Dr. Sue Kaste, an osteopath at St. Jude and one of the researchers. "These are happening at a time when health care providers don't think of breast cancer occurring."

It's ironic that the treatment used to cure cancer also causes it.

Treatment of disease, particularly cancer, by X-ray methods has been in operation since 1896. As a result of radiation therapy, adverse side effects commonly result. These side effects collectively called radiation sickness include: fatigue, prostration, nausea, and vomiting. Doctors who understand what goes on in the body during radiation treatment usually recommend that patients take antioxidant vitamins at the same time. This reduces free-radical damage to normal tissues and lessens side effects which speeds healing.

Whenever we are exposed to X-rays, we undergo some degree of free-radical damage. That's why when you visit the dentist, the technician drapes you with a heavy, lead-like vest and runs out of the room when the pictures are taken. Methods of taking X-rays have improved over the years reducing exposure time, making them much safer than they were just a few years ago.

We are all exposed to varying degrees of radiation every day. We get it from radioactive elements within earth's crust, from cosmic radiation, and industrial and medical sources. Ultraviolet (UV) light, while not as energetic as ionizing radiation, to a lesser extent can also cause the formation of hydroxyl radicals.[8]

Toxins and Pollutants

Besides oxygen, radiation, and heat, there are many other things that can cause or accelerate the formation of free radicals. A variety of toxins and pollutants in our environment, both natural and man-made, can also generate health-destroying radicals.

The air we breathe is full of such pollutants. One of the most common air pollutants is nitrogen dioxide. It is a dense, brown, poisonous gas and a powerful oxidizing agent. It's formed in smoke from burning organic materials and is found at high levels in cigarette smoke.

Radon is a colorless, odorless natural gas that is emitted from rocks. Unlike most natural gases, radon is radioactive. It often seeps into buildings through the ground and, if a home is well insulated, it can accumulate to dangerous levels. Because it is a gas, it is inhaled into the lungs and is believed to cause lung cancer.

Many industrial and household chemicals have strong oxidizing properties. Exposure to certain pesticides in the environment and in our foods can lead to free radical formation. Chemicals used in food processing such as solvents, plastics, and packaging materials are known to migrate into foods.[9] Many food additives can cause free radicals such as nitrites, sulfur dioxide and sulfites, ferric sulfate and iron (added to fortified foods), some food colorings, and polyunsaturated oils.[10]

Several drugs including some tranquilizers, antibiotics, and antiinflammatory drugs create free radicals in the body when the person is exposed to sunlight. These people become photosensitive. Other drugs can cause free radicals without the aid of sunlight. The drug penicillamine is a powerful oxygen scavenger; however, the radicals so generated can attack proteins. This has been suggested to account for the autoimmune symptoms often shown by rheumatoid arthritis patients after prolonged treatment with penicillamine.[11]

Alcohol depletes vitamin E and other antioxidants in cells and increases iron uptake from the gut, both of which increase free-radical activity.[12] Even our water isn't safe. Chlorine is an active catalyst for oxidation reactions. The chlorine which is added to all our drinking water can turn polyunsaturated oils into free-radical terrorists.

Does exposure to oxidizing agents in the environment make all that much of an impact on health? Studies seem to indicate so. In one study conducted in India, the health of people who lived in rural areas was compared with those who lived in urban areas where pollution is much greater. It was found the urban dwellers experienced more oxidative stress in body tissues and had a higher risk of cardiovascular and other degenerative disease. Because factors such as diet and ethnic background of the two groups were very similar, the results were attributed to oxidizing toxins in the environment.[13]

Injury

Another way in which oxidative stress can occur is by tissue injury. When cells are damaged and break open, they release compounds that can cause oxidation and free-radical formation. All forms of tissue injury lead to oxidative stress.[14]

Injured tissues release xanthine oxidase, an oxidizing enzyme that randomly attacks surrounding tissues, as well as free iron which acts as a powerful catalyst for oxidizing reactions.[15]

Mechanisms by which tissue damage can cause oxidative stress include heat, trauma, ultrasound, infection, radiation, elevated O_2, toxins, and ischaemia (tissues deprived of O_2). Ischaemic injury can be caused by stroke, heart attack, frostbite, and shock due to excessive blood loss or low blood pressure.

Any disease that causes tissue injury, consequently, also involves free-radical reactions which further stress the system. In fact, it has been suggested that for many illnesses more harm is done by way of the free radicals it generates than by the disease itself. Many of the symptoms associated with disease are caused by or intensified by free radicals.

For this reason, it has been difficult for researchers to

identify if free radicals actually cause a certain condition to develop or if their presence was just a consequence of tissue injury. For some conditions such as cancer and atherosclerosis (including heart disease and stroke), it is clearly evident that free radicals take an active part in initiating the disease.

Other conditions where free radicals play an important role include cataract, inflammatory bowel diseases (e.g. Chron's disease and ulcerative colitis), autoimmune diseases (e.g. rheumatoid arthritis), allergies, diabetes, shock, Alzheimer's and Parkinson's disease, and traumatic injury to brain and spinal cord.

The brain and spinal cord are very sensitive to free radical attack. Damaged brain tissues undergo oxidation very fast. One reason for this is that some areas of the brain are rich in iron which is very easily released from disrupted brain cells. Iron ions facilitate further damage to surrounding areas by accelerating free-radical reactions. In addition, brain tissue is also very rich in polyunsaturated fatty acids which are highly susceptible to oxidation. The level of antioxidant defense enzymes in the brain is only moderate, and the fluid surrounding the brain (cerebrospinal fluid) has no significant iron-binding capacity, so cannot bind released iron. After a brain injury (e.g. stroke or trauma caused by a blow to the head), free-radical reactions may cause more damage to the brain or spinal cord than the initial injury.

Infections also involve free radicals. Bacteria and viruses can damage cells releasing oxidizing elements. In addition, our own immune system produces free radicals as a means of fighting invading microorganisms. White blood cells use the destructive force of free radicals to kill these organisms by releasing oxidizing chemicals on or near them. This, consequently, can increase the oxidative damage done to surrounding tissues. To limit damage to itself, the body maintains a reserve of antioxidants which quickly stops free-radical chain reactions once they have done their job. This provides an effective way to fight infection so long as the body is supplied with the dietary nutrients to maintain suitable antioxidant protection.

Many nutrients contribute to the antioxidant reserves in our bodies. The most well-known for combating colds and flu is vitamin C. While vitamin C has not been shown to prevent colds, studies have shown that it can reduce its severity and duration.[16]

One of the reasons for the effectiveness of vitamin C against colds is because of its antioxidant properties. As a consequence of the war between our white blood cells and the cold virus, free radicals are strewn about adding to the misery caused by the infection. Vitamin C helps to mop up these radicals, lessening the injury that would otherwise result, thus relieving the intensity of the symptoms and helping to get over the infection sooner.

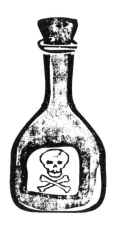

vegetable oil

Oxidation of Polyunsaturated Oils

Oils kill. Most notable are the polyunsaturated oils we add to our foods every day. When we eat foods containing refined vegetable oils, we are opening the door to massive free-radical destruction throughout our bodies. The greatest amount of oxidative damage that we encounter in life is from polyunsaturated oils. Whether they are in our foods or a part of body tissues, polyunsaturated oils are extremely susceptible to oxidation and free-radical formation. Oils kill, but they do it very slowly, so slowly we don't recognize the damage they do and we continue to eat them until we die.

When exposed to oxygen, heat, or light, polyunsaturated oils readily oxidize and become rancid. This is not true with saturated fats. Saturated fats are not easily oxidized and, therefore, generate few free radicals. Rancid fats are carcinogenic and capable of initializing cancer. Eating rancid fat can lead to the development of cancer.[17]

Liquid vegetable oils can be deceiving because they look and taste harmless even after they become rancid. The oil may not smell bad and may look as fresh as the day you bought it, yet be teaming with free-radical terrorists ready to blow holes through your cells as soon as they enter your body.

The oxidation process, which creates free radicals, starts in the factory as soon as oil is extracted from the seed. As it waits in warehouses and on the grocery shelf it continues to oxidize, creating more and more free-radical troublemakers. When you buy vegetable oil from the store, it has already gone rancid!

Oil straight from the bottle is bad enough, but when heated, oxidization is accelerated to an enormous extent. The worst thing you can do to any vegetable oil is to heat it. This sounds ironic since oil is often used in cooking, but heat is one of its worst enemies. On lab animals, heated vegetable oils have shown to cause diarrhea, dermatitis, seborrhea, hair loss, and damage the liver, thymus, testes, and blood vessels.[18] The thymus is known as the master gland of the immune system and, if it is affected, the entire immune system suffers. Damaged blood vessels promote blood clotting and atherosclerosis. The loss of testicular function can lead to low sperm counts which is an alarming trend that has been occurring among human males over recent decades.

Oxidation occurs even at room temperature, but the higher the temperature, the faster oil oxidizes, and the more damage it can do to us. The temperatures used in cooking generate a great deal of free radicals (as well as toxic trans fatty acids). Oil used over and over again for frying, such as they do in restaurants to cook fries, onion rings, chicken nuggets, and such, is extraordinarily unhealthy because this oxidized oil is repeatedly used making it worse over time. Some of these restaurants will heat their oil at high temperatures all day long for several days before it is replaced. One of the most damaging things you can do for your health is to eat greasy fried food. At one time, restaurants used beef tallow, a highly saturated fat, for deep frying, but in order to make their foods appear to be more healthy, many have switched to polyunsaturated and hydrogenated vegetable oils. Beef tallow, being a saturated fat, is more stable under heat and is not as prone to oxidation like vegetable oils, so is by far the healthier oil in view of free radical and trans fatty acid production. *Heated vegetable oils are some of the most toxic foods we eat!*

Some people may say, "Oh, one donut isn't going to hurt me." The effects of a single deep-fried donut may not be outwardly noticeable, but destruction will occur. One donut filled with heat-damaged oil can introduce into your mouth thousands of free radicals, each, in turn, creating free-radical chain reactions that could eventually affect millions upon millions of molecules which make up the cells and tissues in your body. Why is Alzheimer's disease, Parkinson's disease, and other degenerative conditions growing more and more prevalent nowadays? Because many people are saying to themselves "one more donut won't hurt." The effects

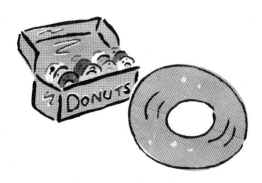

Foods cooked in vegetable oils are dangerously toxic.

aren't immediately noticeable, but creep up on you slowly over time and, before you know it, it's too late; the damage is so extensive there is little hope for recovery.

A single free radical is capable of destroying an enzyme or protein molecule or even an entire cell.[19] Free radicals can easily damage highly sensitive structures such as the DNA of cells which control the cell's function and its ability to divide and multiply. A cell with free-radical damaged DNA that manages to survive may produce mutated daughter cells that are dysfunctional and perhaps even cancerous.

Each of our cells contains tiny organs called organelles—cell organs. Each of these has specific functions just as the organs in our bodies do. One of these organelles is called the mitochondria. The mitochondria is known as the powerhouse of the cell. It takes oxygen and glucose (i.e., blood sugar) and converts them into energy to run the metabolic processes of the cell. The entire cell derives its energy from the mitochondria. Muscular contractions and body movement are powered by the energy released by the mitochondria in each of the muscle cells. The energy for the pancreas to produce digestive enzymes and hormones like insulin comes from the mitochondria in that organ. The energy which powers the production and secretion of digestive juices in our stomachs and peristaltic movement (churning action of muscles in walls of stomach) is powered by mitochondria. Hormone production, body fluid regulation, temperature regulation, acid-base balance of body fluids, and even brain function are powered by the energy released by mitochondria.

The membranes (cell walls) of the cell and organelles, including mitochondria, are made of a variety of fats including polyunsaturated fats and, therefore, are very susceptible to the disruptive and damaging action of free radicals. Free radicals damage the ability of mitochondria to utilize oxygen, thus preventing it from producing energy necessary to carry on its life-sustaining processes.[20] The result is cell degeneration.

The polyunsaturated fats found in every cell membrane readily form free-radical chain reactions in a process that biochemists call lipid peroxidation. "Lipid" is the term biochemists use to designate fat or oil and "peroxidation" means a special type of reaction with oxygen. When oxygen reacts normally with a compound, the compound becomes "oxidized" and the process is called oxidation. However, under certain conditions, oxygen can react in such a way that an extra oxygen atom is involved in the reaction. When this occurs, the compound becomes peroxidized and the process is called "peroxidation." In this book I use the terms oxidation and peroxidation interchangeably when referring to fats.

A polyunsaturated fat in a cell membrane attacked by a free radical will become a free radical and attack a neighboring polyunsaturated fat, likely in the same cell. The destructive chain reaction continues until the cell is severely crippled or utterly destroyed. Random free-radical reactions throughout the body occurring day after day, year after year takes it toll. Is it any wonder why people in affluent countries who eat the most refined vegetable oils have such a high death rate from degenerative disease?

THE FREE-RADICAL THEORY OF AGING

For centuries mankind has sought the fountain of youth. Through the years there have been many claims that a particular type of water, herb, or activity could restore youth. Even today we hear of miracle drugs and dietary supplements. The hormone DHEA was once touted as such a wonder worker not too long ago, and many even now still believe in its power to turn back the clock on aging. Medical researchers have devoted a great deal of time trying to understand the aging process. They reason that if they understand how aging works they would have a better chance of solving the riddle of eternal youth. Up until recently, the causes of aging have remained pretty much a mystery. With the growing knowledge of free-radical chemistry, many researchers now feel they have found the key to unlocking the secret of aging.

Biochemists became interested in radicals only in the 1970s. This interest followed from the discovery in 1968 of an enzyme (superoxide dismutase) that is created specifically by the body to stop free-radical reactions. Scientists discovered that free radicals are involved in most all forms of tissue destruction and degeneration. Without free-radical stress it appeared that the body would experience little deterioration. This led to the proposal of the free-radical theory of aging. This theory states that aging is caused by the slow cumulative oxidation of body tissues over a lifetime.[21]

Oxidation is decay. Decay increases with age. In the environment it is seen as rusting in metal, rotting of meat, rancidity of oils, browning of apples, and hardening of rubber. In our bodies this process is linked with aging—wrinkling of skin, loss of flexibility, stiffening of joints, hardening of arteries, formation of cataracts, poor circulation, fatigue, and various stresses within tissues that cause aches and pains.

We age or slowly deteriorate as we experience more and more free-radical bombardment. Since radicals deteriorate cells and tissues, the entire body slowly deteriorates. In areas of the body where free-radical damage is chronic or extensive (such as old injuries or genetic weaknesses) disease of one type or another develops, causing symptoms (inflammation, aches and pains, high blood pressure, fatigue, etc.) and eventually death.

It appears that free radicals are, at least, partly to blame for the way we look and feel as we get older. Free radicals slowly degenerate body tissues. Aging is a degenerative process. The effects of free-radical degeneration is perhaps most evident in our skin. One of the body tissues damaged most by free radicals is collagen. Collagen acts as a matrix that gives strength and flexibility to our tissues. It is found everywhere in our bodies and holds everything together. It is

The risk of cancer in humans sharply increases with age. Except for a few rare cancers, the incidence of this disease generally increases as people age. The same phenomenon occurs, on a much shorter time-scale, in other mammals such as rats.

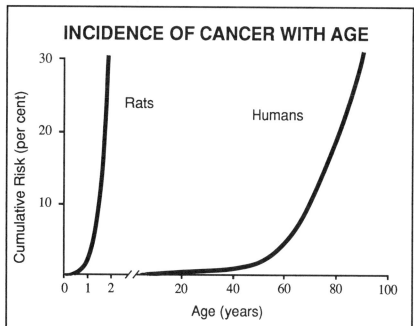

INCIDENCE OF CANCER WITH AGE

The risk of cancer in humans sharply increases with age. Except for a few rare cancers, cancer is generally a disease of older people. The same phenomenon occurs, on a much shorter time-scale, in other mammals such as rats.

Source: Ames, B. *Free Radical Research Communications* 7:122

what keeps our skin smooth, elastic, and youthful. When degraded by free radicals, the skin becomes dry, leathery, and wrinkled—all classic signs of old age.

Free radicals don't just attack the collagen in our skin, but everywhere in our bodies. So as our skin ages and begins to harden and sag, so do the tissues under the skin holding our organs together. The skin is a mirror of what is happening inside your body. Likewise, other tissues are also degraded by free-radical activity and organs become less efficient, so the production of proteins, enzymes, hormones, and other compounds vital to life and health drop off. Even our immune system slows down. When the body functions at a lower level of efficiency, infections become more serious and degenerative diseases are more likely to develop. To get a rough idea of how well your body is aging see the sidebar "How Well Are You Aging."

Have you ever picked up a kitten or other small animal and noticed how

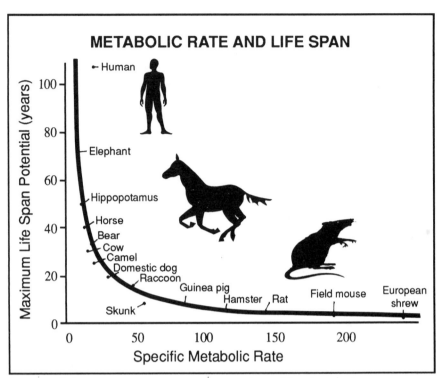

In general the more oxygen consumed, as indicated by the metabolic rate, the shorter the life span.

rapidly it was breathing? The faster an animal breaths, the more oxygen it consumes and the higher its metabolic rate. Many years ago, it was observed that the basal rate of metabolism of animals (i.e., how fast the cells are working when the body is at rest) is approximately inversely related to their life spans. In general, smaller animals consume more oxygen per unit of body mass than do larger ones, and they don't live as long. It is assumed that a major factor in determining the life span depends on the degree of oxidative stress the animal undergoes. Thus, a small animal consumes more oxygen for its size than a larger one and, therefore, experiences a greater amount of oxidative stress, and ages faster and dies sooner.

The maximum human life span is estimated to be about 120 years.[22] Few of us will ever reach this age because we do not live in an ideal world free of health-destroying influences. Most people under the age of 35 die from accidents or violence. Infectious diseases are most common in under developed countries where poor sanitation and malnutrition are of concern. The most common cause of death in most of the world is heart disease and the second is cancer. Our risk for developing either one of these diseases increases with free-radical stress as we age.

It is known that a great deal of free-radical stress can lead to illness very quickly. Exposure to high levels of toxic chemicals or radiation, which accelerate free-radical reac-

tions, can develop health problems within a very short period of time. With lower levels of free-radical exposure—like the kind we experience every day—disease creeps up more slowly.

Both cancer and heart disease are good examples of this process. The incidence of cancer, for example, varies with age. A few cancers, such as leukemia, occur in young people. For most cancers, however, the rate of incidence rises very sharply with age. Thus cancer is an age-related disease. Ordinarily, it takes many years for cancer to develop to a critical stage.

A similar correlation is found in animals, the older they get the greater the risk of cancer and other diseases. The more oxygen an animal consumes the more free-radical damage occurs and the sooner disease can develop. So in rats cancer can develop within 18 months while in humans, who have a lower metabolic rate, it usually takes many years.

Length of life and susceptibly to disease may also depend on the antioxidant defense capability of the organism. Animals with greater antioxidant capacity would fare better than those with less efficient antioxidant defense mechanisms.

If free radicals are the sole cause of aging it could be reasoned that taking antioxidant dietary supplements would slow the aging process. Simply taking antioxidants, while

HOW WELL ARE YOU AGING?

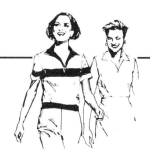

Every day we grow older, but we don't all age at the same rate. A healthy 60-year-old can be "functionally" as young as a 45-year-old while a sickly 40-year-old could have a body comparable to a 70-year-old. The average human life span is about 75 years. Some people live much longer, and those who do are generally free of debilitating disease for most of their lives. They are functionally younger than those people whose bodies degenerate and die before their time. Free-radical destruction is believed to be the major cause of aging and a significant factor in most all forms of disease.

Scientists have identified several biomarkers which give us a way of measuring functional age. By measuring a person's biomarkers, functional age can be determined. There are many types of biomarkers, some involving procedures that require medical supervision. Others you can do yourself. Three self-administered tests are described here so that you can get a general idea of how well your body is holding up against free-radical destruction and the aging process.

Skin Elasticity Test

As we age, our skin loses its elasticity, becoming leathery and wrinkled. This is the result of free-radical destruction and is a sign of degeneration and loss of function. What happens to our skin is also happening to other tissues throughout our bodies. As our skin ages so does our heart, lungs, kidneys, and other organs. The skin, in a sense, serves as a mirror to the health of the rest of our body.

For this reason, the skin is often used as a biomarker. Significant changes in the skin usually occur at

Skin Elasticity Test

Time (sec)	Functional Age (years)
1-4	44 or younger
5	45-50
10-15	60
35-55	70
56 or more	over 70

about the age of 45. The following skin test is a good marker for how the skin and other tissues change after age 45. At younger ages there is only a slight change in the skin.

For this test, pinch the skin on the back of your hand with the thumb and forefinger for five seconds. Let go and time how long it takes for the skin to completely flatten back out. The shorter the time, the younger the functional age of the skin. Compare your results to the table above.

Falling-Ruler Test

This test measures your reaction time. You need a flat 18-inch wooden measuring stick. Have someone hold the stick vertically at the top, by the 1-inch mark. Hold the thumb and middle finger of your right hand $3\frac{1}{2}$ inches apart, equidistant form the 18-inch mark near the bottom of the ruler. Without warning, your assistant will drop the ruler. As soon as you see it fall, catch it between your two fingers.

Falling-Ruler Test

Measurement (inches)	Functional Age (years)
11 or less	20
9	30
8	40
7	50
6	60
5-0	70 and older

Write down the inch mark on the ruler where your finger caught it. Repeat this two more times. Take an average of all three. So, if you caught it at the 10-, 12-, and 8-inch marks the average would be (10+12+8)/3=10. Compare your average score with the table at the bottom of this page.

Static Balance Test

This test is considered the best biomarker among the do-it-yourself measurements. There is a full 100 percent decline with age.

Static Balance Test

Time (sec)	Functional Age (years)
30 or more	20
25	30
16	40
10	50
7	60
5	70

The static balance test measures how long you can stand on one leg with your eyes closed before falling over, For this test you must be either barefoot or wearing low-heeled shoes. Stand on a hard surface with both feet together, close your eyes, and lift your foot about six inches off the ground. If you are right-handed lift the left leg and if you are left-handed lift the right leg. The raised knee should be bent at about a 45-degree angle. Don't move, just stand on one foot with your eyes closed. Have someone time you. When you fall or touch the ground with the other foot, record the time. Do the test three times and take an average. Check your results with the table above.

Source: Bruce Fife, N.D. *The Detox Book: How to Detoxify Your Body to Improve Your Health, Stop Disease and Reverse Aging.*

promising, in humans has not yet been proven. But it can reduce free-radical stress, help prevent disease, and improve the function of organs and tissues, including the immune system which protects us from disease. While free radicals may not be the whole answer as to why we age, they are undoubtedly a very important part of the process, and understanding what they do and how to limit their destructive actions can go a long way in improving your quality of life.

The free-radical theory of aging has received some degree of validation, at least in animals and insects. Scientists injected genes into fruit flies causing them to produce more antioxidants to fight free radicals. The life span of the flies increased by one-third. That's like increasing the human life span from 75 to 100 years of age just by reducing the amount of free-radical reactions occurring in the body. Similarly, antioxidant nutrients fed to laboratory animals have shown to increase life span by 20 to 30 percent.

CARDIOVASCULAR DISEASE

Chances are you will die from cardiovascular disease. Most people do. Sadly, most cardiovascular diseases are preventable. But once the disease has progressed to the point where you know you have it, it's usually too late. Little can be done through conventional treatments to save you. The best protection against cardiovascular disease is prevention. In most cases, it can be prevented.

Cardiovascular disease (CVD) is a general term for all disorders of the heart and blood vessels. Atherosclerosis (hardening of the arteries) is by far the most common cardiovascular disease. It is of great concern because it sets the stage for hypertension (high blood pressure), heart disease, and stroke. Cardiovascular disease is and has been the leading cause of death in Western countries for decades.

The type of oils we use in our foods has a pronounced effect on the health of the heart and circulatory system. Polyunsaturated fats, believe it or not, have a greater impact on cardiovascular health than cholesterol or saturated fat. Recent research has shown that one of the major factors behind the development of atherosclerosis and heart disease is, as you might expect, free radicals.

The recognition that free-radical reactions, particularly lipid peroxidation or the oxidation of fats, are important in the formation of atherosclerosis has been around for many years.[23] At least as far back as the early 1980s heated vegetable oils (rich in free radicals) were found to create a lot of damage in blood vessel walls.[24]

Interest was raised in free radicals' role in the development of atherosclerosis and heart disease when it was found that the cholesterol-lowering drug, probucol, has an antiatherogenic effect which is greater than would be expected from its cholesterol-lowering action.[25] Probucol, like the antioxidant vitamin E, is able to inhibit lipid peroxidation. It is believed that the antioxidant effect is the major mechanism for the action of probucol.

Heart disease has been called a disease of affluence. It is a modern affliction that plunders mainly people in prosperous nations. Until recently, the disease was relatively uncommon in less developed countries. But even less affluent countries have adapted the foods and lifestyles common in more industrialized nations where heart disease has become a major health problem.

Heart disease gives no warning and most people who have heart disease don't even realize it. It has been said that the first sign or symptom of heart disease is a heart attack, a third of which are fatal. Heart attacks can come without any prior symptoms or warning. More people die of heart attacks than any other cause. It is the number one killer worldwide, killing 6.3 million people a year. In the United States someone dies of a heart attack every 45 seconds.

One of the primary functions of the circulatory system is to exchange oxygen, a necessary element to life, with carbon dioxide, a toxic waste product. The transport of oxygen by the bloodstream is of vital significance in cardiovascular disease. Every one of the 70 trillion cells in our bodies demands a continuous supply of life-giving oxygen in order to live. Oxygen is absolutely necessary to power cellular metabolism—the process that keeps us alive and functioning. Of all the elements that the body needs, only oxygen is in such constant demand that its absence brings death in minutes.

When cells are deprived of oxygen, they weaken and die. If circulation is cut off to any particular organ, the cells in the affected area die, which could bring on the death of the entire organ and, consequently, the body. It is the lack of oxygen to the heart that causes heart attacks.

You might think the heart could never suffer from a lack of oxygen. After all, the heart is continually pumping oxygen-rich blood through the body. Blood travels directly from the lungs and enters the chambers of the heart with every beat. The heart, however, is unable to utilize the oxygenated blood in its chambers for its own nourishment. This may seem strange, but take our body as an example. In order to utilize oxygen in the air, we must breathe it into our lungs. If you prevent the lungs from receiving oxygen, the body will die even though it is surrounded by oxygen in the air. Likewise, with the heart, oxygenated blood can be within its chambers, yet be unavailable for its own use. The heart depends on two coronary arteries for its life-giving oxygen and other nutrients.

Normally, blood flows freely through the coronary arteries and the heart receives the oxygen and nutrients it needs

Atherosclerosis

If you asked most people what causes hardening of the arteries or atherosclerosis, they would probably tell you it was from too much cholesterol in the blood. This idea is called the cholesterol or lipid hypothesis. While still loudly proclaimed in the popular press, it has never really fit clinical observation or scientific studies and has since been replaced with the response-to-injury hypothesis.[27]

Cholesterol doesn't simply come dancing freely down the artery and suddenly decide to stick somewhere. In fact, cholesterol isn't even necessary for atherosclerosis or the formation of plaque. Contrary to popular belief, the principle component of arterial plaque is not cholesterol but protein. Some atherosclerotic arteries contain little or no cholesterol.

According to the response-to-injury hypothesis, atherosclerosis initially develops as a result of injury to the inner lining of the arterial wall. The injury can be the result of a number of factors such as a virus, toxins, or free-radical damage. Free radicals are believed by many to be the main cause of arterial damage.

Injury from any source triggers platelets to clot and arterial cells to release protein growth factors that stimulate growth of the muscle cells within the artery walls. A complex mixture of scar tissue, platelets, calcium, cholesterol, and triglycerides are incorporated into the site to heal the injury. The fibrous tissue, not cholesterol, forms the principle material in plaque. Calcium deposits harden the plaque which is a characteristic of atherosclerosis.

When cells are injured, they release ions from their cytoplasm which generate more free radicals. This, in turn, causes further injury to surrounding cells, perpetuating the cycle which causes abnormal growth and inflammation to build up plaque.

Plaque isn't plastered along the inside of the artery canal. It grows *inside* the artery wall itself. Arterial walls contain a layer of strong circular muscles which prevent the plaque from expanding outward. As the plaque grows and expands, it begins to push inward and close the artery opening. The growth has only one way to expand and that is by protruding into the opening of an artery. The artery slowly narrows, choking off blood flow.

Platelets gather at the site of injury to form blood clots, plugging the holes in the damaged vessel. But if the injury persists or if the blood is prone to clotting (thick blood), clots may continue to grow to the point where they can block the artery. An artery already narrowed by plaque can easily be blocked by blood clots. When this process occurs in the coronary artery of the heart, it is commonly referred to as heart disease.

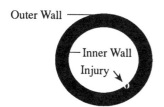

Injury occurs on the inside surface of the artery.

Plaque begins to develop inside artery wall.

Plaque buildup causes the wall of the artery to bulge inward restricting blood flow.

to function. If one of the coronary arteries, or one of its branches becomes clogged, restricting flow of blood, even though the heart's chambers are full of oxygenated blood, the part of the heart which is denied blood will suffocate and die. This is a heart attack. If only a small part of the heart is affected, the victim may survive. The dead tissue will gradually be replaced by scar tissue. But if a larger part of the heart is deprived of oxygen, the entire function of the heart will cease, thus causing death.

Although heart attacks can occur suddenly, without warning, they don't just happen. The conditions that lead to a heart attack build up slowly over many years. Heart disease, as well as many other serious cardiovascular disorders, is usually a consequence of atherosclerosis.

Healthy arteries are flexible, have smooth linings, and can easily carry a steady stream of blood. Atherosclerosis is a process in which fatty material mixed with fibrous tissue and hardened calcium are deposited on the inner walls of the arteries. These walls become rough and thick, like rust in a water pipe. Atherosclerotic deposits, called plaque, gradually enlarge and become hardened. This is why atherosclerosis is often referred to as hardening of the arteries. As plaque builds, the passageway within the arteries narrows and blood flow becomes restricted.

Normally, the arteries are flexible and expand to accommodate the increased volume of blood that occurs with every beat of the heart. Arteries hardened and narrowed by calcified plaque cannot expand, as a result, blood pressure rises. The increased pressure puts a strain on the heart and causes tiny lesions or tears to form on the artery walls. At these damaged points the plaque forming process is accelerated. As pressure builds up in an artery, the arterial wall may weaken and balloon out forming an aneurysm. An aneurysm can burst in a major artery causing massive bleeding and death.

Small proteins in the blood, known as platelets, cause clots to form when they encounter an injury to blood vessels. Clotting is necessary to stop bleeding and facilitate healing. Arteries damaged by atherosclerosis and high blood pressure encourage platelets to spontaneously clot onto the walls of the artery.

A clot once formed may remain attached to a plaque in an artery and gradually enlarge until it shuts off the blood supply to that portion of the tissue supplied by the artery. A clot can also break loose and be carried by the blood into smaller vessels where it can become lodged, blocking the flow of blood. Arteries already narrowed by plaque are easily clogged by clots.

Circulation can be blocked anywhere in the body, sometimes with fatal results. When a blood clot lodges in the coronary artery or one of its branches, a heart attack is the result. If an artery feeding the brain becomes clogged, a stroke results. Like heart attacks, strokes can occur without warning. A stroke can affect mental and physical ability, causing permanent disability and even death. Clogging other arteries can lead to kidney failure, lung disease, and gangrene.

Next to heart attacks and cancer, strokes account for more deaths worldwide than any other disease. Over four million people die each year from strokes. In the United States (and most other industrialized nations) more people die from cardiovascular disease (which includes heart attacks, strokes, and other conditions caused by atherosclerosis) than all other causes of death combined. During your lifetime you have at least a 50 percent chance of dying as a result of cardiovascular disease.

The major risk factors that are associated with atherosclerosis and heart disease include: gender (being male), glucose intolerance (diabetes), heredity (history of CVD prior to age 55 in family members), high blood cholesterol, hypertension, lack of exercise, obesity, smoking, and excessive stress. Consumption of excess sugar and alcohol has also been associated with cardiovascular problems. None of these risk factors, however, actually causes heart disease. As many as 40 percent of the people who die of heart attacks don't have any of these risk factors.[26] So the cause of heart disease lies somewhere else. One of the keys to solving the riddle of heart disease is to understand why it is the predominante cause of death in industrialized countries, yet relatively rare in other parts of the world. This will be discussed more fully in later chapters.

Chapter 3

VEGETABLE OILS

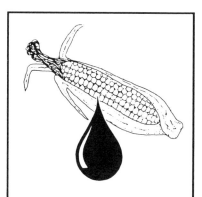

SALADS COULD BE HAZARDOUS TO YOUR HEALTH

When you go out to eat, have you ever chosen the tossed salad because you considered it a healthier choice? After all, what could be so bad with a bunch of fresh raw vegetables? Many health-conscious people do not eat meats and dairy products so as to avoid saturated fat. They often eat lots of fresh vegetables in the form of salads. You would think this would make a healthy meal, but it can be just as bad or even worse than a greasy hamburger. Yes, you read that right, eating salads may be hazardous to your health!

I can hear the meat lovers among you cheering! Health experts often promote eating "live" foods—fresh, raw fruits and vegetables. We all know that vegetables are packed with vitamins and minerals that are supposed to be good for us, so why would a bowl of raw vegetables be harmful?

Actually, it's not the vegetables that are bad, it's the salad dressing that is the culprit. When we eat salads we always have to have salad dressing on it to "make it taste good." Admittedly a salad without dressing is rather bland. But what are salad dressings made of? The primary ingredient of most salad dressings is vegetable oil.

What's so bad about that, you may question? Vegetable oils are perhaps the worst food you can put into your mouth! They're worse than eggs, beef stake, or sugar. There are many "vegetarians" who stopped eating meat to avoid the detrimental effects of saturated fat and cholesterol, yet they come down with heart disease and cancer anyway. Why is that? One reason is because they eat a lot of polyunsaturated oils. Vegetarians who eat vegetable oils with little regard to the quantities they consume would be better off eating meat and lard instead. I don't advocate eating these foods necessarily, but want to stress the dangers of vegetable oils. That is the focus of this chapter.

POLYUNSATURATED VEGETABLE OILS

For years now we've been told that vegetable oils were good and saturated fat and cholesterol were bad. The truth is that vegetable oils are even a worse health hazard than other oils. Polyunsaturated vegetable oils have been favored as healthier substitutes for saturated fats and cholesterol primarily due to industry sales propaganda.

Before the Second World War, industrial and household paints and varnishes were made of soy, safflower, and linseed (flaxseed) oils. When chemists learned

"Diets high in polyunsaturated fats increase the risk of cancer, speed up aging and degeneration of tissues, and may aggravate inflammatory diseases and immune-system disorders."

—Andrew Weil, M.D.

"Oil easily combines with oxygen. This combination is either slow or rapid. In the first case rancidity is the consequence, in the second inflammation."

—Jean Antoine Claude Chaptal (1791)

"It is possible to assemble an impressive arsenal against vegetable oils rather than in favor of them insofar as coronary heart disease is concerned."

—Paul B. Addis and Gregory J. Warner, University of Minnesota how to make cheaper oil-based paint from petroleum, the seed oil industry found itself facing a dwindling market.

In the late 1940s chemicals were used to suppress the thyroid function of pigs, so that they would become fatter while on the same amount of food. These chemicals were found to be carcinogenic. They discovered that corn and soybean oil had the same antithyroid effect, causing the animals to be fattened at lower cost.[1]

At about this same time, farmers were experimenting with different ways to make their animals fatter on less expensive feed. Dietary fats and oils seemed to show promise. Fat contains twice as many calories as carbohydrate or protein and a high fat diet encourages weight gain. By increasing the fat content of the animal's feed they would gain more weight and bring bigger profits with the less expense. The seed oil industries began marketing their products as an additive to animal feed.

According to Dr. Joel Wallach, a veterinarian who turned to natural medicine, although the cattle grew larger with the addition of vegetable oils in their diet, they also developed tumors and other degenerative health conditions.[2] Since diseased cattle had severe economic consequences, the meat industry stopped using vegetable oils and turned to animal fat from fish and the carcasses of dead cattle which were ground up into meal and added to their feed. The fat from the carcasses of dead animals, although high in saturated fat and cholesterol, did not produce the adverse health effects as the vegetable oils did. They also focused on using soybeans and other plants with a high fat content.

The vegetable oil producers, confronted with dwindling sales and the rejection from the farming industry, began a new marketing strategy. They began to push their products for human consumption. With the negative publicity saturated fat was beginning to receive at that time, vegetable oils high in polyunsaturated fatty acids seemed like a sensible solution. The problem is that vegetable oils are doing the same thing to us as they did to the farm animals and making us sick!

People don't see an immediate cause-and-effect relationship. We don't eat an oil and immediately develop symptoms. So we are led to believe we are doing ourselves good by eating vegetable oils in place of saturated fats. Degenerative disease, which is painfully evident in our society, is a product of modern food processing and diet. While there are many factors involved, one of the primary culprits is vegetable oil consumption.

Look at the ingredient labels in the foods you buy. Consider the amount of cooking oil, shortening, and margarine you use. Vegetable oils are in almost all our foods nowadays. We consume them for breakfast, lunch, and dinner, every day, day in and day out. If the farm animals developed hideous degenerative diseases eating this stuff, what do you expect it to do to you!

The most common vegetable oils are safflower, sunflower, corn, soybean, cottonseed, peanut, and canola. All of them are high in polyunsaturated oil. The thing that makes vegetable oils toxic is the *unsaturation*. It doesn't matter if the oil is refined at high temperatures, cold pressed, or consumed as part of the living plant, they are *all* toxic. It is not the processing, refining, or any special industrial treatment that makes them toxic. The vulnerable double carbon bonds in the molecule of the polyunsaturated oil is what causes them to be toxic. These chemical bonds are highly susceptible to oxidation and free-radical formation.

If polyunsaturated oils were chemically stable they would not be so toxic. They become toxic when they are oxidized. This is what causes rancidity. The double-bonded carbons which are missing hydrogen atoms are most susceptible to oxidation reactions. Therefore, the more unsaturated the oil is the more rancid it can become and the greater damage it can cause the body. Rancidity occurs when oils are exposed to oxygen, heat, light, or free radicals, in the bottle or in our bodies. Oxidation causes harmful free radicals to be formed. The longer a bottle of oil sits, the more opportunity for oxidative damage. Oil stored in clear plastic bottles is exposed to damaging radiation from light. Any oil which is heated becomes oxidized. The higher the temperature, the greater the degree of oxidation. Cooking foods at high temperatures accelerates oxidation. Numerous studies, in some cases published as early as the 1930s, have reported on the toxic effects of consuming heated oils.[3]

Seeds provide a rich source of polyunsaturated oil. The vast majority of our cooking oils come from seeds such as cottonseed, sunflower seeds, safflower seeds, rapeseed (canola) are typical examples, but even grains (e.g., corn) and legumes (e.g., soybeans and peanuts), and nuts (e.g., almonds, walnuts) are seeds.

Oils spontaneously oxidize when they are warmed and exposed to oxygen. Seeds naturally contain a small amount of vitamin E to delay rancidity. Seeds are designed to germinate in early spring before hot oxidizing temperatures appear. When oils are extracted from the seeds, they are immediately exposed to oxygen and what vitamin E was present is quickly used up, as heat, light, and oxygen bombard the oil. By the time we buy the oil in the store it is already rancid.

Researchers have pointed out that polyunsaturated oil provides a substrate for free-radical attack within our bodies, resulting in loss of function in membrane structure and as eicosanoid (hormone-like chemicals) precursors as well as causing damage to other cellular constituents, contributing to disease.[4]

Oils are masters of deception. You can't tell a rogue from a saint. They all pretty much look alike. The most toxic vegetable oil can appear as sweet and pure as those that are freshly extracted.

Jurg Loliger, Ph.D. of the Nestle Research Center in Switzerland, states in the authoritative book *Free Radicals and Food Additives* that primary oxidation products of vegetable oils have no objectionable flavor or taste, but the secondary degradation products are generally very potent flavor modifiers and can modify the structure of the product.[5] So, pure vegetable oil may be very rancid, but give no indication of this because it doesn't affect taste or smell. You can eat rancid vegetable oil and not realize it. If mixed with other substances, the free-radical reactions may cause these substances to produce an unpleasant smell and taste. The disagreeable odor of soured milk is a result of rancid fats affecting proteins and other milk components. When the proteins in the milk are damaged by free radicals they produce a most putrefying smell.

How long does milk stay fresh? If kept cold in the refrigerator, it may last five or six days. If left on the countertop unrefrigerated, it will not last a day before going rancid. The warmer the room temperature, the quicker the milk spoils. What causes milk to sour? It starts with the polyunsaturated fat content of the milk. The polyunsaturated fats in the milk oxidize quickly. When they go bad, they create free radicals that spread out, contaminating the proteins which, likewise, become oxidized. This produces the "sour" smell and taste. The oils themselves do not create any noticeable taste or smell.

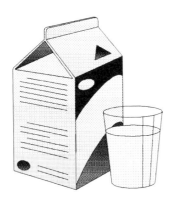

The same oils that go rancid in milk in a few hours are doing the same thing in a bottle of pure vegetable oil. Storing vegetable oil in a cupboard is just as bad as leaving milk on the counter to sour. How long has that vegetable oil been sitting on the store shelf before you bought it? If it were a bottle of milk would you buy it? I would hope not, it would be foul smelling. Just because we can't see or taste any difference in rancid oils does not mean they are safe.

The polyunsaturated fats in pure vegetable oil act the same way as the oils in milk. While the vegetable oils are stored in warehouses, transported in hot trucks, and sit on the store shelves, they are going rancid. They are not refrigerated. They are usually bottled in clear containers where light can penetrate and create more free radicals. These oils may sit around for months exposed to warm temperatures and light before they are sold. How long would a bottle of milk last under these conditions? The polyunsaturated fats in milk become rancid within one day! So do the vegetable oils you buy at the store. But because pure vegetable oil does not produce any noticeable signs of rancidity, we assume them to be safe. All vegetable oils are rancid by the time they reach the store. So, when you buy them, it's like buying milk that has been sitting unrefrigerated for a month or two and in some cases up to a year. Would you drink milk this old?

To make matters worse, the vegetable oils we buy sit on our kitchen cupboards for months. And when we use them they are almost always cooked with our food. The cooking accelerates the oxidizing process making the oil even more rancid and unhealthy. Cooking also creates toxic trans fatty acids as well. Whenever you eat vegetable oils, whether on a salad or in a cooked dish, you are eating one of the most toxic foods modern technology has ever created.

WHERE'S THE EVIDENCE?

You might be thinking: "So where's the evidence? If vegetable oils are so bad for us, wouldn't there be research to substantiate it?" Yes, there should be and there is. Lots of it! Theoretically, we can see how the more unsaturated a fat is the more susceptible it is to oxidation. Since oxidation causes destructive free-radical chain reactions that lead to degeneration of body tissues, the use of polyunsaturated oils should lead to the development of degenerative disease. Indeed it does, and the more unsaturated the oil the greater the danger.

Studies have shown that polyunsaturated oils promote the growth of tumors.[6, 7] This fact is well known among researchers and is not even contested. It is interesting to note that where refined vegetable oils are routinely eaten, cancer rates are high. Where they are not normally eaten, cancer rates are usually much lower.

Consuming vegetable oils lowers our resistance to infectious disease by depressing the immune system. This fact is so well known that vegetable oil emulsions with water are used for intravenous injection, for the purpose of suppressing immunity in patients who have had organ transplants.[8] One of the ways unsaturated fats hinder the immune system is by killing white blood cells.[9] The white blood cells, which defend us against harmful microorganisms, are the primary component of our immune system.

When the immune system is depressed, the entire body is subjected to a greater degree of harm from microorganisms and toxins, including free radicals. Unsaturated oils have been linked to numerous degenerative conditions. Some researchers feel that cancer won't even occur unless there are unsaturated oils in the diet.[10] Others claim that alcoholic cirrhosis of the liver cannot occur unless there are unsaturated oils in the diet.[11] Heart disease has also been linked to unsaturated oils. This is of particular interest because most people associate saturated fat with heart disease, not vegetable oil. Studies have shown that heart disease can be produced by unsaturated oils, and prevented by adding saturated oils to the diet.[12] We are discovering that polyunsaturated oils are more to blame for heart disease than saturated fat or cholesterol.

Researchers have found that the consumption of polyunsaturated oil exceeding 10 percent of total calories can lead to blood disease, cancer, liver damage, and vitamin deficiencies.[13] In an eight-year experiment conducted at a Los Angeles veterans' hospital, a group of patients whose diet contained four times as many polyunsaturates as a second group had 60 percent more cancers.

This list of diseases sounds more like what we would expect of saturated fat rather than unsaturated vegetable oil. Studies have shown that saturated fat can stimulate cancer.[14] That's the type of news we often hear about, but what we don't hear is that polyunsaturated oils stimulate cancer formation *more* quickly than do the saturated fats![15, 16]

In one study done at the University of Western Ontario, ten different fats of varying degrees of saturation were used to determine which ones would produce the most cancers.[17]

Table 3-1
Incidence of Cancer with Different Oils

(Diet containing 20% fat)			
Type of Oil	Saturated	Mono	Poly	Total Cancers
Rapeseed oil	6	62	32	62
Coconut oil	83	15	2	69
Tallow	52	44	4	70
Butter	66	30	4	79
Lard	41	47	12	91
Soybean oil	15	24	61	101
Corn oil	13	25	62	105
Olive oil	14	77	9	109
Cottonseed oil	27	19	54	122
Sunflowerseed oil	11	20	69	124

Table 3-1 Survival Rate

(Number of rats alive after 28 and 30 months)		
Fat	Percent alive after 28 months	Percent alive after 30 months
Lard	70.8	45.8
Olive	58.3	37.5
Corn	47.8	13.0
Safflower	29.2	12.5

Coconut oil is the highest in saturated fat, comprising at least 83 percent, and lowest in polyunsaturated fat, only 2 percent. The other highly saturated oils included tallow, butter, and lard. All the vegetable oils are very low in saturated fat, comprising no more 15 percent. With one exception, rapeseed oil*, the cancer rate for the vegetable oils were significantly higher among the unsaturated vegetable oils (see table 3-1).

Generally it appears that the more unsaturated the fat, the greater its ability to stimulate cancer. Why do oils cause cancer and why does polyunsaturated oil cause more cancer than saturated oil? All oils are subject to oxidation. The double-carbon bonds in unsaturated oils are especially vulnerable. The more double bonds, the greater the chance and degree. A portion of the polyunsaturated oil that comprises soybean oil, for example, has three double bonds making it three times more susceptible to oxidation and cancer formation than butter.

In one study, the effect of the amount or degree of unsaturation of dietary fat on mortality rate for rats was demonstrated. The amount and type of fat were the only significant variables used. The type of oil included lard (saturated), olive oil (monounsaturated), corn oil (polyunsaturated), and safflower oil (very polyunsaturated), listed in order of increasing amount of unsaturation (see table 3-2).

When fat intake was low (5-10%) the degree of unsaturation did not have a significant effect on the mortality rate. However, when fat intake was high (20%), the mortality rates increased with the degree of unsaturation.[18]

All rats in the unsaturated groups died by the 36 month. Experiment terminated at 38 months with 4.2 % of rats still surviving in the group highest in saturated fat (lard).

The oils used weren't special, but were the same kind sold in stores for human consumption.

The fact that polyunsaturated oils are unhealthy is not new. Researchers have known about their destructive effects

*The explanation proposed for the uncharacteristically low cancer occurrence with rapeseed oil even though it is primarily unsaturated, is that it was believed to be significantly fresher than the other oils used in the study and, therefore, created fewer free radicals than expected.

for decades. One area in the body that free radicals have a pronounced effect on is the central nervous system—the brain and spinal cord. Free-radical destruction can age the brain faster than the body. Alzheimer's and Parkinson's diseases are examples. These conditions, once rare, have now spread like a monstrous plague. Some people believe the culprit is vegetable oil. Since the introduction of vegetable oil into our food system, these diseases and other nerve disorders like meningitis and multiple sclerosis have become common.

One possible means of decreasing the rate of degeneration in the central nervous system and elsewhere, would be to decrease the ingestion of vegetable oil.[19]

The central nervous system is more susceptible than the rest of the body to accumulative degenerative changes that lead to dementia and other central nervous system disorders. Several studies have shown the relationship between vegetable oil consumption and free-radical damage to the central nervous system.

In one study, the effect of varying degrees of unsaturation on the mental ability of rats was determined by analyzing their maze-learning abilities. Different oils were added to the rats' feed. The study was initiated after rats had aged considerably, allowing enough time for the effects of the oils to become measurable. Rats were tested on the number of maze errors they made. The more errors, the greater the deterioration of mental function.

The test was designed to test effects of the amount of fat in the diet and the type of fat. The results showed that the number of maze errors increased as total dietary fat increased. It also showed a clear increase of errors with degree of unsaturation.[20] Those animals receiving the most fat in their diet had the greatest decrease in mental ability. All the rats, regardless of the amount of oil given, showed increasing loss of mental ability as the degree of unsaturation increased. The ones given lard retained their mental capacities the longest. The ones given polyunsaturated safflower oil lost them the quickest.

Studies have clearly shown that as unsaturation of dietary oil increases, cancer rate increases, heart disease increases, mental ability diminishes, and in fact, the entire body deteriorates from the onslaught of massive free-radical damage.

So why hasn't the public been informed about the dangers of unsaturated fat? A few people have voiced concern about the vegetable oils, but the food and supplement industry have been so successful in condemning saturated fat and promoting their products as healthy alternatives, we've all become brainwashed.

The fact of the matter is, researchers know about it, but the consumer doesn't. The reason is that information is

VEGETABLE OILS AFFECT YOUR HEALTH

There are those who still urge the public to use more polyunsaturated fat despite the fact that most persons have already tremendously increased their vegetable fat intake. Unfortunately, this recommendation is made with the promise that heart disease may be prevented or treated.

It is true that exchanging polyunsaturated fat for saturated fat will cause a slight decrease in serum cholesterol levels, but this has never been proven to prevent or treat heart disease.

In fact, the National Heart and Lung Institute admits that any relationship, between diet (insofar as saturated vs polyunsaturated fats are concerned) and heart disease, is strictly "intuitive" and based only on personal impressions and fragmentary conclusions rather than on scientific proof. The Food and Drug Administration has gone on record as saying that it is a violation of the law to make any claim that polyunsaturates can prevent or treat heart disease.

Several years ago I counseled a 48-year-old female patient who really believed in polyunsaturated fat. She used polyunsaturated margarine, mayonnaise, oils; in fact, almost all food which she cooked or purchased had to contain some polyunsaturated fats. Margarine went on the bread, vegetables, and potatoes; mayonnaise went on all salads and sandwiches. She considered oil to be a medicine, and therefore, almost everything had to have a generous helping of polyunsaturated fat. This lady looked older than her stated age, and she had many physical complaints, but her overriding concern was her constant weakness and lack of energy. I advised her to remove all refined, polyunsaturated fats from her diet. She was allowed to use natural foods that contain polyunsaturated fats (olives, avocados, nuts and seeds), sparingly. Lean white meat was also allowed, but only 3-4 oz a day. All other visible animal fats, including butter, were restricted. After several weeks, I saw her again, and the change in her was significant. She appeared cheerful and energetic, and with a smile on her face, she told me how well she was feeling. This is not an isolated incident, but is the usual result seen in a patient who has removed refined, oily and greasy products from his diet.

—Zane R. Kime, M.D.
 Sunlight Could Save Your Life

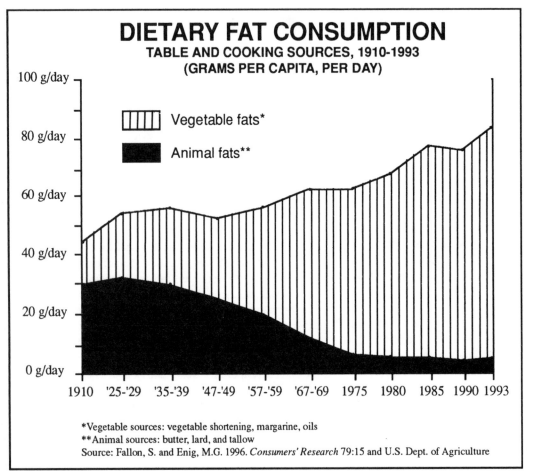

DIETARY FAT CONSUMPTION
TABLE AND COOKING SOURCES, 1910-1993
(GRAMS PER CAPITA, PER DAY)

Vegetable fats*

Animal fats**

*Vegetable sources: vegetable shortening, margarine, oils
**Animal sources: butter, lard, and tallow
Source: Fallon, S. and Enig, M.G. 1996. *Consumers' Research* 79:15 and U.S. Dept. of Agriculture

Since the beginning of the 20th century vegetable oil consumption has steadily increased. Animal fat consumption has decreased. During the same period of time heart disease, cancer, diabetes, and a host of other degenerative diseases have increased along with the rise in vegetable oil consumption. It is evident that animal fat consumption does not correlate with disease rate but vegetable oils do.

disseminated by the advertising and marketing efforts of big food and drug industries. Even the health food industry conveniently ignores unfavorable findings and emphasizes the favorable in such a way as to make a "questionable" product appear better. All businesses do this to some degree. The food industry is no different. Look at how the tobacco and alcohol industries have misled consumers about the health effects of their products in order to protect their sales.

We hear all the good things about vegetable oils, but not the bad. The food industry will tell you a certain oil is "good" for you because it doesn't, for example, cause as much platelet stickiness as some saturated fats. What they don't tell you is that not all fats do this and the supposedly "good" oil, although might not contribute as much to platelet stickiness as some fats, may contribute more to cancer, diabetes, arthritis, and a host of other degenerative conditions. Any advertiser is going to promote *only* the good aspects of his product and conveniently ignore any and all bad effects. That's simly the way business is run.

Why isn't the bad effects more widely advertised? The reason is because there isn't any money in it for anybody.

The food industry wants to sell a product, so they will naturally publicize any positive research. There is no significant industry that sells a product because of negative research of a product. The studies showing the negative effects of oils are buried in scientific journals which are only read by other scientists. Consequently, no one ever hears about the detrimental effects of vegetable oils. Even medical doctors and other health care professionals are generally unaware because they don't have the time to search through hundreds of research journals every month to find the information. They need to spend their time making a living. They often rely on promotional material from food and supplement manufactures (a highly biased source) for their information. Many, but not all, books on health are written by people who are misinformed. They've been brainwashed by the media and the marketing propaganda from the food industry.

My father was a medical doctor and a nutritionist. He believed strongly that diet affects our health and taught his family to eat healthfully. He, like most everybody else, fell into the trap of condemning all saturated fat as unhealthy and promoting all vegetable oils as a better alternative. So we grew up avoiding butter, lard, and other animal fats. In their place we ate what he thought were "healthy" vegetable oils including margarine and shortening. We now know that these oils are harmful, especially margarine. My father died of heart disease, diabetes, and Alzheimer's disease. It was a slow lingering process that extend several years and was pure torture for him. He suffered through operations, daily insulin injections, and senility. When he died, his family felt relieved because it released him from the pain he was suffering as a consequence of these degenerative conditions.

From 1965 to 1972 total fat consumption increased by 11 grams per person per day. Ten of the 11 were vegetable fat, one was saturated fat.[21] Since 1909 the per capita consumption of unsaturated vegetable oils has greatly increased. Between 1970 and 1995 total added fat (that added to food) in pounds per person per year in America increased from 55 to 68. Margarine and butter consumption remained steady with margarine consumption over twice that of butter. Lard decreased slightly and shortening and vegetable oils increased from 15 to 25.

The chart on previous page shows the per capita consumption of vegetable fat as compared to animal fat. No-

tice that animal fat consumption since 1910 has decreased while vegetable oil consumption has greatly increased. If animal fats are supposed to be so unhealthy, then this decrease in saturated fat consumption should have brought about a much improved level of health. But it hasn't. As vegetable oil consumption has increased so has heart disease, cancer, diabetes, and a host of other degenerative diseases. The disease rate has risen in correlation with vegetable oil consumption. Saturated fat consumption shows no correlation with disease rate.

MONOUNSATURATED OILS

For years most all types of oils were considered bad, contributing to many disease conditions particularly of the cardiovascular system. We were told that the more fat we ate, the higher the health risk. People started eating leaner cuts of meat and choosing foods with lower fat content. However, it was noticed that some people did not fit the proposed model. People with diets high in fat did not always develop cardiovascular disease. This was particularly true for those living in southern Europe around the Mediterra-

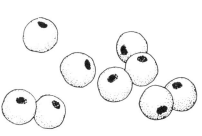

Cold pressed oils involve only pressure to squeeze the oil from the fruit. Higher pressures, heat, and chemical solvents are added to extract additional oil from both the fruit pulp and pits. This gives rise to a great deal of variety in the quality of olive oils. The International Olive Oil Institute has created a set of labeling terms in an effort to provide a uniform grading system. The most common grades are presented below.

Extra Virgin Olive Oil is drawn from the first cold pressing of olives. The result is a pure oil that is very low in acid (about 1 percent), quite mild and full of aroma. Its most pronounced characteristic is its distinctive fruity fragrance, which varies from brand to brand. You can't tell the grade of the oil just from the color. Extra virgin oils can range from pale shades of straw to the most intense greens. Generally speaking, the darker the shade, the richer the flavor.

OLIVE OILS

Virgin Olive Oil is also from a first pressing, but contains a higher acid level (typically 2 to 3 percent), which gives it a little more of a bitter flavor.

Fino Olive Oil is a blend of extra virgin and virgin olive oils.

Olive Oil formerly known as "pure olive oil" combines both refined (pomace olive oil) and extra virgin or virgin olive oils. Flavor is more mild than virgin or extra virgin olive oils. This grade is usually used in the making of flavored oils such as garlic and roasted pepper olive oils.

"Pomace" or "Pomage" Olive Oils may be extracted from the ground olives or pits that have been mechanically ground, crushed or solvent-extracted. Highly refined and tasteless. Used as an all purpose oil when a mild flavor is desired.

"Light" Olive Oil is a marketing gimmick. It has the same amount of calories and fat as other grades. But "light" versions are literally, lighter. They're paler not only in color but also in flavor and fragrance. This oil is highly refined to remove natural flavor and color.

nean Sea. The most striking aspect of the so-called Mediterranean Diet was the high fat consumption. Some villagers got as much as 40 percent of their calories from fat. Studies found that the Mediterranean Diet was not just high in fat, but it was high in fat derived from olive oil—primarily a monounsaturated fat. Before heading out to the fields, some Greek farmers were chugging glasses of olive oil for breakfast. Consumption of saturated fat was moderate to low, and especially low in polyunsaturated fats. Polyunsaturated vegetable oils weren't used much because olive oil was the vegetable oil of choice. The people did eat meat and dairy so they got moderate amounts of saturated fat.

This led to the discovery that monounsaturated fats did not possess the negative health consequences attributed to other fats..[22] Because olive and other monounsaturated oils did not appear to contribute significantly to cardiovascular disease, they gained the status of "healthy" dietary oils.

Olive oil is not the only source for monounsaturated fatty acids. Oils containing a high percentage of monounsaturated fatty acids include avocado, canola, almond, hazelnut, and apricot. Most high monounsaturated oils are over-processed, clear, odorless, and tasteless, meaning they have had all nutritive value stripped away except for the fatty acids. This process usually involves high temperatures and chemical solvents. Avocado oil, in particular, must undergo harsh extraction and chemical treatments to remove its displeasing flavor and is, therefore, always highly processed and unfit to eat. Canola oil is much the same. Canola oil contains an undesirable fat known as erucic acid.* Erucic acid is a very long chain monounsaturated fat (22:1) that has been found to be highly toxic to the heart muscle.[23] Normally, canola oil contains as much as 45-50 percent erucic acid, making it very dangerous. Because of erucic acid's toxic effects, laws limit the amount of this fatty acid in oils used for human consumption. Through modern agricultural science, varieties of rapeseed containing less than 1 percent erucic acid have been developed. This is the type used to make the canola oil used in food. Although the amount of this toxic fatty acid in canola oil is small, any amount is really undesirable.

Olive oil is much better than any other high monounsaturated oils because it is commonly cold pressed and unadulterated by chemical additives. There are different grades of olive oil. Extra virgin olive oil is cold pressed without any additional processing. It retains all its flavor, color, aroma, and vitamins and minerals and is the best type to use. The more processing the oil receives, the more degraded it becomes. Other types of olive oil are less healthy because they will contain more chemical additives and are more oxidized.

Although olive oil is often called a "heart healthy" oil, it does not promote any particular benefit to the heart. With the possible exception of omega-3 fatty acids (found most abundantly in fish and flaxseed) *all oils*, including olive oil, promote platelet stickiness.[24] Platelet stickiness promotes blood clotting and encourages hypertension, both of which are risk factors for atherosclerosis and heart disease. But olive oil has a much lower effect that other oils and is often considered benign in this respect. It is considered heart healthy because its adverse effects on the heart and circulatory system are much less than that of other fats. Replacing other vegetable oils with olive oil will reduce negative effects on the heart and the body in general and, therefore, in that respect is considered heart healthy. But keep in mind that olive oil still raises blood fat and body fat levels.

Monounsaturated fat is more stable than polyunsaturated oils and, therefore, is not affected by oxidation and free-radical activity as much. A polyunsaturated oil that has two double-carbon bonds is twice as susceptible to oxidation as monounsaturated oil. Our own body tissues favor monounsaturated fat. Olive oil is 77 percent monounsaturated fat, 14 percent saturated fat, and only 9 percent polyunsaturated fat, which makes it the most stable vegetable oil common in kitchen use.

Another interesting fact about olive oil is that it is very similar in composition to our own body fat profile. The predominante fatty acid in olive oil is oleic acid—an 18-carbon chain monounsaturated fat. This is also the predominante fatty acid found in human tissues. The second most abundant fatty acid in olive oil is palmitic acid—a 16-carbon chain saturated fat. Palmitic acid is also the second most abundant fatty acid in the human body. The third fatty acid of significance in olive oil is linoleic acid—an 18-carbon chain polyunsaturated fat. Likewise, it is the third most abundant fat in human tissue. The relative quantity of each fat is roughly comparable in both olive oil and the human body. This correlation suggests that olive oil is compatible to human needs.

_____

*borage and blackcurrant oils also contain erucic acid.

Chapter 4

ESSENTIAL FATTY ACIDS

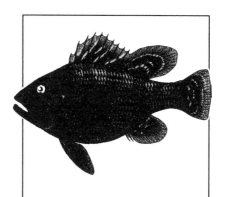

ESSENTIALLY

For hundreds of years sailors on long ocean voyages forced to subsist on diets limited to salted meat and biscuits were plagued with a disease called scurvy. Health often improved once the sailors were given fresh fruits and vegetables, but the cause was completely unknown. It wasn't until the early 20th century that the cause of scurvy was identified as a deficiency in a compound known as vitamin C.

Beriberi was a disease which ravaged Asia soon after the custom of polishing rice became common. Medical researchers thought the illness was caused by a bacteria or virus and spent years looking for the culprit. They searched in vain. Eventually they discovered that it wasn't an infection at all, but a vitamin deficiency brought on by eating a diet dominated by white rice. The rice was nutrient deficient as a result of having its vitamin-rich outer layer polished or rubbed off. Discoveries like these led researchers into seeking other nutrients that were essential to health.

Under controlled conditions, animals were fed diets lacking in certain nutrients, and symptoms, if any, were noted. If symptoms abated when the missing nutrients were added back into the food, it was determined that the nutrient was a necessary component of a healthy diet. As a result, several nutrients have been classified as essential.

Essential nutrients are defined as substances that the body cannot make for itself, or cannot make in sufficient quantities to meet its needs. We must, therefore, get these nutrients directly from the foods we eat. Just because a particular substance is not considered "essential," however, does not mean it isn't important. Nonessential nutrients are still necessary, but can be manufactured in our bodies from other nutrients.

By the 1920s researchers had identified several vitamins and minerals that were considered essential. Carbohydrate and some amino acids, which make up protein, were also added to this list. Fats, as yet, had not been shown to be essential. Part of the reason was the problem in synthesizing a food completely devoid of all fats. Fats in one form or another are found in all foods. Removing them requires special preparations under controlled laboratory conditions.

Dr. G.O. Burr was the first researcher to feed lab animals diets completely devoid of all fat in an attempt to determine the importance of fatty acids on health. On a totally fat-free diet, the rats developed skin lesions and reproductive abnormalities. When he gave them vegetable oil, it prevented or reversed these conditions. His findings were published in the *Journal of Biological Chemistry* in 1929.[1] This landmark study provided the basis for the essentiality of fats in our diet. Veg-

"It ain't what we don't know that gives us trouble. It's what we know that ain't so that gives us trouble."

—Will Rogers

etable oils are composed of a mixture of saturated, monounsaturated, and polyunsaturated fats, and it was not known if they were all of equal importance in preventing deficiency symptoms. Research by Dr. Burr and others demonstrated that saturated and monounsaturated fats could be synthesized in the body from other nutrients and, therefore, although important, were not considered "essential" nutrients. Polyunsaturated fatty acids, however, seemed to fit the definition of essentiality.

The first polyunsaturated fatty acid to be identified as being essential was linoleic acid—a member of the omega-6 group of fats. Later, alpha-linolenic acid, a member of the omega-3 family, was also given the same status.

Early studies demonstrated that the exclusion of all fats from the diet produced a variety of symptoms such as growth retardation, reproductive failure, skin abnormalities, visual problems, and kidney and liver disorders. Adding fat back into the diet corrected these symptoms. Omega-6 fatty acids prevented or corrected all of these symptoms. Omega-3 fatty acids appeared to be at least partially effective in correcting symptoms. So both are now considered essential.

Added support to the claim of essentiality is the observation that large amounts of DHA (an omega-3 fatty acid) have been found in the brain and eyes. In one experiment, female monkeys were fed diets low in DHA during pregnancy. Their offspring suffered from eye defects until their diet was supplemented by DHA.[2]

It has been generally believed that animals, including humans, cannot make the polyunsaturated fatty acids belonging to the omega-6 or omega-3 families from any other nutrients; nor convert any members of the omega-6 family to an omega-3 fatty acid or vice versa. The shorter linoleic acid molecule (18-carbon chain), which is a member of the omega-6 family of fatty acids, can be converted into larger molecules in the same family (20- and 22-carbon chains). Likewise, the smaller alpha-linolenic acid molecule (18-carbon chain), which is a member of the omega-3 family of fatty acids, can be converted into larger molecules in the same family. Therefore, if we need a fatty acid of either family, we must have, if not the very fatty acid, then another one of that family.

More recently, the question of essentiality has resurfaced. Studies show that linoleic and alpha-linolenic acid can, in fact, be synthesized in our bodies from other fats present in the diet. This is evidenced by the absence of clear symptoms of essential fatty acid deficiency in healthy adults when these fats are limited in the diet.[3]

Common foods adequately supply all the fatty acids the body needs. Fats are also easily stored in body tissues so they are available if not consumed in the diet for an extended period of time. It has been 70 years since the publication of Dr. Burr's research, and in that time clear deficiencies in humans have not been noted. The only evidence of possible essential fatty acid deficiencies have been observed in those people eating laboratory prepared foods which may have lacked other important nutrients as well. For instance, in infants fed formula lacking fatty acids and in hospitalized patients who have been fed intravenously for prolonged periods of time through a formula that provides no polyunsaturated fatty acids.[4]

Researchers have noted examples of animals living generation after generation without unsaturated oils in their diets and human cells growing in culture-dishes without polyunsaturated fats, exhibit no noticeable ill effects on health.[5] This, combined with the fact that the addition of those oils disrupts the body's function in many ways, has raised questions about the essentiality of these oils. Still, most scientists continue to accept them as being essential, at least to some degree. But the amount we need, if we do need them, may be much smaller than what many adherents have suggested.

Furthermore, using essential fatty acids to treat illness has been a disappointment. Psoriasis is recognized as one of the characteristic symptoms of essential fatty acids deficiency, but in clinical studies when patients are treated with essential fatty acids, no improvement is noted. If a true fatty acid deficiency existed, improvement would be expected when the fats were added to the diet.

Since more recent studies have shown that we can produce the so-called essential fatty acids (EFA), the question is: can enough be synthesized to meet the body's needs? This probably depends on the physiological state of the individual. EFAs are more necessary during pregnancy, lactation, and periods of rapid growth.

The Food and Agricultural Organization (FAO) and the World Health Organization (WHO) suggest that a minimum of 3 percent of total calories should be from essential fatty acids in adults, and 5 percent in young children and pregnant and breast feeding women.[6] This is a very small amount that is easy to obtain just from eating a normal diet.

How important are fats? We know they must be important to health because nature has included them in a wide variety of foods. Like carbohydrate, both saturated and unsaturated fatty acids are so abundant in nature that it's virtually impossible not to get enough so long as you consume a reasonable quantity of wholesome food.

THE FISH CONNECTION
The Greenland Eskimos

The initial nutritional studies on vegetable oils focused on linoleic acid (omega-6) because most vegetable oils are

predominantely of this type. The importance of the omega-3 family of fatty acids did not become apparent until the second half of the 20th century.

By the 1960s linoleic acid was generally recognized as an essential nutrient. Omega-3 fatty acids had not gained as much interest and were still under study. At this time, saturated fat and cholesterol were pegged as the culprits in causing cardiovascular disease and for the high rate of death due to heart attack. The cholesterol hypothesis of heart disease was reaching its zenith. Because of the marketing efforts of pharmaceutical companies and the sensationalism of the news media, everybody, except for many researchers, believed that dietary cholesterol and saturated fat (which was easily converted into cholesterol by the liver) were the cause of heart disease.

Studies seemed to show that those countries where people ate the most meat, eggs, and milk—all high in saturated fat and cholesterol—also had the highest incidence of cardiovascular disease. The more fat consumed, the greater the disease rate. The evidence seemed clear, however, there were many notable exceptions to this observation. Several groups of people, particularly the Eskimos of North America and Greenland who ate a diet extremely high in saturated fat and cholesterol were completely free from heart disease and atherosclerosis.

The Greenland Eskimos' diet included almost a pound of whale and seal meat a day including blubber and intestines, plus fish and game. The meat and fish were eaten baked or raw mostly without any greens. According to the cholesterol hypothesis the Eskimos should be reeking with heart disease. The Eskimos were clear examples of a group of people who defied the cholesterol hypothesis of heart disease. To find out why, researchers headed to Greenland to study the Eskimos' diets, lifestyle, and health.

Danish researchers visited Greenland in 1970 and, judging from the Eskimos' diet, expected to find rampant heart disease. They found just the opposite. When the researchers studied health records from 1963 to 1967, they found that only two cases of atherosclerotic heart disease had occurred among the 1,300 inhabitants in an Eskimo settlement—one in a 78-year-old man, the other in someone suffering from rheumatic heart disease. Death from heart disease constituted only 3.5 percent of all deaths among Greenland Eskimos, whose average life span at the time was over 60 years.[7] In 1982 the American Heart Association estimated that nearly one million Americans died of some form of cardiovascular disease, or over half of all deaths for the year. The researchers also observed that arthritis and other chronic inflammatory diseases were almost unknown among the Eskimos.

They noted one other curious thing—the Eskimos tended to bruise easily and bleed for a longer time when injured. When samples of their blood were analyzed, it was found to be low in fats, especially triglycerides (the main substance found in the fat tissue of the body and the main dietary fat) and lipoproteins, and in cholesterol. The researchers also found that the Eskimos bled more freely because something was affecting the normal functioning of their platelets—tiny disk-shaped cells that float in the blood and help in clotting. Their platelets appeared to be less sticky and didn't clump together as readily as those of other groups of people. The major cause of death among the Eskimo was cerebral hemorrhagic stroke caused by bleeding in the brain. When the body loses its ability to clot, arteries weaken and bleed and, because clotting ability is depressed, bleeding can become excessive and deadly. This mode of death was essentially the opposite of the type typical in Europe and America. Coronary heart disease and stroke due to cerebral thrombosis and cerebral embolism, which are the most common forms of cardiovascular disease in Western countries, are caused by excessive blood clotting.

Because coronary heart disease is the leading cause of death in most Western countries, the diet of any society that shows a low level of heart disease is bound to attract attention. Researchers returned to Greenland several times to verify the findings, but the results were the same. The big question many asked was did the Eskimos have a genetic resistance to heart disease. That was ruled out when it was found that Eskimos who settled in Denmark had just as much heart disease as native Danes. The researchers concluded that the large amounts of fatty marine food that the Eskimos were eating somehow protected them from heart disease.

It was noted that in Japanese fishing villages and other parts of the world where seafood comprised a major part of the diet, the people also demonstrated some degree of protection against the circulatory diseases commonly found in Western countries.

In may 1985 the *New England Journal of Medicine* created a stir in the medical world by publishing the results of a study which said that eating fish was possibly beneficial to human health. Especially significant was a 20-year prospective Dutch study, which began in 1960 and involved 852 middle-aged Dutch men initially free from heart disease. Their cooperative wives kept track of what their husbands ate for all those years. During the study, 78 men died of coronary artery disease. The death rate was more than 50 percent lower among those who consumed at least 30 grams of fish per day then among those who did not eat fish. And it made no difference whether the fish was lean or fatty. Thus, not eating fish at all turned out to be a risk factor for heart disease in this group. The authors concluded that eating as little as two fish meals per week may help prevent coronary artery disease.[8]

In another study published by the *New England Journal of Medicine*, researchers from Oregon Health Sciences University used 20 subjects who had high blood fat levels. The group went on a strict low-fat and low-cholesterol diet, containing salmon oil and a commercial fish-oil concentrate, and enriched with polyunsaturated vegetable oils. The levels of fat and cholesterol fell in every patient. According to the cholesterol hypothesis, lowering blood fat levels would also reduce risk of heart disease.

The component of fish oil that seemed to be having the most impact on the circulatory system were the omega-3 polyunsaturated fatty acids, particularly eicosapentaenoic (EPA) and docosahexaenoic (DHA) acids.

The major role they play in heart disease is in decreasing platelet stickiness, thus reducing the blood's tendency to clot. Blood pressure is also reduced. The advantage is that decreased stickiness and decreased blood pressure means fewer clots, less atherosclerosis and, possibly, less heart disease.

Precautions

As great as all this sounds, a few words of warning are in order. Although studies have shown that those who eat fish may have less heart disease than those who don't, what they don't show is whether the fish eaters have a greater prevalence of other types of disease. This is a very valid concern. Because of omega-3's tendency to reduce blood clotting, Eskimos had trouble with excessive bruising and healing from injuries and suffered heavily from hemorrhagic stroke which was their most common cause of death. This suggests that a little may be good but a lot may not.

Research has also shown that the good effects of omega-3 fatty acids last only as long as they are consumed. The same type of action that occurs when you take drugs to treat an illness. Omega-3s are only a temporary fix that do not cure the problem but only mask the symptoms. Nor is there presently any good scientific evidence that consum-

ing fish oils will reverse any preexisting cardiovascular disease. And while thinner blood and longer clotting time may be great for the heart and the arteries, for many of us it could be a serious complication in the event of an accident or emergency surgery.

Adding a little fish to your diet appears to provide some health benefits. Deep-water ocean fish may be safe to eat, but fish caught nearer shore may contain pollutants, such as lead or polychlorinated biphenyls. Shellfish may be exposed to naturally occurring environmental contaminants or sewage, so it's important to buy only from dealers whose fish are harvested from safe waters. Rainbow trout raised commercially or fished from clear mountain streams generally are safe.

Some people don't want to eat fish. Another way to get the benefits of omega-3 fatty acids without eating fish is to take fish oil supplements. Some commercial fish oil preparations (commonly sold in concentrated capsule or emulsion forms) may also pose hazards. Though they contain omega-3 fatty acids, they may also contain substances that can be harmful. Since most chemical residues concentrate in the liver and fatty tissues, it's possible that fish oils derived from fish livers and parts of fish not normally consumed may be contaminated with pesticides or other potentially dangerous toxins.

Fish Oil Supplements

Promising studies on fish and fish oil in the 1980s generated a flood of omega-3 dietary supplements onto the market. Everybody wanted the oil that would protect them from heart disease. Those who are most active in telling everyone to rush out and buy fish oil concentrates or other omega-3 supplements are the ones who manufacture or distribute these products. Many doctors and nutritionists were also caught up in the craze being persuaded by manufacturer's sales and promotional literature.

Initial studies on omega-3 fatty acids showed promising results in the treatment of a variety of conditions including arthritis, atherosclerosis, cancer, high blood cholesterol, diabetes, eczema, psoriasis, migraines, and hypertension. Supplement distributors began making claims their products could help protect against these conditions. And many people believed them. Sales skyrocketed.

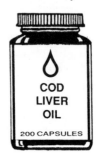

The Food and Drug Administration (FDA) stepped in, having completed an extensive review of the evidence and stated, "There is inadequate scientific evidence to support any health claims on fish oils," and ordered off the shelves all fish oil supplements with labels that promised to cure, prevent, or mitigate disease. This didn't stop distributors, it only modified the way they promoted their products.

Mixed Results

The health benefits of fish-oil supplements are far from proven. While initial studies showed some benefits with fish oil, later studies reported that they may not do everything earlier studies suggested they might.

Anyone who still buys the distributor's claims hook, line, and sinker should consider the results of a study conducted at the Minneapolis Veterans Affairs Medical Center. When some 40 men with moderately high blood cholesterol took fish oil capsules for a period of 12 weeks, their cholesterol concentration *increased* by about 5%. They suffered loose stools, belching and abdominal distension as well. Other potential risks of taking omega-3 supplements: blood that becomes too thin to clot in the case of an accident, and higher blood sugar levels for people with diabetes.[9]

Many studies have reported findings showing that omega-3 fatty acids are anything but the panacea they are made out to be. In a study performed at the University of California, San Diego, the cholesterol levels of 6 diabetics given fish oil remained unaffected. What really stood out from this study was not the lack of influence on cholesterol, but was that control of the subject's blood sugar deteriorated. This deterioration in blood sugar control evidently occurred because fish oil stimulated the liver to release more glucose into the bloodstream than it usually does.[10] It appears that fish and omega-3 fatty acids are *not* good for those people with blood sugar problems. This presents a problem for diabetics because they are at high risk of cardiovascular disease. While omega-3's may provide some protection against heart disease, it may also aggravate problems associated with diabetes.

Some studies have shown that fish oils can lower blood cholesterol. Other studies show little effect and some showed it can raise blood cholesterol. At the Kalamazoo Clinical Investigational Complex in Michigan researchers studied the influence of fish oil on blood cholesterol. Investigators gave fish oil to subjects with cardiac risk factors. Of the 31 subjects with high cholesterol levels, 13 were given fish oil and the others a placebo. Cholesterol levels *rose* even higher when fish oil was given and returned to normal when it was stopped.[11]

Doctors at the University of Wisconsin confirmed studies showing large doses of fish oil supplements can, at least

initially, lower blood fats. This study continued over a longer period of time than earlier ones and included lower-dose maintenance therapy. After six months, however, the initial fat-lowering effect of fish oil in patients with high levels almost disappeared.[12]

Another study cast doubt on the benefits of omega-3 oils for heart patients. Angioplasty is a medical treatment for heart disease in which a balloon is inserted in clogged arteries to reopen them. Because fish oil reduces blood clotting, researchers reasoned it would help keep open such arteries, which are at risk of becoming clogged again.

Three small studies reported positive results, but a larger study from Harvard Medical School and Beth Israel Hospital proved otherwise. In the Harvard study, 137 angioplasty patients got fish oil and 67 got olive oil. The fish oil patients actually had a higher rate of recurrent narrowing of the arteries and even a slightly higher heart attack rate. Another smaller study conducted in Australia reported that fish oil was no better than corn oil (high in polyunsaturated fatty acids) for angioplasty patients.[13]

A study from Wales published in the *Lancet* found a 29 percent reduction in mortality in men who ate fish three times per week following a heart attack. The total number of heart attacks, however, did not change.[14] A more recent study using data from the Physicians Health Study, which began in 1982 and involved 20,551 doctors between the ages 40 to 84 showed similar results. While cardiac death rate was reduced by eating fish, the total number of heart attacks remained unchanged.[15]

The results of studies on fish consumption have been mixed. Some studies have shown a relationship between lower cardiovascular death and fish consumption.[16, 17, 18] Other studies show no relationship.[19, 20, 21, 22] It appears that eating fish oil or whole fish may provide temporary benefit for people with heart disease, but not cure the underlying problem.

When taken in capsule form, which is more concentrated than in foods, fish oil has a drug-like rather than a nutritional effect.[23, 24, 25] Like drugs, fish oil supplements may have adverse side effects. As more studies have been performed it has become clear that eating whole fish, rather than taking concentrated fish oil supplements, provides the most benefit. One of the most obvious effects of taking too much omega-3 fatty acids is a serious reduction in the blood's ability to clot and prolonged bleeding time.[26]

A recent study reported in the *Journal of the American Medical Association* found that those who ate fish at least once a week had a 52 percent lower risk of sudden cardiac death than those who ate it less than once a month. Eating more than one fish meal a week did not provide any significant additional benefit.[27] The authors estimated that a single 4- to 6-ounce serving per week did the job. People who have one fish meal a week cut their risk of sudden cardiac death in half. This has been consistent with other studies.[28] This showed that only a small amount of fish, or fish oil if that was indeed the active ingredient that brought about the benefit, was needed to provide protection.

In this study it was also noted that lean fish, the ones that had the *least* amount of oil, were the *most* beneficial. Dark meat fish, which has the most omega-3 gave the least protective effect. The Study's author noted, "If omega-3 fatty acids are indeed the active agent, this result is somewhat surprising, because this type of fish has the highest omega-3 fatty acid content." This observation led the researchers to suspect that there might be some "unidentified nutrient" other than the omega-3 fatty acids that is actively involved in reducing cardiac death. The presence of such a nutrient would possibly make eating whole fish better than just taking fish oil supplements, which may not contain this other nutrient.

Studies show that fish, and not necessarily fish oil, reduce risk of coronary heart disease. John La Rosa, M.D., of George Washington University School of Medicine and a former chair of the American Heart Association nutrition group stated, "Encouraging people to eat fish is one thing, but there is very little evidence of effectiveness in taking fish oil capsules." (See the sidebar on page 158.)

PROSTAGLANDINS

In the 1930s a Swedish scientist by the name of von Euler discovered a unique hormone-like compound in seminal fluid. Believing it to be from the prostate gland he called it prostaglandin. Later it was discovered that this new substance wasn't unique to men, woman also had prostaglandins and they were present throughout the body.

Prostaglandins are a class of eicosinoids—hormone-like substances synthesized from polyunsaturated fats in our food. They have a pronounced effect on how our bodies function and, for this reason are very important. They have influence on such things as blood pressure, cholesterol synthesis, inflammation response, and platelet aggregation (clotting ability of the blood). Because prostaglandins affect so many vital functions of the body, an imbalance can cause serious health problems and, as you will see later in this chapter, many of the degenerative diseases so common today are directly correlated to them and their precursors— the polyunsaturated fatty acids.

All prostaglandins are synthesized in the body from fatty acids. The synthesis of prostaglandins involves a series of steps controlled by special enzymes. These enzymes cause oxidation reactions to take place in just one particular way to make a particular type of prostaglandin. There are at least 30 different prostaglandins that have been identified. All of the prostaglandins fall into three families or series, depending on the fatty acid from which they were made.

The series 1 and 2 prostaglandins come from the omega-6 family, with linoleic acid (LA) as the starting point. Linoleic acid is converted in the body to gamma-linolenic acid (GLA), then to dihomogamma-linolenic acid (DGLA) and then to arachidonic acid (AA). The series 1 prostaglandins are made from DGLA. The series 2 prostaglandins are made from arachidonic acid.

The series 3 prostaglandins are made from the omega-3 family, with alpha-linolenic acid (ALA) as the starting point. Alpha-linolenic acid is converted to stearidonic acid, then to eicosatetraenoic acid, then to eicosapentaenoic acid (EPA). The series 3 prostaglandins are all made from EPA (see diagram on next page).

Each of these prostaglandins have different effects on the body. Some exert a greater influence on bodily function than others. In general, series 2 prostaglandins (PGE2) exert a stronger influence than series 1 prostaglandins (PGE1), and series 3 prostaglandins (PGE3) have a stronger influence than either PGE2 or PGE1. So, in general, the larger the number in the series, the stronger its effects on the body.*

Series 1 prostaglandins (PGE1) have several important functions in different tissues in the human body. It keeps blood platelets from sticking together, and thereby helps to prevent heart attacks and strokes caused by blood clots in the arteries. In the kidneys, it helps to remove fluid from the body, acting as a diuretic. It opens up blood vessels, improving circulation and relieving angina (chest pain). It helps insulin work effectively. It also slows down cholesterol production and inhibits inflammation.

Series 2 prostaglandins (PGE2) made from arachidonic acid (AA) has almost the opposite effect. It promotes platelet aggregation (stickiness), which encourages clot formation. It induces the kidneys to retain salt and constricts the blood vessels leading to water retention and increased blood pressure. It also encourages inflammation.

Series 3 prostaglandins (PGE3) are made from eicosapentaenoic acid (EPA). This prostaglandin is much like PGE1 in its effects. It has potent platelet anti-stickiness effects, reduces inflammation, slows the synthesis of cholesterol, and dilates blood vessels.

---

*The degree of influence is evidenced in the fact that consuming only linoleic acid (omega-6), the precursor to both PEG1 and PEG2, will create symptoms of excess PGE2. Adding just one third to one tenth as much alpha-linolenic acid (omega-3), the precursor to PGE3, will balance the effects from linoleic acid (omega-6), the precursor to PGE1 and PGE2.

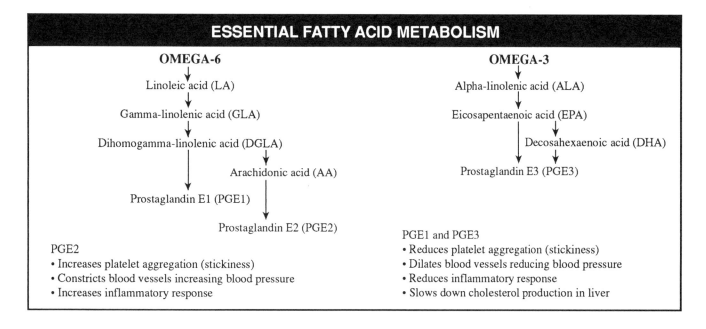

Omega-6 fatty acids are found abundantly in the foods we eat, coming from both plant and animal sources. They are most abundant in vegetable oils. Corn, safflower, cottonseed, and soybean oils consist predominately of omega-6 fatty acids (linoleic acid). Gamma-linolenic acid (GLA) which is also a member of this family is most abundant in black currant oil, borage oil, and evening primrose oil, but make up less than 10 percent of the total oil content. Arachidonic acid, the direct precursor to PGE2, is found in very small quantities in meats. Most of the arachidonic acid in our bodies is synthesized from the linoleic acid we get in vegetable oils.

Prostaglandins have been used pharmaceutically for various purposes, such as to affect blood pressure, to decrease platelet stickiness, and stimulate uterine contractions to induce abortions. But they must be injected into the body in relatively large doses to achieve these effects. Taken orally they are broken down by stomach acids and rendered useless. For this reason, omega-3 and omega-6 fatty acids are given orally so that the body can manufacture its own prostaglandins.

One of the problems of taking omega-3 and omega-6 fatty acids orally is that it is easy to build up an excess in the tissues and experience toxic side effects. Since fatty acids are fat-soluble, they accumulate in body tissues rather then simply wash out of the body like many other nutrients.

Vegetable oils contain both linoleic and alpha-linolenic acids. Even margarine and shortening, which are made from hydrogenated vegetable oil, have been recommended as sources for essential fatty acids. When these oils are hydrogenated, their chemical structure is altered. Natural fatty acids are known as cis-linoleic and cis-alpha-linolenic acids when they are hydrogenated they are transformed into trans-linoleic and trans-alpha-linolenic acids and *cannot* be utilized by the body to make prostaglandins of any type. Trans fatty acids have absolutely no biological value and, therefore, are worthless except that they can be broken down to some extent to provide energy.

LINOLEIC ACID (OMEGA-6): ESSENTIAL NUTRIENT—MODERN MENACE

Linoleic acid is the precursor to all the other omega-6 fatty acids. This is the most plentiful fatty acid in the human diet. Omega-6 fatty acids include: gamma-linolenic acid, dihomogamma-linolenic acid, and arachidonic acid, all of which can be synthesized from linoleic acid. Linoleic acid is found naturally in most all fruits, vegetables, grains, meats, eggs, and dairy products. It is virtually impossible to eat a diet lacking in this nutrient.

When scientists first determined the essentially of fatty acids in the diet, they had to create foods devoid of all fats. The only way to do that is to carefully prepare food under controlled conditions in a laboratory. Omega-6 fatty acids are so abundant in nature and in our modern foods that it is virtually impossible not to get enough of them with a normal diet.

The problem we face in most Western countries today is not a lack of omega-6, but an excess! This is a very important fact and has considerable health consequences. It is the reason that linoleic acid has become a modern menace.

With the exception of olive oil, most every vegetable oil we commonly use in cooking and in salads is composed predominantely of omega-6 fatty acids. Vegetable oil consumption has increased dramatically over the years, replacing those high in saturated fats such as butter and lard. As a consequence, our society is suffering from omega-6 toxicity. Many of the degenerative diseases that have become prominent over the past few decades can be linked to the overconsumption of omega-6 fatty acids.

There is a great deal of conflicting information about the need and importance of essential fatty acids. Some research supports the need for them while others show little need. You probably have not heard anybody say that essen-

tial fatty acids are not that important or that they may be even detrimental to health. Why? Because there is no industry that can profit from *not* selling these oils. But you do hear a lot about the benefits and need for them by the vegetable oil producers and others who are trying to sell products. Any salesperson is going to portray his product in the most favorable light, even stretching the truth and ignoring negative attributes in order to make sales. For this reason, the oil industry has hyped up the importance for fatty acid supplementation. Because of the marketing efforts and publicity of the oil industry, we all assume and believe these fatty acids are important to good health, but what we don't hear is that they also can cause serious health problems.

THE "OMEGA" IN FATTY ACIDS

Ω-9

Ω-6

We often talk of the essential fatty acids as being omega-6 or omega-3. What does the "omega" stand for anyway? Alpha-linolenic acid is called an omega-3 fatty acid and linoleic acid an omega-6 fatty acid. Omega-3 and omega-6 fatty acids are actually groups or families of fatty acids each consisting of several members. Alpha-linolenic acid is only one member of the omega-3 family. Linoleic acid, likewise, is only one member of the omega-6 family. Both represent the starting point or first fatty acid in the family and from them other members can be synthesized.

Fatty acids consist of linear chains of carbon atoms with two ends. One end is designated the methyl (CH3) end and the other the acid (COOH) end. The number associated with omega fatty acids is determined by the position of the first double carbon bond from the methyl end. In omega-3 fatty acids the first of its double carbon bonds is *three* carbons away from its methyl end. Omega-6 fatty acids have the first of

its double bonds *six* carbons from its methyl end. Oleic acid, which is an omega-9 fatty acid, has its first carbon bond nine carbons from its methyl end. Saturated fat does not have any double carbon bonds so it does not have an omega designation.

Linoleic acid, gamma-linolenic acid, dihomogamma-linolenic acid (DGLA), and arachidonic acid (AA) are all omega-6 fatty acids. Alpha-linolenic acid, eicosapentaenoic acid (EPA), and docosahexaenoic acid (DHA) are omega-3 fatty acids. The major differ-

ences between each of these polyunsaturated acids in their respective family is the length of their carbon chains and number of double bonds (degree of unsaturation). Linoleic acid has 18 carbon atoms and two double bonds. Arachidonic acid has 20 carbon atoms and four double bonds. Alpha-linolenic acid has 18 carbon atoms and three double bonds. EPA has 20 carbon atoms and five double bonds. DHA is the longest with 22 carbon atoms and the most unsaturated with six double bonds.

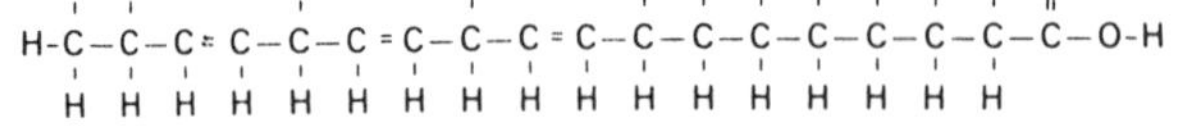

Prostaglandins are synthesized from omega-3 and omega-6 fatty acids having chain lengths of 20 carbons. So DGLA and arachidonic acid, both 20 carbon omega-6 fatty acids, are converted to PGE1 and PGE2 respectively. EPA, a 20 carbon omega-3 fatty acid, is converted to PGE3. The human body cannot make DGLA, arachidonic acid, or EPA, so we must get them directly from our food or from their precursors—linoleic acid and alpha-linolenic acid.

Alpha-linolenic acid (omega-3)

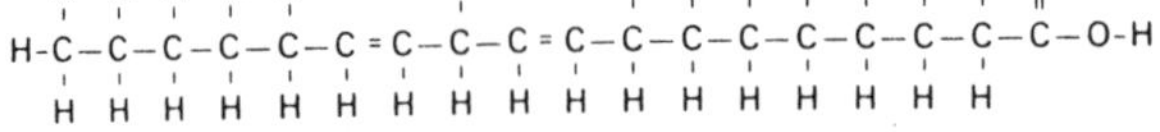

Linoleic acid (omega-6)

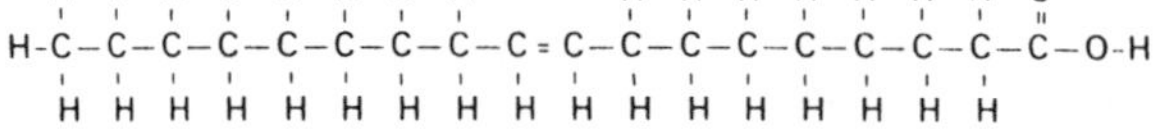

Oleic acid (omega-9)

Obesity

You might question that if omega-6 fatty acids are essential to good health, how can they cause disease? The philosophy that if a little does you good than a lot will do you a lot more good, is not true for most nutrients and it's definitely not true for omega-6 fatty acids.

Next time you go to the grocery store, look at the ingredient labels on all the packaged, canned, and frozen foods. You will find in almost every case one or more of the following: safflower oil, corn oil, soybean oil, cottonseed oil, sunflower oil, peanut oil, canola oil, margarine, and shortening. All of which have a high percentage of omega-6 fatty acids. Plus many of the foods we eat are cooked in vegetable oil. Add to that the fact that most all foods including meats and dairy naturally contain omega-6 fatty acids, and you can see that we are consuming a huge amount of this type of oil. Researchers have estimated that we need the equilivent of only about a half tablespoon a day. This amount is easily obtained from fresh produce and whole grains without adding any vegetable oil, margarine, or shortening. Packaged foods are loaded with fat. A typical diet supplies up to 20 times the amount we need.

Excessive fat, from any source, is stored as body fat. This contributes to weight problems. Being overweight increases your chances for developing arthritis, gout, high blood pressure, high cholesterol, respiratory problems, varicose veins, diabetes, atherosclerosis and heart disease, cancer, gallbladder disease, and gynecological irregularities. According to insurance companies' reports, overweight people die younger from a host of causes.

Free-Radical Free-for-All

Another problem with consuming omega-6 fatty acids is that because they are polyunsaturated, they are also highly susceptible to oxidation which initiates free-radical generation. When you eat these oils you are feeding your body millions of free-radical terrorists that are tearing the molecules in your cells apart. Would you purposely swallow a box of tacks? No, of course not because they would rip your intestinal lining to shreds. But that is just about the same effect you get whenever you eat polyunsaturated oils.

The biggest danger from free radicals comes from packaged or precooked foods. Processing causes oils to form free radicals quickly. Cooking any polyunsaturated oil also accelerates the free-radical cascade. If you use vegetable oil, margarine, or shortening in cooking or baking, you are eating an enormous amount of free radicals (as well as toxic trans fatty acids).

Most cooking oils are used for that purpose—cooking. But heating polyunsaturated oils makes them even more toxic. The literature on the toxicity of heated oils is extensive. Heated oils have been found to induce damage to interstitial tissues and blood vessel walls, and cause numerous organ lesions.[29] Heating accelerates free-radical formation, creating a very toxic substance.

Omega-6 fatty acids which are naturally found in unprocessed foods, such as fresh fruits, vegetables, and whole fish, do not easily generate free radicals. Whole foods, like these, are rich in antioxidants such as vitamins C and E and, because they are not cooked, cut, or mutilated in any way, they are not exposed to the oxidative damage caused by oxygen or pollution in the air.

The more processing food undergoes, the more likely it is to generate free radicals. If the food contains a high percentage of oil either naturally or added, it will create a great deal of free radicals. In packaged foods the oils have already been highly oxidized before you even carry them out of the grocery store. To slow down the free-radical process, food manufacturers add antioxidants. Most of these antioxidants are chemically synthesized in a laboratory and are just more toxic products our bodies must remove from the foods we eat.

All vegetable oils and oil supplements undergo some degree of free-radical damage before they ever leave the store shelves. The longer they sit on a store shelf or at home in the cupboard, the more damage occurs. If the oil is stored where it is exposed to light (from the sun or indoor lighting), warmth (even room temperature encourages oxidation reactions), and oxygen (every time it's opened, fresh oxygen has a chance to attack it) oxidation and free-radical generation proceeds even faster. How old is the oil sitting in your kitchen...three months...six months...a year?

Even dietary oil supplements, which are processed more carefully than cooking oils, undergo oxidative degeneration while they sit in the bottle. In one study, oil supplements were tested for oxidation of the polyunsaturated fatty acids. The researchers found that oxidation was already present when the products were freshly received by the lab and increased through time during the testing period. *All* the products they tested showed some oxidation. Those with chemical preservatives showed less oxidation than those preserved with vitamin E or other natural preservatives/antioxidants.[30]

Prostaglandin Overdose

Still another problem with consuming too much omega-6 fatty acids is that they are converted by the body into PGE2—prostaglandins that increase stickiness of the blood, raise blood pressure, and increase inflammatory response, all of which encourage atherosclerosis. Too much PGE2 can contribute directly to cardiovascular disease causing heart attacks and stroke—two of the world's biggest killers.[31]

So why does the body produce a substance that is so detrimental to our health? Actually, we need PGE2 to maintain optimal health. That is why omega-6 fatty acids are important in our diet. Nature knows this and has put these fatty acids in almost every food we eat. If we didn't have PGE2 to thicken the blood and help form blood clots, the tiniest cut or scratch could become deadly. Without the ability for the blood to clot, we would bleed to death with even a minor injury. A normally harmless bruise could turn fatal. Inflammation is another process that is important to our health. Through the process of inflammation, injuries and infections are flooded with blood which carries disease-fighting white blood cells and accelerates the clotting process to repair injury. For these reasons, PGE2 is vital to our health. But too much can contribute to disease. Researchers have found that some people suffering from certain diseases have elevated levels of linoleic acid in their bodies.[32, 33, 34]

Too much linoleic acid leads to the production of too much PGE2 and blocks the production of PGE3, which is derived from alpha-linolenic acid. This can create an excess of PGE2 and a deficiency of PGE3. That, combined with the free-radical damage caused by too much linoleic acid, can lead to numerous health problems.

Excessive linoleic acid and the overproduction of PGE2 have been strongly linked to intestinal and other forms of cancer and have been shown to promote breast tumors.[35, 36] The more omega-6 fatty acids in the diet, the greater the chance of cancer.[37] Many studies have shown that when polyunsaturated fats are added to the diet cancer rate increases.[38] The carcinogenic effects of vegetable oil is a well-established fact. However, most of us are unaware of this because it is still being recommended by many as a "healthy" alternative to saturated fat.

Polyunsaturated vegetable oil is also linked to the development of allergies (most notably asthma, scaly dermatitis, and psoriasis),[39, 40, 41, 42] defective blood glucose

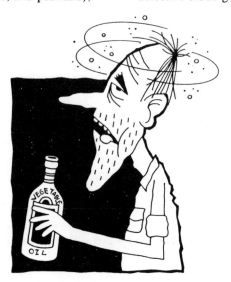

regulation,[43, 38] visual problems,[44] migraine headaches,[45] and a variety of autoimmune and inflammatory conditions including rheumatoid arthritis,[46, 47] irritable bowel syndrome,[48] multiple sclerosis,[49] lupus nephritis,[50] and certain inflammatory kidney conditions.[51]

The type of fatty acids in our diet determine the type of materials that go into building the cells in our brains and nervous system. Sixty percent of our brain is compose of fat, most of which is cholesterol. Too much or too little dietary fat can result in alterations in membrane fluidity, enzyme activities, and the binding of neurotransmitters and hormones to membrane receptors. When this happens, it can impair brain functions such as learning ability, memory, cognitive functions, and behavior.[52, 53] This may explain, at least in part, the increase over the past few decades in diseases that affect the brain such as Alzheimer's disease, Parkinson's disease, senile dementia, dyslexia, and attention deficit disorder (ADD).[54, 55, 56]

A little linoleic acid appears to be necessary for optimal health. Even our immune system depends on it. Too much, however, is detrimental and will *suppress* the immune system.[57] The health of the immune system is vital to protecting the body from invading organisms and cleaning metabolic waste, diseased cells, and other toxic substances. When the immune system is depressed, we open ourselves up to disease of all types, and many detrimental health conditions can progress much faster than they could otherwise.

Diets high in the kinds of polyunsaturated fat prominent in corn, safflower, and soybean oils disrupt the immune system. This impairment of immune system function may increase the risk of developing infections and even cancer. According to Dr. John Kinsella, a lipid biochemist at Cornell University, high levels of dietary polyunsaturated fat fosters the growth of tumors. This may help explain the finding in several large clinical studies that diets high in polyunsaturated fats increased the death rates due to cancer and other causes.[58]

The increasing rate of diabetes may also be due, in part, by overconsumption of polyunsaturated vegetable oils. In the 1920s, Dr. S. Sweeney produced reversible diabetes in all of his medical school students by feeding them a high vegetable oil diet for forty-eight hours. None of the students had previously been diabetic.

ALPHA-LINOLENIC ACID (OMEGA-3): NATURE'S EQUALIZER
Benefits of Omega-3

Alpha-linolenic acid, the precursor to the omega-3 fatty acids DHA and EPA, has been hailed as our newest wonder nutrient. Hundreds of studies have shown promising ef-

Diabetes in Children Rising With Obesity Rate:
Type 2 Becoming Epidemic in Kids

On a recent Friday, Tyshon Young, 13, and a nutritionist strolled the aisles at Fairway in Harlem for a little comparison shopping.

He picked up a box of butter cookies. She pointed to graham crackers. He picked out frosted flakes. She said Special K was a better choice. He picked ice cream. She told him to get the low-fat brand.

High-fat, high-carbohydrate snacks like that have made Tyshon obese, which has triggered a form of diabetes once considered rare among people his age. The trip to the grocery store was part of an elaborate effort to coax him into a new regimen of exercise and healthy eating that could save his life.

At 5 feet 6 inches and 216 pounds, Tyshon represents an alarming new health trend: the sharp increase in the number of youngsters with Type 2 diabetes, also known as adult-onset diabetes, and incurable and progressively damaging disease that can cause kidney failure, blindness and poor circulation, which, in turn, can lead to amputation. Doctors long believed the disease occurred only during middle age of later.

There have not been any national surveys documenting the rise of this form of diabetes in children, though several small-scale studies have found that such cases have more than tripled in the past five years, and, anecdotally, doctors across the country say they have observed similar trends among their own patients. In the past month, officials at the Centers for Disease Control and Prevention convened a meeting to discuss the problem, and the American Diabetes Association has appointed a new task force.

"Ten years ago, we were teaching medical students that you don't see this disease in people under 40, and now we're seeing it in people under 10," said Dr. Robin Goland, co-director of the Naomi Berrie Diabetes Center, which opened in October at Columbia University's College of Physicians and Surgeons in Manhattan. Goland said Type 2 diabetes was diagnosed in 10 percent to 20 percent of the center's new pediatric patients, compared with less than 4 percent in the hospital's clinics five years ago.

Children with Type 2 diabetes look a lot like their adult counterparts. Most are black or Hispanic, with a particularly high rate found among children of Mexican decent. Most of the Type 2 children have close relatives with the disease, and almost all are obese.

In fact, doctors said, the spiraling rate of childhood obesity in America—declared an epidemic last month by U.S. Surgeon General David Satcher—is the most significant factor in the rising numbers of children with this form of diabetes.

Researchers speculate that the rise in reported cases of Type 2 diabetes in children results form both an increased incidence of the disease and an increased awareness of it by primary-care physicians. Until the past few years, Goland said, the correct diagnosis was likely to have been missed in some children.

Diabetes, which affects about 16 million Americans and is the sixth-leading cause of death by disease in the United States, results form a breakdown in the body's system for absorbing sugar.

If the disease is left undiagnosed or untreated, however, life threatening complications, caused by damage to blood vessels, can develop within 10 years to 20 years.

"If we aren't detecting this disease in children because we aren't looking or it," Goland said, "then we are going to start seeing complications in people in their 20s that we would normally associate with people in their 60s and 70s."

Source: *The New York Times*, Dec. 14, 1999

fects attributed to the omega-3 family of fatty acids. Omega-3 fatty acids from flaxseed and fish oil supplements have been added to many vitamin formulas because they are now considered to be as vital to good health as vitamin C or calcium. They are recommended therapeutically for a wide variety of physical conditions ranging from cancer to dermatitis. It's a wonder how the human race ever existed at all without these dietary supplements.

This brings up an interesting question: how did we survive before omega-3 supplements were available? The richest source of omega-3 fatty acids is fish, but not all people eat fish. Some cultures never eat it. Flaxseed is not exactly a common source of food, even among those people who cultivate it. They use the plant primarily for the tough fibers to make rope and cloth. So how has the human race survived for so long without all the degenerative diseases that omega-3 fatty acids are suppose to prevent?

The rural peoples of Africa who subsist on diets composed entirely of native foods do not experience ulcerative colitis, intestinal cancer, diabetes, heart disease or any of the degenerative diseases that have become so common in the Western world. The same is true for the villagers of South

America and Asia and many other underdeveloped areas of the world. It can't be because they eat flaxseed oil, because they don't. It's not because they eat fish, because many of them don't.

Their native foods don't contain any more omega-3 fatty acids than our own. And our own doesn't have much. So what protects them? Their secret, and the secret our ancestors shared with them, is the fact that the food they ate was full of vitamins, minerals, and antioxidant phytochemicals, and relatively *low* in omega-6 fatty acids. Our ancestors didn't add vegetable oil to their foods, they didn't eat potato chips, French fries, and oil-soaked donuts. They never heard of hydrogenated vegetable oil or margarine. They did, however, eat lots of butter, raw whole milk, and lard, but no refined vegetable oil. Butter, raw milk, and lard contain many vitamins and minerals, but processed vegetable oils are stripped of most all nutrients except the fatty acids, of which omega-6 is by far the most predominant.

If you look at the dietary history of the world and at nonindustralized cultures in more modern times, what common elements are found among those who have the best health? Many researchers have analyzed the lifestyles and dietary habits of these people to discover the secret to long life and good health. When the healthiest people are compared, there is really little in common. The type of foods they eat all differ. Some eat little or no meat, others eat a great deal of meat. Some eat no dairy at all while for others it's a major part of their diet. They eat both cooked and raw foods. They live in all types of climates both cold and hot, dry and wet. Religious beliefs, social behavior, and customs vary greatly. But there is one thing that is common among them all. The common denominator among all cultures that have had and do have a long, healthy life relatively free from the diseases so common among Western nations, is that they don't consume highly processed foods like vegetable oil. Their diets consist entirely of foods grown locally without modern processing and packaging, and without any added

vegetable oils! What oils they do eat are usually of animal origin—the ones we consider to be the most unhealthy. Could our thinking on oils perhaps be backwards?

Foods rich in omega-3 fatty acids aren't common among all these people. So, where does omega-3 fatty acids fit in to all of this? Why have omega-3 oils all of a sudden become important? The first clue to the usefulness of omega-3 fatty acids came as a result of the fish studies. Omega-3 fatty acids help to protect us against heart disease, which is caused, in part, by excessive consumption of omega-6 fatty acids. Omega-3 also helps against autoimmune and inflammatory diseases, which are again promoted by omega-6 fatty acids. Do you see a pattern forming here? The power behind omega-3 fatty acids are their ability to dilute or balance the effects of the overconsumption of omega-6 fatty acids.

Balancing Act

In many ways the effects of omega-6 and omega-3 fatty acids oppose each other. The essential fatty acids are a perfect example of the concept of yin and yang practiced in Chinese medicine. Yin and yang represent two opposites such as hot and cold, wet and dry, up and down. Health is maintained so long as all factors that influence it are in balance. Too much of one element or the other creates an imbalance in the body which leads to disease. Too much of anything, even things we consider good, such as vitamins or fatty acids, can cause imbalances in the body which lead to disease.

Too much linoleic acid (omega-6) produces prostaglandins that can cause high blood pressure and increase a tendency to form blood clots and increase risk of heart attack. Prostaglandins from omega-3 fatty acids, which have the opposite effects, can reduce or eliminate these symptoms and lower the risk of heart attack. But too much omega-3 fatty acids can also be detrimental to health.

Essential fatty acid consumption has only become an issue in recent years. You don't see deficiencies in primitive cultures that eat native foods (so long as they have enough food to eat). It's only found in Western countries who eat a large amount of oil, specifically vegetable oils rich in omega-6 fatty acids.

We are told that we need essential fatty acids, especially alpha-linolenic acid (omega-3), in our diets or we will suffer from any number of deficiency symptoms. Oil supplement sales have skyrocketed over the past few years as a result of this public awareness and industry marketing effort.

We don't want to be deficient in these important nutrients. However, we eat more omega-6 and omega-3 fatty acids now than our grandparents and great-grandparents did,

> "You should also minimize intake of polyunsaturated oils and products made from them. I do not eat safflower oil, and I recommend that you do not either. Safflower's history as a food plant in the Western world is very recent; mostly we have grown it as a natural dye. We do not eat safflower seeds as we do other oil sources. The plant is native to India, and ancient medical texts from that country warn against using the plant as food."
>
> —Andrew Weil, M.D.,
> *Natural Health, Natural Medicine*

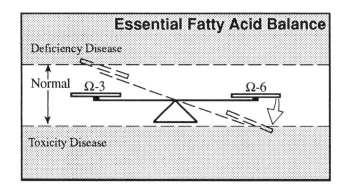

Omega-3 and omega-6 oils must be consumed in the proper ratio to maintain chemical balance within the body. When balanced the ends of the scale illustrated on the left lie within the "Normal" health zone. Too much of either one will tip the scale creating a toxicity of one and a deficiency of the other. The dashed line illustrates the shift in balance when there is too much omega-6, leading to symptoms of omega-6 toxicity and omega-3 deficiency. To eliminate symptoms all that is needed is to reduce comsumption of omega-6 or increase omega-3.

so how can we suddenly be deficient in either one? Over the past 100 years, vegetable oil added to our food per person has increased from nearly zero to over 80 grams a day. [see graph on page 38] This is equivalent to 6 tablespoons worth.

The amount we need is actually very small. Although an exact figure has not been determined, it is estimated that we need about 1 gram of omega-3 and 3 to 9 grams of omega-6 per day to satisfy the body's requirements.[59] How much is a gram? A half a tablespoon equals 7 grams. So a half a tablespoon of linoleic acid (omega-6) and just a fraction of that of alpha-linolenic acid (omega-3) is needed each day. This amount is easy to get in the foods that are available to us every day. We need 7 grams of linoleic acid and 1 gram of alpha-linolenic acid, but we already consume 80 grams of vegetable oil, do we need to add more?

The threat most of us face is not from a true deficiency of either one of the essential fatty acids. The real danger is a "relative" deficiency or imbalance caused by excessive consumption of one over the other. This is easy to do with our abundance of vegetable oils and dietary supplements.

In the process of making prostaglandins, both essential fatty acids compete with one another for the body's enzyme reserves. Too much of one will prevent the synthesis of the other. So, excessively high intakes of one will create a deficiency of the other.[60, 61, 62, 63]

Since essential fatty acids are readily available in our diet, the real concern is not the total amount we get, but that we obtain a balance between the two.[64] What is this balance? Each is required in different amounts by the cells in the body and serve different functions. So what is the optimal ratio of omega-6 to omega-3 fatty acids? No one knows for sure, but researchers believe it is somewhere between 3:1 and 9:1 because that is what is normally found in our tissues.[65]

The foods that naturally contain the most omega-3 fatty acids—fish, flaxseed, and leafy green vegetables are not eaten to any great extent by most of us. Because omega-6 fatty acids are found everywhere and more is added to many

of our foods during processing and cooking, we typically we get a ratio of linoleic acid to alpha-linolenic acid that is between 10:1 and 20:1.[66] It's no wonder "deficiency" symptoms for omega-3 fatty acids are common.

Sources

Eating fish has proven to be a safe and reliable way to afford some degree of protection against heart disease. The American Heart Association currently recommends eating fish every three or four days.[67] Recent research from Harvard Medical School has shown sufficient benefit with just one fish meal a week.[68] We can get EPA from all types of seafood, including shrimp, lobster, and clams. The fish with the highest percentage of fat supply the greatest amount of omega-3 fatty acids. The fatty fish include herring, sardines, mackerel, tuna, trout, and salmon. These fish store most of their fat in their muscle tissue; in contrast, lean fish, such as cod, flounder, and haddock store their fat in their livers. Protection can be provided by either type of fish regardless of fat content.[69]

Fish liver oil, particularly cod liver oil, has been used for years as a rich natural source of vitamins A and D. They also provide a concentrated source of essential fatty acids. For people who don't eat fish often or don't like fish, taking cod liver oil or an oil supplement in capsule form allows them to add essential fatty acids to their diet.

In the past, fish liver oil may have been a safe and reliable way to supplement the diet. Nowadays, with our water polluted with garbage and industrial waste, it isn't recommended. The liver is the detoxification organ of the body and as such, accumulates high quantities of heavy metals, pesticides, and other contaminants. Oil made from fish liver may be heavily contaminated. A better source for EPA (the omega-3 fatty acid that is converted directly into PGE3) that has appeared on the market in recent years is fish oil derived, not from the liver, but from the skin. Oil extracted from salmon skin is becoming popular.

If you've ever tasted cod liver oil you, like me, cringe at the thought of eating any fish oil supplement, even in capsule form. The aftertaste can come back and haunt you for hours. Many people, some being strict vegetarians, avoid meats of all types, including fish. For people wanting to avoid fish and fish byproducts, seaweed is an option. Seaweeds such as nori, dulse, and wakame contain a fair amount of EPA and are commonly used as food. Rice rolled in dried nori is used to make sushi which is a popular food in Japan and Korea.

A seaweed salad may not be your idea of an appetizing meal. Most people in Western countries are not accustomed to eating seaweed and don't eat it. Quite frankly, most seaweed tastes like, well...seaweed. It has a strong fishy flavor. Besides fish, fish oil supplements, and seaweed, there are no good sources for EPA. There are, however, plant sources for alpha-linolenic acid, another omega-3 fatty acid. Alpha-linolenic acid can be converted by the body into EPA.

Many of the foods we eat contain alpha-linolenic acid, but few of them contain it in any appreciable amount. The foods that supply the richest source are green leafy vegetables which include spinach, chard, beet tops, mustard greens, kale, turnip greens, bok choy, collards, purslane, and dark green lettuce. Although iceberg lettuce is considered a green leafy vegetable, it doesn't have an appreciable amount of any nutrient, including the fatty acids. Among the green leafy vegetables, the one with the most alpha-linolenic acid is purslane. Purslane is eaten extensively in soups and salads in Greece, Lebanon, and other parts of the Mediterranean. This vegetable, although commonly grown in other parts of the world, is not ordinarily seen on the dinner table. Those who are familiar with it usually consider it a troublesome weed. Purslane grows just about anywhere and commonly invades flower beds and vegetable gardens. It grows very rapidly, hugging the ground. Leaves are small but thick and spongy.

Whole grains and beans have a small amount of omega-3 fatty acids as do many seeds and nuts. It's from these sources we get our vegetable oils. Most vegetable oils and even animal fats contain 1 or 2 percent alpha-linolenic acid. The ones with the most are walnut oil, soybean oil, canola oil, and flaxseed oil. Soybean oil contains 7 percent alpha-linolenic acid and canola oil 10 percent. Flaxseed oil has by far the most with 57 percent alpha-linolenic, 25 percent linoleic, 18 percent monounsaturated fat, and about 10 percent saturated fat.

Because flaxseed oil contains such a high percentage of alpha-linolenic acid, it has become the premiere plant source for omega-3 fatty acids. Flaxseed oil is readily available as a dietary supplement in liquid form or in gel capsules.

Contrary to popular belief, in and of itself, alpha-linolenic acid has not been shown to be a necessary nutrient.

Researchers have found it difficult to ascribe any specific nutritional role for alpha-linolenic acid aside from being a precursor to EPA and DHA.[70] It's EPA and DHA that the body needs and alpha-linolenic acid is important only in that it can be converted into these forms by our bodies. It is for this reason that fish and fish oil are considered by far the best sources for EPA. Seaweed is also a good source, but few people make a habit of eating it.

The prostaglandins (PGE3) derived directly from EPA are what affects body functions in countering cardiovascular disease. Alpha-linolenic acid cannot be converted directly into PGE3, but must go through a series of steps before it is transformed into EPA. Only a small fraction of the oil actually completes the conversion from alpha-linolenic acid to EPA to PGE3, the rest being broken down, oxidized, or stored as body fat.[71] Fish oil, on the other hand, is better utilized by the body and has a stronger effect because it takes fewer steps for conversion into PGE3. Therefore, the omega-3 in fish oil (EPA) is much more readily converted into PGE3 than the omega-3 in flaxseed (alpha-linolenic acid).

Too Much of a "Good" Thing

Omega-6 fatty acids are present in meat, poultry, fish, and most all vegetables, nuts, seeds, and grains. In fact, omega-6 fatty acids are so abundant in the foods we eat it is nearly impossible not to get enough. In order to have a deficiency you would need to live on a diet specially prepared in a laboratory—such as the foods fed to rats in order to determine deficiency effects. Omega-6 fatty acids may be essential, but their abundance in nature assures us that the chances of ever suffering a deficiency is essentially zero.[72] The only way a person could experience a deficiency outside the laboratory is if he were severely malnourished and, in that case, he would be deficient of all nutrients.

In contrast, foods rich in omega-3 fatty acids (fish and green leafy vegetables) are not frequently eaten by most people. Taking omega-3 fatty acid supplements is promoted as the solution to achieving the balance our bodies need. But taking supplements can create an imbalance depending on the types of food you eat. Blindly taking supplements because you read from some popular magazine that they were good for you, isn't wise. Too much omega-3 fatty acid can cause serious health problems.

The overconsumption of omega-3 fatty acids can lead to excessive bleeding and interfere with wound healing. Spontaneous bleeding can be a problem. Often people complain of getting a bloody nose for no apparent reason or having a minor bump develop into an ugly bruise or experience bleeding gums while brushing their teeth. Many people who take flaxseed supplements notice the development or an increase in liver spots—a dark pigment that commonly develops in skin. These are signs that you may be getting far too much omega-3 fatty acids. You also run the risk of hemorrhagic stroke—the number one killer among the Eskimos.

Another potentially serious problem with taking omega-3 fatty acid supplements is that it is a highly polyunsaturated oil as much as two to three times more vulnerable to free-radical destruction than linoleic acid (omega-6). Omega-3 fatty acids are very easily oxidized. No matter how fresh a supplement is, it will have undergone some degree of oxidation. The longer it sits on the store shelf or on your cupboard or in your refrigerator, the more it oxidizes. The more it oxidizes, the more free radicals it forms, and the more internal damage it can do to you. Of all the oils commonly found in our food, omega-3 is the most easily oxidized and, therefore, holds the most potential for free-radical damage. The effects resulting from free radicals can penetrate every corner and crevice of the body, causing premature aging and tissue degeneration.

Cod liver oil is a rich source of omega-3 fatty acids and often used as a supplement. Fifty years ago, researchers found that a large amount of cod liver oil added to foods fed to dogs increased their death rate from cancer over a certain period of time from the usual 5 percent to 100 percent![73]

There are many adverse effects to getting too much of the essential fatty acids. More and more researchers are speaking up publicly against the use and abuse of essential fatty acid supplementation. Dr. Ray Peat, an endocrinologist, states that "The essential fatty acids suppress metabolism and promote obesity; are immunosuppressive; cause inflammation and shock; are required for alcoholic liver cirrhosis; sensitize to radiation damage; accelerate formation of aging pigment, cataracts, retinal degeneration; promote free-radical damage and excitoxicity; cause cancer and accelerate its growth; are toxic to the heart muscle and promote atherosclerosis; can cause brain edema, diabetes, excessive vascular permeability, precocious puberty, progesterone deficiency, skin wrinkling and other signs of aging."[74] Diabetics need to be especially careful about omega-3 fatty acids. Several studies have demonstrated that they can disrupt metabolic control by raising blood sugar levels or insulin requirements.[75]

Although still considered to be essential by most authorities, these fatty acids exert powerful effects both good and bad. The biggest problem we face is getting too much of one and not enough of the other to maintain a healthy balance.

ARE YOU GETTING ENOUGH EFA?

The essential fatty acids (EFA), linoleic acid and alpha-linolenic acid, are generally recognized as important el-

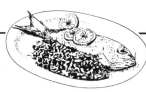

Fried Fish

A Canadian study reported in the *American Journal of Preventive Medicine* compared diets of people who lived near the Atlantic Ocean with those who lived farther inland. In the Atlantic provinces people eat fish twice as often as their neighbors in the inland prairie provinces do. Based on their fish consumption they should have a lower rate of heart disease. But the fish those near the Atlantic eat is almost always served fried. As a consequence, heart disease mortality rates are actually higher among people in the Atlantic provinces than they are among their landlubber neighbors. Fried fish provides little or no protection against heart disease dispite the fact it contains omega-3 fatty acids.
Source: Barnett, R. and Barone, J. 1989. The fish nobody knows. *American Health* 8(5):104

ements in a healthy diet. As with all essential nutrients, a legitimate concern is knowing if we are getting enough.

Essential fatty acids are often recommended as dietary supplements to treat a wide variety of symptoms. We are almost becoming conditioned to look at them as miracle cures for every disease that ails us. Do we really need to supplement our diets with essential fatty acids?

If you eat a typical westernized diet of processed, packaged, convenience foods and use vegetable oil, including margarine and shortening, when cooking than *you are getting far too much linoleic acid.* Even if you think you eat healthfully, if you add *any* vegetable oil to your foods you probably get too much. We can get all the essential fatty acids our bodies need directly from unprocessed foods—fruits, vegetables, and grains.

Vegetable oils have become an essential part of daily food preparation. As a consequence, we eat far too much of it. The amounts we eat are contrary to the basic physiological makeup of our bodies. Humans and animals were not meant to eat refined vegetable oils. It's unnatural. Our bodies were not designed to process 80 grams of oil a day. We do much better with about 8 grams—the equilivent of half a tablespoon.

It is interesting to note that olive oil has been considered the healthiest of the vegetable oils because those who eat it, in place of other vegetable oils, have much better cardiovascular health and fewer heart attacks. Please note that olive oil has *very little* of either of the essential fatty acids. It consists of 77% monounsaturated fat and 14% saturated fat with only 8% linoleic acid and 1% alpha-linolenic acid. A total of only 9% of it is composed essential fatty acids. It has more saturated fat (14%) than polyunsaturated fat (9%). Its ratio of 8:1 linoleic to alpha-linolenic acid is also within the range considered to be ideal. It's no wonder why people who eat olive oil instead of other vegetable oils have such better health.

William Lands, Ph.D. of the University of Illinois, Chicago, said we are consuming well in excess of the documented 3 percent calories needed to prevent essential fatty acid deficiencies.[76] William Connor, M.D., Oregon Health Sciences University, Portland said, "We probably ought not to have any more omega-6 polyunsaturated fat in our diet than we have now because of the possible carcinogenic effects and influence on the eicosanoid system. We need to establish a balance between the two."[77]

As we have seen earlier in this chapter, consuming too much linoleic acid (omega-6) encourages the conditions that lead to heart disease and other health problems. Alpha-linolenic acid (omega-3) has the opposite effect and thus provides some degree of protection. Our typical diet provides too much linoleic acid resulting in a relative deficiency in alpha-linolenic acid. The result? A society of people with cardiovascular disease and a host of other health problems. That's exactly where we are today.

The simple solution to an excess of linoleic acid in the diet is to either reduce consumption of vegetable oils or increase the amount of alpha-linolenic acid (omega-3) we consume. You can do one or the other or both to counter the effects of too much linoleic acid (omega-6). Most of the emphasis we hear is on increasing the amount of alpha-linolenic acid in the diet. Supplement manufacturers who pro-

Is Thin Blood Good?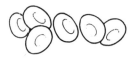

The words "blood clot" can send chills up our spines. Blood clots are one of the primary mechanisms responsible for heart attacks and strokes. We have become so paranoid about blood clots and the damage they can do that we tend to look for any means possible to prevent them from occurring. In this frenzy to "thin" our blood to reduce chances of clotting, we can go too far. When this happens we create equally severe health problems from an inability to produce clots when needed. Dr. Dean Ornish in his book *Dr. Dean Ornish's Program for Reversing Heart Disease* explains it this way:

"It has been known for a long time that aspirin interferes with blood clot formation. For many years, this was viewed simply as a troubling side effect of aspirin when it was given to reduce pain. Doctors then began to wonder is aspirin could reduce the incidence of heart attacks by helping prevent blood clots from forming inside the heart.

"A large clinical trial was established to see if aspirin prevented heart attacks. The Physicians' Health Study,

as it was called, randomly divided over 22,000 doctors into two groups; one group took an aspirin every other day, the other group took a placebo. Until the study was completed, only an independent data monitoring board knew who took which. (Bristol-Myers, maker of buffering aspirin, helped to fund this study.) Neither group was asked to make lifestyle changes.

"After five years of follow-up, the group that took aspirin had 44 percent fewer nonfatal heart attacks than the placebo group. For ethical reasons, the study was stopped early, news was made, and it seemed that everyone should start taking aspirin.

"A closer look at the results of that study revealed that while aspirin did reduce the incidence of heart attacks, it increased the risk of hemorrhagic strokes: bleeding into the brain. The group that took aspirin had over twice the incidence of moderate to severe hemorrhagic strokes when compared with the placebo group. Also, the incidence of sudden cardiac death was almost twice as high in the aspirin group, and the incidence of gastric and duode-

nal ulcers was almost twice as high in the aspirin-treated group. Although the group taking aspirin had fewer heart attacks, overall, there was no difference between he two groups in number of deaths resulting from heart disease from all causes of death. Similar results were found in the British Doctors' Trial."

"Fish oil capsules also interfere with blood clotting. It has long been known the Greenland Eskimos have relatively low rates of coronary heart disease even though their diet is high in fat. Scientists learned that the fatty fish they consume is rich in omega-3 fatty acids...Television and magazine advertisements began to appear, showing Eskimos sitting around a fire, eating blubber, while the announcer promoted fish oil capsules. What these advertisements failed to mention is that Eskimos have among the highest rates of hemorrhagic stroke in the world. Also, fish oil capsules tend to raise cholesterol levels." ♥

Source: Dean Ornish. *Dr. Dean Ornish's Program for Reversing Heart Disease*

FATTY ACID CONTENT IN COMMON OILS

The percentage of saturated, monounsaturated, and polyunsaturated
(linoleic and alpha-linolenic) fatty acids in common oils.

Oil	Saturated	Monounsaturated	Polyunsaturated	
			Linoleic (omega-6)	Alpha-Linolenic (omega-3)
Flaxseed oil	9	19	14	58
Canola oil	6	62	22	10
Soybean oil	15	24	54	7
Butter	66	30	2	2
Corn oil	13	25	61	1
Olive oil	14	77	8	1
Chicken fat	31	47	21	1
Beef fat	52	44	3	1
Lard	41	47	11	1
Safflower oil	10	13	77	trace
Sunflower oil	11	20	69	0
Peanut oil	18	49	33	0
Palm oil	51	39	10	0
Coconut oil	92	6	2	0

The exact percentage of the oil components of each source varies. For example the saturated fat content of coconut oil can vary from 83 to 92 percent and the monounsaturated portion from 15 to 6 percent.

duce the alpha-linolenic acid (omega-3) products and who advertise and disseminate most of the information on this subject, focus exclusively on adding more omega-3 fatty acids. This is natural, because there is money to be made from selling these products. Since adding omega-3 fatty ac-

Dietary Lipids: Fatty Acid Analysis

Carbon Number	Safflower (%)	Lard (%)
14	0.5	1.7
16	6.7	26.5
16:1	0	2.1
18	1.6	12.1
18:1	11.1	49.8
18:2	79.7	10.3
20 to 22 acids	0.1	2.4

You can see the safflower oil is 80 percent 18-chain polyunsaturated oil this is the omega-6 fatty acid. The lard is 40 percent saturated and 51 percent monounsaturated. This difference in saturation makes the difference in free radical formation and effects on health. What does this say? For one thing, over consumption of essential fatty acids can be detrimental to your health!

ids to our diet is all we ever hear, this is the only option most of us know about.

One obvious problem with taking omega-3 fatty acid supplements to dilute or counter the effects of too much omega-6 fatty acids is knowing how much to take. Too much omega-3 fatty acids can be just as bad as too much omega-6 fatty acids. Excessive omega-3 fatty acids will lead to the overproduction of PGE3 which can cause blood to become too thin and lose its clotting ability, resulting in a very dangerous situation if injury occurs. It may also cause spontaneous bruising and inability of the body to respond properly to injury or infection. A minor viral infection can drag on much longer than it otherwise should and can even turn into a life threatening situation.

The other solution to counter the effects of too much omega-6 fatty acids, rather than taking additional omega-3 fatty acids, is to simply *reduce your intake of vegetable oils.* This is by far the better solution. The less vegetable oil you consume, the less omega-6 fatty acids will be in your body and the less omega-3 fatty acids you will need to balance the two. This is easy to do and definitely cheaper and ultimately much healthier than increasing your intake of omega-3 fatty acids. But there is no money to be made by not eating certain foods or not taking certain supplements, so you

never hear about this
lifesaving option. This
is one of the most im-
portant concepts this
book presents and one
of the prime reasons
for which this book
has been written. This
small piece of advice
can save your health
and your money at the
same time.

The reason it is
safer to simply reduce
your vegetable oil
consumption rather
than add omega-3
supplements to the
diet is because:

Unsaturated Fatty Acids Found in Natural Fats

Unsaturated Fatty Acid	No. of Carbons	No. of Double Bonds	Common Source
Palmitoleic (omega-9)	16	1	Butterfat
Oleic (omega-9)	18	1	Olive oil
Linoleic (omega-6)	18	2	Vegetable oil
Alpha-linolenic (omega-3)	18	3	Linseed oil
Arachidonic (omega-6)	20	4	Lecithin
Eicosapentaenoic (omega-3)	20	5	Fish oils
Docosahexaenoic (omega-3)	22	6	Fish oils

Note that all unsaturated fatty acids are long-chain molecules, that is they have 14 or more carbon atoms. Although chains shorter than 16 and longer than 20 exist they are much rarer. This means that all dietary unsaturated fats are packaged in lipoproteins thus increasing total blood fat levels. Note also that omega-6 and omega-3 fatty acids have two and three double bonds on carbons, each a potential site for oxidation, especially omega-3 fatty acid. The more double bond present the greater the vulnerability to oxidation and free radical formation.

(1) Any oil added to your food increases the number of calories you consume, which in turn contributes to weight problems. All fats, even omega-3 fatty acids, have more than twice as many calories as carbohydrate or protein. A gram of flaxseed oil or fish oil is over twice as fattening as a gram of pure sugar.

(2) Alpha-linolenic acid (omega-3) is a polyunsaturated fatty acid and, therefore, highly susceptible to oxidation and free-radical generation. The more of this oil you eat, the more destructive free-radical chain reactions will occur in you body, breaking down the cells and tissues.

Linoleic acid and alpha-linolenic acid compete with each other for enzymes involved in conversion to arachidonic acid and EPA—the precursors to the eicosanoids PGE2 and PGE3. Too much of one inhibits the production of the other. But if the amount of each of the essential fatty acids were reduced to such a point where there are ample enzymes to go around, there would be far less of a chance of developing deficiency symptoms from either one.[78, 79]

We have been given the impression that if we eat a lot of "bad" fat, all we have to do is eat more "good" fat. It doesn't matter how much you eat of one, just so long as you get enough of the other to balance it out.

The effects of PGE2 produced by linoleic acid (omega-6) are beneficial, up to a point. The same is true with PGE3 produced by alpha-linolenic acid (omega-3). They, too, are beneficial, up to a point. Too little or too much of either one can have *drastic* health consequences.

The difference between the amount the body needs and too much can be very little. Iodine, for example, is an es-

sential trace mineral necessary in minute quantities to maintain optimal health, but an excess even in tiny amounts can become toxic. With essential fatty acids, even one pill or half a spoonful may be too much. Time after time, people who are actually getting enough in their diet from seafood, fresh vegetables, and vegetable oils also take omega-3 or omega-6 supplements. They're overdoing it and may develop any number of symptoms. Just consider the amount of dressing that is placed on a green salad. Most dressings are nearly all oil. A single bowl of salad will contain two or three tablespoons of dressing. This amount is far more than what the body needs.

Because of the negative health effects of eating too much of either of the essential fatty acids, it is advisable to limit consumption of both while keeping the ratio or balance between them. This can be done by eating whole natural foods and eliminating vegetable oils entirely. Will eating just foods supply enough of the essential fatty acids the body needs? Yes. They will supply all you need without overtaxing your body or depleting your enzyme reserves.

Just because these fatty acids are considered essential nutrients doesn't mean you need a lot or that you can't get all you need from your foods. Carbohydrate is also an essential nutrient, but we rarely worry about getting enough because it is so plentiful in the foods we eat. Likewise, with the essential fatty acids. There is plenty in our foods, so we don't need to add any more. What we need to do is eat more of the types of foods that supply omega-3 fatty acids (e.g., leafy green vegetables and fish) and cut down on foods that have too much omega-6 fatty acids (e.g., vegetable oils and processed foods).

Chapter 5

THE FACTS ON FLAX

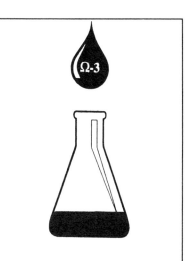

GOOD AND BAD

Studies have shown that people who eat as little as one fish meal a week can reduce their risk of dying from cardiac arrest by fifty percent.[1] Fish is without question the best source for omega-3 fatty acids, because it supplies EPA, the direct precursor to PGE3, the compound that initiates protective mechanisms against heart attack. Fish oil supplements are believed to provide the same degree of protection as eating seafood, but many nutritionists do not recommend oil from fish liver because of the possibility of contamination.

Many people nowadays are avoiding all types of meat and meat byproducts, including fish. These people prefer a vegetable source for omega-3 fatty acids. Alpha-linolenic acid, which the body can convert into EPA, is found to some degree in many plants. Flaxseed contains the highest percentage of alpha-linolenic acid (57%) of any commercially grown plant. Because of its high alpha-linolenic acid content, flaxseed oil has become the leading supplemental source for this essential fatty acid.

Over the past several years we have witnessed a flaxseed revolution. A few years ago no one ever heard of flaxseed, nowadays it's considered a new super nutrient. It's been hailed as a panacea for many ills. No respectable health food store would be caught dead without a half dozen assorted varieties available for sale.

Both good and bad can be said about alpha-linolenic acid and flaxseed oil in general. Unfortunately, the bad is ignored in preference to promoting only the good. This has created the misconception that flaxseed oil provides great benefits with little risks. In reality, there are many risks.

Studies suggest that alpha-linolenic acid may be useful in treating numerous conditions. The most notable being: cancer, arthritis, irritable bowel syndrome, hypertension (high blood pressure), heart disease, phrombosis, dermatitis, lupus nephritis, and in lowering total cholesterol. If it can do all this, isn't that proof that flaxseed is a useful dietary supplement? It can appear that way, but if you understand how flaxseed oil works, you would consider it a dangerous drug to be used with extreme caution just as you would other powerful drugs, rather than look at it as a harmless dietary supplement.

The best thing that can be said about alpha-linolenic acid is that it has a neutralizing or balancing effect against the overconsumption of linoleic acid found in vegetable oils. Since vegetable oil consumption can lead to numerous health problems, alpha-linolenic acid can be useful in reversing or preventing these problems. The reason why flaxseed oil has been shown to be useful for so many health prob-

"A desire to take medicine is perhaps the great feature which distinguishes man from other animals."
—William Osler, M.D.

"Any substance that interferes with the natural workings of the body is a toxin—food included!"
—Dr. M. Ted Morter, Jr.
Your Health, Your Choice

lems is because vegetable oils cause so many. Flaxseed can counterbalance these effects. In so doing, however, the body must suffer the ravages of internal warfare.

So in one respect, flaxseed oil can be very useful. But as a consequence, the body must suffer with side effects that can be every bit as destructive as a prescription drug. In most cases, alpha-linolenic acid supplementation is unnecessary because there are other ways to bring the essential fatty acids in our bodies into balance without causing further harm.

Since alpha-linolenic acid is extracted from flaxseed, it is considered a "natural" substance and, therefore, regulated as a dietary supplement. Supplements, for the most part, are relatively harmless. But because flaxseed oil is readily available to anyone, and because it is recommended for the treatment of just about every ailment from stomach ulcers to kidney disease, it is easy to take too much, and instead of suffering from an excess of omega-6, like most everyone else, you may suffer from an excess of omega-3. The effects can be just as bad, if not worse.

DANGERS OF FLAXSEED OIL
Heart Disease
There is a great deal of evidence on flaxseed oil which suggest that it isn't the best thing to be eating in its concentrated, refined state.

Alpha-linolenic acid from flaxseed affects the liver's ability to process certain nutrients. For example, it inhibits the production of enzymes necessary to synthesize cholesterol. Some people may consider this a positive effect because it lowers the body's total cholesterol level. Others question any substance that stifles the body's normal metabolic processes. Cholesterol which is formed in the liver is not the same as the cholesterol that clogs the arteries. So inhibiting the liver's production of cholesterol does not affect cardiovascular health. The cholesterol that contributes to plaque in the arteries is *oxidized* cholesterol. Non-oxidized cholesterol does not clog arteries, but is used in cell membranes, nerve tissue, and as part of the brain, and therefore is an important and necessary component of our bodies.

Our intestines absorb fats from the foods we eat and package them together into small bundles called lipoproteins. Lipoproteins are then released into the bloodstream and transported throughout the body. As they are carried through the circulatory system, fat is dispersed and picked up by our cells.

Polyunsaturated oils, including flaxseed oil, are easily oxidized. When it oxidizes it kicks off a series of free-radical chain reactions that affects all molecules around it. Millions of molecules can be destroyed or oxidized by the generation of a single free radical. Cholesterol that is in close proximity to a polyunsaturated oil that is becoming oxidized, as is the case in lipoproteins, will also become oxidized. These oxidized, free-radical damaged oils are absorbed into the lining of the artery walls and contribute to the formation of plaque. Non-oxidized fats are incorporated into the cells as they should be, and do not end up as plaque deposits. Here is the warning: even though alpha-linolenic acid may lower total cholesterol, it actually contributes to atherosclerosis and all forms of cardiovascular disease. It does this by causing the oxidization of cholesterol and other fats, both of which are components to arterial plaque.[2]

All polyunsaturated oils provide a source of free radicals which can damage arterial walls which initiates the plaque-building process. PGE2 derived from vegetable oils constricts blood vessels and increases platelet stickiness, which raises blood pressure and causes further damage to arterial walls. When injury occurs to the artery in this type of environment, oxidized fat is attracted to and incorporated into the injury site. Because platelets become sticky, blood clots easily form on injured artery walls. These clots can grow big enough to block an artery or break off and float down and lodge into a smaller artery. When an artery is clogged, cells are deprived of much needed oxygen, causing tissue death. In the heart it can cause a heart attack; in the brain it can cause a stroke. Studies show that lipid peroxides (oxidized vegetable oils) are associated with coronary heart disease, caused by enhanced free-radical formation.[3]

It is interesting to note that the countries that consume the most vegetable oils are also the ones that have the highest death rate from heart attack and stroke.

The effects of free-radical damage and plaque buildup are partially offset by the fact that PGE3 from the alpha-linolenic acid in flaxseed oil makes platelets in the blood less sticky and diminishes vasoconstriction (widens artery passageways), so positive results could be deducted. The stickiness of the blood and widening of the artery passageways are temporary benefits that occur only as long as PGE3 is in the blood. PGE3 has a short life so must be replenished continually to retain benefits. Plaque, on the other hand, represents long-term damage that won't just go away once the cause has been removed. In brief, what I'm saying here is that flaxseed oil can have short-term benefits, but because it is highly susceptible to free-radical generation, in the long run it can actually contribute to cardiovascular disease. It's ironic that a substance recommended to help prevent heart disease can actually contribute to it!

This may be difficult for some people to believe because many people who are at high risk of having a heart attack have been able to reduce their symptoms (such as lower blood cholesterol and blood pressure) after taking flaxseed oil. One well-known nutritionist* who promoted the use and benefits of omega-3 fatty acids as healthy for the cardiovascular system and even wrote a popular book about it, suffered a heart attack himself. He was considered an expert on the health benefits of flaxseed oil. He ate very little meat, avoided saturated fat like the plague, and faithfully took flaxseed oil supplements every day for many years. But it didn't work. Flaxseed oil helped to keep his cholesterol level and blood pressure within normal ranges, but he still developed cardiovascular disease and suffered a heart attack. The flaxseed oil only masked the symptoms, it did not prevent the disease. It is interesting to note that he ate a heart-healthy diet full of fresh fruits and vegetables and low in animal fats. But he continued to supplement his diet with vegetable oils, particularly flaxseed oil. If it didn't protect him, how can we expect it to help us?

Keep in mind that I am referring primarily to oxidized flaxseed oil, the type that is usually sold as a dietary supplement and not fresh oil. Some brands of flaxseed oil are preserved with natural antioxidants such as vitamin E which will prolong their shelf life. But even they will oxidize if too old or not stored or handled properly.

The oil industry tries to downplay the danger of free-radical damage that can be caused by flaxseed and other polyunsaturated oils. They admit that oxidation of their products poses a potential problem, but stress the benefits outweigh the risks. They have done a great deal of research and have accumulated a long list of health conditions for which flaxseed and other oils have shown to be of benefit. Many of these degenerative conditions, as you have seen, are a result of too much linoleic acid from vegetable oils rather than from a deficiency in alpha-linolenic acid. Just simply reducing the intake of vegetable oils is all that is needed to reestablish the body's balance.

A Safe and Natural Product?

One of the loudest claims we hear for the use of flaxseed oil is for its cancer-fighting ability. Cancer is the second leading cause of death in Western countries. If alpha-linolenic acid from flaxseed oil can prevent or cure cancer it would be a very valuable remedy. Many studies have been undertaken which show alpha-linolenic acid has potent anticancer properties. There is no question in this regard, the studies are clear. Because alpha-linolenic acid comes from flaxseed oil, which is considered a "natural" product, the health food industry and natural health care practitioners have embraced it as a miracle worker.

*Name of this person, with whom I am personally acquainted, is not included so as to protect privacy.

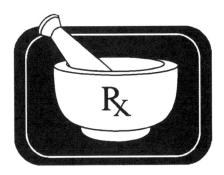

There are some problems, however. Flaxseed oil can hardly be classified as a "natural" product. It is highly processed and refined, making it no more natural than white sugar (or even aspirin which originally came from the bark of the white willow tree). Many of the synergistic elements of the whole plant are removed to obtain a pure oil, just as all the phytochemicals, vitamins, and minerals are removed from sugar beets to make sugar (or the willow plant to refine aspirin, although nowadays aspirin is synthetically manufactured). The oil resembles a drug more than a food. Depending on your viewpoint of medicine, this isn't necessarily bad, but it certainly can't be considered natural.

I classify flaxseed oil as a drug, because that is how it works against cancer. Most people who hear that flaxseed oil has anticancer properties assume it to be a safe natural product without harmful side effecs that will protect them from cancer. Many start taking it regularly just as a precaution. What they don't know, and what the oil industry doesn't publicize, is that the anticancer properties of flaxseed oil are a result of free-radical damage to cancerous tissues and not to any healthful properties of the oil itself!

Flaxseed oil and other polyunsaturated oils create so many destructive free radicals in the body that they can actually kill cancer cells.[4, 5, 6, 7, 8, 9, 10, 11]

The theory behind this process is that cancer cells are diseased and, therefore, weakened. Free-radical reactions will further weaken and kill these cells. Although free radicals affect the entire body, including healthy cells, the weakest cells will die off first. This is the same type of process that happens in chemotherapy.

Chemotherapy drugs are highly toxic and affect the entire body. The cancer cells, being abnormal, are less capable of resisting these drugs, are the first to die. The entire body is poisoned in the process, but normal cells are better able to withstand and recover from the drugs. Flaxseed oil is used in exactly the same manner and is, therefore, no different than chemotherapy drugs.

The most obvious drawback to chemotherapy are the side effects. While chemotherapy drugs attack the entire body, the strongest effects take place where cells grow the fastest such as the bone marrow, the intestinal lining, the hair

follicles, and the mouth, sometimes causing a variety of severe side effects. The side effects from flaxseed therapy can
be just as damaging. This is not a harmless nor a natural
remedy for cancer.

The effects of free-radical damage from flaxseed oil
are not immediately evident. Your hair doesn't fall out after a couple of months of treatment like it might with chemotherapy. The damage caused by free radicals may not surface for several years. By this time, the effects of degeneration may be attributed to any number of factors and thus
divert the blame away from the real cause.

Researchers know that it's the free-radical chain reactions that kill the cancer because when antioxidants, such
as vitamin E, are given at the same time, flaxseed oil has
no anticancer effects. The vitamin E stops the oxidation of
the oil within the body and thus prevents the formation of
free radicals. Without free radicals roaming around inside
the body tearing up the cells, the cancer remains unharmed.[12, 13]

It's interesting to note that vitamin E is also known to
have anticancer properties. But it works in a totally different way, supporting the body's natural healing mechanisms
rather than poisoning it.[14] Our cells naturally contain antioxidants to protect them against renegade free radicals, but
if free-radical exposure is excessively high, as it can be when
large amounts of vegetable oils are consumed, they will ex-
haust the cells antioxidant reserves and cause cellular damage.[15]

While polyunsaturated oils can be used to fight cancer, they have also been shown to cause it as well. Studies
have shown that oils rich in linoleic acid (omega-6) promote
the growth of cancer cells while fish oils can depress or
stimulate tumor growth depending on the dose.[16] Too many
omega-6 derived prostaglandins (PGE2) encourage breast
cancer.[17, 18]

Free-Radical Cures

The concept of using free radicals from polyunsaturated oils to fight cancer has been applied to other pathologic
conditions. Flaxseed oil has been used successfully to kill
the microscopic parasites which cause malaria. It has been
noted that individuals who have low antioxidant reserves,
for one reason or another, are known to be more resistant
to malaria. Exposure to substances that produce free radicals provides ammunition to attack and kill the parasites.
While having an antioxidant deficiency is not desirable because it allows free radicals to damage cells, it also allows
those same free radicals to destroy troublesome microorganisms. In people who do not have an antioxidant deficiency,
flaxseed oil can generate enough free radicals to overcome
the body's reserves and kill the parasites which cause malaria.[19]

Polyunsaturated fat-induced free radicals have also
been shown to be toxic to other microorganisms. Researche-
ers have shown it to inhibit the growth of Helicobactor pylori bacteria which is credited with causing 90 percent of
all stomach ulcers.[20]

Take a moment and consider this: if free radicals can
kill rapidly growing cancer cells and microorganisms roaming around our bodies, what do they do to our own cells? It
is assumed that normal cells are not affected by free radicals because they contain antioxidant bodyguards. But these
reserves can be quickly depleted by repeated free-radical attack. It is assumed that cancer cells lack adequate antioxidant defenders and so are more susceptible to the destructive action of free radicals. The lack of antioxidants in diseased cells, however, may have been one of the reasons why
cancer developed in the first place. Free radicals can inter-
rupt the cell's ability to function normally, causing it to become cancerous. This may be one reason why linoleic acid
from vegetable oil promotes cancer (see references above).
Flooding the body with more free radicals to treat any illness seems crazy. It may provide some help immediately,
but in the long run it could cause serious physical degeneration and illness.

Inflammatory Disease

Flaxseed oil has also been recommended as an aid in
treating a variety of inflammatory diseases. Since PGE3,
which is synthesized in the body from flaxseed oil, has an
anti-inflammatory effect, it makes sense that it would also
help reduce inflammation caused by inflammatory illnesses.
Some of the inflammatory conditions that flaxseed oil has
been recommended for include arthritis, allergies, psoriasis,
chronic bronchitis, and colitis.

Inflammation in itself is not a disease; it is a natural
and essential process in the body's effort to fight disease and
speed healing. The inflammatory process is an important part
of our body's system of healing itself. Normally, inflammation speeds healing.

Chronic inflammation is caused by a chronic health
problem. Inflammation is the body's healing response to that
problem. Inflammation, however, promotes swelling and the
buildup of pressure which increases pain. Reducing inflammation reduces the pain, but it also hampers the body's ability to heal itself. Anti-inflammatory medications do nothing to heal the condition, they only lesson the pain. It's nice
to reduce pain, since most of us don't like it, but in doing
so you also reduce the body's ability to heal itself. Also,
since pain is removed there is a tendency to overuse the injured tissues causing further damage and encouraging more
inflammation. More anti-inflammatory medications are
needed and the cycle continues with the diseased or injured

Sequence of Events in Inflammation

Injury to tissue
(heat, infection, trauma, radiation, etc.)
↓
Increased blood flow in area
(causing heat and redness)
↓
Blood vessels become leaky
↓
Fluid leaks out of blood vessels
(causing swelling)
↓
White blood cells leave blood vessels and enter inflamed
area to remove the cause of irritation
↓
System returns to normal

Inflammation is a normal, healing response to tissue injury. Some diseases, such as arthritis and colitis cause persistent irritation which leads to chronic inflammation. Chronic inflammation is often viewed as an illness, but it is really only a natural symptom of an illness.

tissues getting worse and worse. The reason anti-inflammatory medications are used is because there isn't anything else medically that can be done to relieve the symptoms. So it's a catch-22 situation.*

The production of PGE3 is only part of the reason why flaxseed oil reduces inflammation. A far stronger anti-inflammatory mechanism is actually at work here. The effectiveness of flaxseed in suppressing the body's inflammatory response mechanism is related to the destructive action of free radicals.[21, 22]

Yes, free radicals again. Much like its effect on cancer, free radicals attacking the cells will suppress the body's ability to respond to injury and disease, thus reducing inflammation. Contrary to popular opinion, researchers have shown time and time again that flaxseed oil and other polyunsaturated oils *depress* the immune system and hamper the body's ability to heal.[23, 24, 25, 26, 27]

Flaxseed oil and other polyunsaturated oils (i.e., linoleic acid, gamma-linolenic acid, DGLA, AA, EPA, and DHA) suppress the production and activity of our white blood cells—the work force of our immune system. In fact, these oils can even kill them.[28] These are the cells that attack and clean out invading microorganisms, cancer cells,

*There are many natural and dietary treatments that are very effective against inflammatory disease. One of which is the Antioxidant Health Plan outlined in chapter 14.

toxins, and other harmful substances from our bodies. They are vital to our health and must be present in large enough numbers to repel attack from viruses and bacteria. When we get an infection, the body's inflammatory response kicks in, stimulating the increased production of white blood cells to fight the invaders. The more white blood cells we have surging through our veins, the stronger will be our defense and the quicker our recovery. Vegetable oils, therefore, slow our recovery from both acute infectious illness as well as from chronic disease. Inflammation is reduced, not by PGE3, but primarily by this destructive action of free-radical stress on the immune system. It suppresses the body's ability to heal itself and in so doing, inflammation response is reduced.

Depressed Immunity

Oil manufacturers and the health care providers who believe their propaganda claim that flaxseed oil and other polyunsaturated oils will stimulate the immune system. They may even be able to cite studies to prove their position. Sounds good, but it's only partly true.

Polyunsaturated oils have both a stimulatory and depressive effect on the immune system. We never hear about the depressive effects—that doesn't sell products. The stimulatory effects aren't that wonderful either, and can be misrepresented as being beneficial. Let me explain.

Studies show (see references above) that essential fatty acids interfere with the normal production of certain substances produced by the white blood cells in the process of fighting an illness. It's like a prankster turning the water hose off while firemen are spraying down a raging fire. These oils hamper the normal function of the white blood cells. In this respect they depress the immune system's ability to function at the level for which it was designed.

At the same time these oils also act as a stimulant, the same as any toxin or disease-causing germ might. The body recognizes a harmful substance and is stimulated into feverish activity to protect itself. This is how polyunsaturated fatty acids "stimulate" our immune system. They are not strengthening the immune system, *they are stressing it!* Why would the white blood cells start producing substances to protect the body when they encounter polyunsaturated oil? Think about it. What causes the immune system to kick into high gear? It does so in response to a threat to health. When the body senses a threat from any toxic substance it signals the immune system into increased activity. To say flaxseed oil is good for you because it stimulates the immune system is like saying small pox and bubonic plague are good for you because they, too stimulate the immune system.

When we consume polyunsaturated oils, it is like eating a group of arsonists who run around our bodies lighting little fires (starting free-radical chain reactions). The fire department, or our immune system, is called into action to douse these potentially lethal fires. The firemen (the white blood cells) are stimulated into action, but if their hoses are turned off by free-radical pranksters, they are ineffective in accomplishing their mission.

To credit flaxseed oil for stimulating the immune system is like crediting arsonists for calling out the fire department and then sabotaging their water hoses. The overall effect of eating any polyunsaturated oil is to burden and depress the immune system.

The immunosuppressive effects of vegetable oils have been known for many years. Ray Peat, Ph.D., explains that "Vegetable oil is recognized as a drug for knocking out the immune system."[29] At one time "vegetable oil emulsions were used to nourish cancer patients, but it was discovered that the unsaturated oils were suppressing their immune systems. The same products, in which vegetable oil is emulsified with water for intravenous injection, are now marketed specifically for the purpose of suppressing immunity in patients who have had organ transplants. Using the oils in foods has the same harmful effect on the immune system."[30] Unsaturated fats not only suppress the immune system but can even kill white blood cells.[31]

You have to be very careful when someone tells you some substance "stimulates" the immune system. Does it stimulate it like bubonic plague or small pox or does it *support* it like vitamin C? There is a world of difference. The first stimulates it into action to defend itself while the second does not "stimulate" it but *strengthens* it, making it work more effectively.

Vitamin E Deficiency

Another threat that can result from the overconsumption of flaxseed oil and as well as other polyunsaturated vegetable oils is vitamin E deficiency.[32] Polyunsaturated oils, because they are extremely vulnerable to oxidation and free-radical formation, quickly devour our vitamin E reserves. Vitamin E acts as an antioxidant that stops free-radical chain reactions. In the process, vitamin E is consumed. The most obvious consequence of depleted vitamin E reserves is that we lose our most important bodyguard against free-radical destruction. Without sufficient vitamin E reserves, free-radical chain reactions and damage can wreak havoc on our bodies, allowing free-radical wrecking crews to roam through our bodies with little restraint. Since free radicals are involved in numerous degenerative conditions and accelerated aging, this can have a pronounced effect on overall health and put a heavy burden on the immune system.

When the body loses vitamin E, it causes the breakdown and destruction of red blood cells, producing anemia. People who are anemic may believe their condition is due to lack of iron when it is really caused by a lack of vitamin E resulting from the consumption of too much flaxseed or vegetable oil. Very few people are actually deficient in iron, especially nowadays with vitamins readily available and so many foods being fortified with this mineral.

Vitamin E is necessary for healthy nerves and muscles. A lack of the vitamin can cause degeneration and weakness which can make walking difficult, even causing severe pain in calf muscles and a loss of coordination.

Breast lumps and cancer can also result in the depletion of vitamin E reserves.[33] The most common cause of breast lumps is fibrocystic breast disease. In recent decades, fibrocystic breast disease has become a very common affliction among women in Western countries. Although the majority of these tumorous masses are benign, as much as 20 percent may be malignant.

Some manufacturers add vitamin E to their oil supplements. They don't do this to help you prevent deficiency necessarily, they do it to preserve the oil because they know it is oxidizing while it is sitting in the warehouse and on the store shelves. By the time you eat it, the vitamin E has been used up so it provides you no nutritive value from this vitamin.

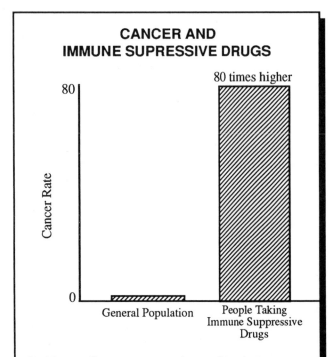

**CANCER AND
IMMUNE SUPRESSIVE DRUGS**

Incidence of cancer among those taking immune suppressive drugs (including vegetable oils used for this purpose) is 80 times greater than normal.

MONEY TALKS

True blue flaxseed fans will find the statements made in this chapter hard to accept because they have heard over and over again how good flaxseed is for us. Of course you hear this; it comes from the people selling the product and from people brainwashed by marketing propaganda. I didn't make up these facts. The research has proven it. You never hear about the negative aspects of these oils because the dissemination of research information is done by the food and supplement industry. They are naturally biased in the material they publicize. Nobody is going to spend money publicizing negative information, because there is no profit in it. You can't make money by not selling a product. So all you ever hear are the positive things. You hear flaxseed is good against cancer and inflammatory disease, but you never hear why it is. We just assume that because flaxseed is a so-called "natural" product, it must be good for us.

I must clarify one point. Flaxseed can be useful just as any drug can be for certain conditions. But like other drugs, it has serious side effects. The damage caused by vegetable oils works slowly so the effects may not manifest themselves for years. By that time the physical deterioration caused by free-radical damage will be credited to age, genetics, or some other cause. If you believe in using drugs, then go ahead and use flaxseed oil. If you want to avoid drugs and prefer to use natural, harmless, remedies, you don't want flaxseed or any other polyunsaturated oil supplements. Flaxseed oil supplements can be useful like any other drug, but they are not natural and they are not harmless!

While I've focused on flaxseed oil in the above discussion, when I refer to vegetable oils I am referring to all vegetable oils, both those used in cooking and those sold as supplements. You hear a lot about evening primrose, black currant, and borage oils. These oils are predominantely composed of linoleic acid (omega-6) and affect the body in the same way as cooking oils do. Since most of us consume far

> "How could a poisonous substance possibly be able to enter the body and not affect any healthy tissue while finding and destroying unhealthy tissue? That would be the same thing as dropping a bomb in wartime on a city and expecting only the enemy to be killed while the sympathizers to your cause are left unscathed. The absurdity of such thinking is totally beyond sane logical reasoning, yet this method of 'healing' is being attempted every day. If you have been led to believe in the truthfulness of such an outrageous supposition, you will also be shocked to know that the moon is *not* made of green cheese."
>
> —Harvey Diamond

too much linoleic acid as it is, taking this oil in supplemental form just compounds the problem. Like flaxseed oil, they generate free radicals, suppress the immune system, etc. Researchers have expressed caution in their use.[34, 35, 36, 37]

If someone recommends that you take flaxseed oil, evening primrose oil, or any other oil supplement, ask them why? What will it do for you? They may say it lowers cholesterol, reduces inflammation, or whatever. Then ask them how it works? Ask them what is the mechanism that makes the oil do what it is supposed to do? Listen to their answer. Chances are, they don't know. Most people, including health care practitioners, don't have any idea how the oils work. They just take it on faith from what they have heard or read somewhere. Many health care practitioners get their information from marketing materials distributed by drug and supplement companies. Many authors who write health books and magazine articles get their knowledge from the same sources. These aren't reliable resources! They're advertisements and, therefore, very biased, and at times, misleading. After all, their purpose is not to educate, but to sell a product.

Will you take these oils to reduce inflammation even if you know free radicals are the primary reason they work and that they are destroying cells throughout your body at the same time? Will you take them to reduce cholesterol even though you know they inhibit normal liver function and may cause liver stress or even damage? That is the decision you must make. If you had a sliver in your finger, would you chop off your finger to prevent infection? No, there are simpler, safer methods of dealing with the problem.

The fact that omega-3 and omega-6 fatty acids can be detrimental to your health goes contrary to most of the things you hear about these oils. Again, this is because the food and drug industry has brainwashed us into believing this.

In writing this book I've avoided company propaganda and gathered all my facts directly from scientific and medical journals and from first-hand observation and clinical studies. This book was written to awaken the public to the plain facts on oils and health.

PRECAUTIONS FOR USE OF FLAXSEED OIL

Despite the health hazards of flaxseed oil, there may be incidences where it can be useful for a limited amount of time under the supervision of a knowledgeable health care professional. For example, if your blood pressure is dangerously high, it can help to lower it quickly. But it should be used only as a temporary measure while other, safer but slower methods, such as diet and lifestyle changes, have time to take effect.

Like linoleic acid (omega-6) from vegetable oil, alpha-linolenic acid (omega-3) from flaxseed oil is polyunsaturated. What this means is that it readily oxidizes to form destructive free-radical chain reactions. In this respect, alpha-linolenic acid is worse than linoleic acid because it is even more polyunsaturated and, therefore, more susceptible to oxidative damage. Linoleic acid has two carbon double bonds—the sites where free-radical reactions occur. Alpha-linolenic acid has *three* carbon double bonds. While linoleic acid is twice as likely to be degraded by oxidation as oleic acid (a monounsaturated acid like olive oil), alpha-linolenic acid is three times more susceptible to oxidation.

Because flaxseed oil oxidizes very easily you must keep it tightly closed and stored in the refrigerator. Never buy flaxseed oil that is not refrigerated or not stored in a dark bottle. Oxygen, heat (even room temperature), and light break down flaxseed oil very quickly. Flaxseed oil should be used within a month or so after purchasing. It should not taste like turpentine or household paint, but have a mild, pleasant taste. If it tastes bad, it's far too oxidized and you are doing more harm to your health than good by eating it. The biggest problem with many flaxseed oil supplements is that they are too old, even before you buy them. After they are manufactured and bottled, they sit in warehouses, trucks, and store shelves for who knows how long. Most flaxseed oil is rancid, even those in capsule form.

The flaxseed itself, rather than the oil, would be a better source for alpha-linolenic acid because the oil in the seed remains fresh, for the most part, until the seed is broken (ground) or heated, and retains all the natural antioxidants, vitamins, and minerals found in the seed.

FLAXSEED MEAL AND FIBER

Because flaxseed oil supplements are often degraded by oxidation, they become a health hazard. Some of the alpha-linolenic acid will still be converted into PGE3, but a lot will just cause destructive free-radical chain reactions. A much safer source for alpha-linolenic acid from flax is through the seed itself.

The seed eaten whole or ground into a meal provides health benefits unrelated to its oil content. Many of the health claims you hear attributed to flaxseed oil are not really a product of the oil, but of the fiber in the seed.

Flaxseed is high in fiber, particularly lignans. This fiber helps to move digested food particles through the digestive tract, increasing bowel movements, pulling toxins and cholesterol out with it, and thus promoting intestinal health. Because of its ability to remove carcinogenic substances, it is useful in the prevention of colon cancer.[38]

Flaxseed ground into a meal and added to flour and then baked into muffins has shown to lower total cholesterol. This is due to the ability of the fiber to bind with cholesterol-rich bile acid and carry it out of the body.[39]

Lignans have antioxidant effects that help to keep the oil in the seed from oxidizing before and after it's been eaten and helps to support the antioxidant processes in our bodies.

Intestinal bacteria convert some of the lignans into hormone-like compounds called phytoestrogens. These phytoestrogens, or plant estrogens, bind to estrogen receptors in the cells and produce estrogen-like effects which influence hormone production, metabolism, and biological activity. This process provides protection against some types of cancer, particularly breast, colon, and prostate cancer.[40, 41, 42]

These phytoestrogens also exert some degree of protection against the loss of calcium and so have been considered of possible benefit in treating osteoporosis.[43]

The greatest degree of protection comes to those who have a healthy digestive tract because the type of flora present will affect the production of the phytochemicals.

Keep in mind that it's the fiber content in the flaxseed that produces these benefits and not the oil. In fact, flaxseed oil in some cases can have the opposite effects. Some studies show that too much of the oil can contribute to calcium loss in bones.[44]

In order to get the most benefit from the lignans and other fibers in flaxseed, as well as the oil, flaxseed must be ground before eating. Whole flaxseed can be eaten, but it simply goes through the body without doing much. Flaxseed should be eaten as soon as possible after is has been ground into a meal. Once the seed has been broken, it is exposed to oxygen, and the enzymes and antioxidants that have kept the oils fresh now rapidly disintegrate. The longer the meal sits before it's eaten, the more oxidation or free-radical damage occurs. It's just like an apple. The inside will stay fresh and white for weeks, but after it is cut and exposed to oxygen in the air, it takes only a few minutes to turn brown. The brown is caused by oxidation just as oxidation affects the exposed oils in the flaxseed.

Fresh flaxseed contains antioxidants such as vitamin E. The antioxidants are necessary for the stability of the oil both in the seed and in the body. When oil is extracted and refined, the natural antioxidants disintegrate rapidly. The oil loses its protection and quickly becomes rancid.

Flaxseed meal can be added to any baked or cook dish—breads, muffins, pancakes, casseroles, etc. You should *not* eat it raw! Raw flaxseed contains a toxin called thiocyanate—a cyanide-like compound. This toxin can be found in the blood after eating raw flaxseed. Cooking neutralizes this compound, making it harmless.[45, 46] By far the best way to eat flaxseed oil is in its natural state by grinding the seed into meal and adding it to a cooked dish.

Chapter 6

THE POLY-UNSATURATED COW

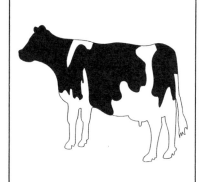

BUILDING BLOCKS

You are not the same person you were ten years ago. You may look and feel the same but your body is different. The cells that made up your body then are not the same ones that you have now. Our cells are continually changing. They live and die and are replaced by new cells on a continual basis. For example, the skin that covered your body ten years ago is long gone. It has been entirely replaced by new cells. The rate of cellular replacement varies within the body. Red blood cells live for only 120 days. The cells lining your digestive tract are replaced every three days. Those in the long bones of the arms and legs are completely replaced every seven years or so.

The building blocks for new cells come from our foods. The protein we eat is broken down and incorporated in the building of the protein within our own body tissues. Fats, likewise, are taken from our food and reassembled into body tissues. And so it is with all the compounds that make up every cell in our bodies. Our foods also supply our bodies with the energy we need to fuel metabolism, reproduce, and make vital substances such as antibodies, hormones, and enzymes, all of which are necessary for life.

It's like building a house. The quality of the house depends on the quality of the materials being used and the labor force doing the work. If you use cheap materials, the house will break down sooner and become less functional. Also, if you don't have enough labor and they are overworked to meet deadlines, corners are cut to save time and work may become sloppy. Even though materials used may be of good quality, if they were not put together properly, they too will break down quickly. The materials for the house can be compared to the proteins, fats, minerals and other compounds that make up the cells and tissues of our body. The work force is the energy necessary to use the raw materials in a constructive way. If we do not eat the foods that supply the proper building blocks or energy-producing compounds, our cells will be built like a second-rate house ready to crumple long before its time.

We need some 90 different nutrients in order to maintain optimal health. These nutrients include water, amino acids (from protein), fatty acids (from dietary fats), carbohydrates, vitamins, and minerals. When these nutrients are lacking in our diet, new cells either cannot be made or are restricted with what materials are available, which may make the resulting molecule dysfunctional and a burden to the rest of the body.

"Man is what he eats."
—Goethe

"The purpose of life, as I see it, is to be happy and the only way to be happy is to be healthy or at least free from physical suffering, and the only way to be healthy is to obey the laws that Nature has laid down for building the human body."
—Dr. Eugene Christian

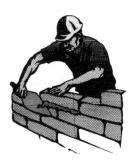

In order to build a house, you need all the right materials at the right time. It does no good to have 10 tons of bricks but no mortar to hold them together, or have a stack of lumber but no nails. A brick house might be built without mortar by just stacking the bricks one on top of the other, but such a house will not hold up for long. Our bodies, like a house, needs a variety of nutrients so that we have all the materials necessary to build healthy cells.

Protein synthesis is a good example of the need for all the right materials at the right time. When the body signals a need to build any type of protein (muscle, skin, tendons, blood, hormones, enzymes, etc.), it uses amino acids from the diet. There are 20 amino acids important to human nutrition. At least nine of these are classified as being *essential*, which means the body cannot manufacture them from other nutrients so we must get them directly from the foods we eat. When the body attempts to build a particular protein, say, for example, an enzyme necessary for digestion of dietary protein, it may need several different essential amino acids to complete the job. If all of these amino acids are available except for just one, the enzyme will *not* be made. And the other amino acids will not be stored until the missing one eventually comes along. So because one amino acid is missing, all the other amino acids necessary to make that particular enzyme will be broken down and discarded in the urine. Amino acids are not stored in the body like fat or some vitamins are; therefore, we must have them in our diet continually. Now, since the digestive enzyme is not made, this leads to an enzyme deficiency that hampers the digestive process, limiting the absorption and availability of additional nutrients. A vicious cycle can easily emerge. Without the enzyme necessary to digest protein, essential amino acids that are derived from dietary protein and necessary to build more enzymes cannot be made, and the situation goes from bad to worse.

Our bodies, at times, will attempt to build certain molecules even when all the right materials are not available.

Iron is an important constituent in the construction of red blood cells. If your diet is insufficient in iron, and your iron reserves become low, the body will use another element in its place when building new red blood cells. If lead, which is a common contaminant in our environment and our food, is available, our bodies will use it in place of iron in the manufacture of blood. Lead renders the newly formed cells incapable of carrying and delivering oxygen to the rest of the body—a potentially fatal situation even in tiny amounts.

A more common problem is the body's use of chemically altered foods in place of natural ones. The use of trans fatty acids provides a good example. Trans fatty acids are dietary fats that have been chemically altered for commercial reasons. They are made by taking unsaturated vegetable oils and saturating them with hydrogen atoms under high heat. This process is called hydrogenation. It is done so the oil can remain solid at room temperature and to extend shelf life. Margarine and shortening are hydrogenated oils. All hydrogenated and partially hydrogenated oils are damaging to the body.

Hydrogenation changes the shape of unsaturated fatty acid from their natural horseshoe configuration to one that is straight. This is important. Most all of the cell membranes (cell walls), in our bodies, as well as many other cellular structures, are composed of fatty acids. The cells get the raw materials to construct their membranes from the fatty acids in our diet. If hydrogenated oils are eaten, trans fatty acids from these oils are used as building blocks when cell membranes are made. This is where the shape is important. Normal fatty acids link together in a tight bond because of their horseshoe shape. Trans fatty acids cannot link together or to other fatty acids in the proper manner. This weakens the cell wall and hampers or even destroys normal cellular function.

Trans and Cis Fatty Acids

Bear with me for a moment and let me explain in some detail what happens when trans fatty acids are formed and then incorporated into our bodies. This is important to gaining an understanding of how chemically altered fatty acids can adversely affect your health. Hydrogenation affects only *unsaturated* fatty acids. In the hydrogenation process, hydrogen atoms are attached to fatty acid molecules. Since saturated fats already hold as many hydrogen atoms as they possibly can, they are not affected by hydrogenation and remain unchanged. Monounsaturated and polyunsaturated fatty acids are affected because they can accept additional hydrogen atoms whereever they have double carbon bonds and in so doing they become more saturated—saturated with hydrogen atoms. A monounsaturated oil can accept two pair of hydrogen atoms and become a saturated fat. A polyunsaturated oil can accept two or more pairs of hydrogen atoms on its double bonds and become either a monounsaturated or saturated fat in the hydrogenation process.

Hydrogen atoms are attached to the unsaturated fatty acids wherever there is a double carbon bond. When a pair of hydrogen atoms are missing, a double carbon bond is always formed. Hydrogenation forces hydrogen atoms to attach themselves at these sites in unsaturated fats.

Now here is the problem. A pair of hydrogen atoms can either attach themselves on the same side of the fatty acid molecule or on opposite sides. The normal way in which fatty acids are structured in nature is called a cis configuration where the two hydrogen atoms are on the *same side* of the double bond. In the trans (called a transformation) configuration, which is rarely found in nature, the hydrogen atoms are positioned on *opposites sides* of the double bond. During hydrogenation, both cis and trans bonds are formed as hydrogen atoms are attached to double bonded carbon atoms in the fatty acid molecule. The cis configurations or cis fatty acids do not cause any problems as they are exactly the same as other fatty acids found in nature. The trans fatty acids are the troublemakers.

Although the chemical makeup of the trans fatty acid molecule is exactly the same as a cis fatty acid, their shape is distinctly different and this is extremely important biologically. When both hydrogen atoms are on the same side of the fatty acid, as it is with cis configurations, it causes the molecule to bend because the hydrogen atoms have the same electrical charge and repel each other. This is the form they should have. When the hydrogen atoms are on oppo-

site sides, as in the trans configurations, the fatty acid becomes straight. A straight molecule gums up the works. Its like building a brick house using relatively soft Styrofoam bricks. They may stack up like normal bricks, but they create some serious weaknesses that can destroy the entire house.

When we eat hydrogenated oils, our bodies cannot tell the difference between the cis and trans fatty acids. It will, therefore, grab a trans fatty acid and use it like it would any other fatty acid. The consequences can be serious.

The membranes that make up the covering of all our cells and the organelles within the cells are composed predominantly of fatty acids. Trans fatty acids are incorporated into the body's cell membranes as if they were cis fatty acids. In the process, your cells become hydrogenated. Once in place, trans fatty acids with their misplaced hydrogen atom, wreak havoc with cell metabolism.

Like the skin covering our bodies, the membrane covers each cell and each organelle within the cell. Its unique design is carefully balanced chemically and structurally to keep out harmful toxins and disease-causing microorganisms, yet allow oxygen, glucose, hormones and other vital compounds in and at the same time expel carbon dioxide and other waste products. Any disruption of the membrane's function can seriously affect the health and function of the cell. If our own skin lost its ability to keep out bacteria, we would be helplessly exposed to a host of dangerous organisms that otherwise would pose little threat to us. Likewise, with our cells. If the cell's membrane loses its ability to carefully monitor the absorption and excretion of nutrients, wastes, and harmful microorganisms, it degenerates and loses its ability to function as it should. A person full of damaged or poorly manufactured cells creates a degenerative sickly body prone to frequent illness and premature aging.

Research is beginning to find correlations with trans fat consumption and the incidence of disease. For example, a report from the European Community Multicenter Study on Antioxidants, Myocardial Infarction, and Breast Cancer some stated that women with breast cancer have higher levels of trans fatty acids in their bodies than other women, suggesting—but not proving—that eating trans fats may raise the risk of this disease. The researchers measured trans and other fats in tissue samples taken from the buttocks of 291 women with breast cancer and 407 similar healthy women in Germany, Ireland, the Netherlands, Japan, and Switzerland. Those women who had eaten higher levels of trans fats were almost four times more likely to have breast cancer than the women who had eaten less.

If you eat margarine, shortening, hydrogenated and partially hydrogenated oils (found in most processed and convenience foods), or eat heat-processed refined vegetable

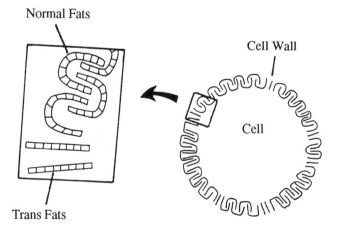

Normal Fats

Cell Wall

Cell

Trans Fats

Trans fats incorporated into cell walls causes distortion adversely affecting cellular function (Source: Zane R. Kime, M.D., Sunlight Could Save Your Life.)

oils, then you are consuming trans fatty acids! Keep in mind that heating or cooking vegetable oils, whether they are hydrogenated or not, also creates trans fatty acids.

If people tell you that these types of oils are not harmful, don't listen to them. If they want to eat these toxic fats let them, but you can avoid a lot of health problems in the future by staying as far away from them as possible.

Free radicals can also cause similar effects as those of trans fatty acids. Free radicals attack the polyunsaturated fatty acids in the cell membrane, distorting their shape and rendering the cell membrane dysfunctional. Free radicals are even worse than trans fatty acids because they not only attack the cell membrane but any molecule or cellular component anywhere, including the DNA. The more polyunsaturated fats you eat, the more of them are incorporated into your cells and the greater the chance and degree of free-radical damage. The more saturated and monounsaturated fats in our bodies the less chance there is for free-radical damage. Nature isn't stupid, that is why our bodies are naturally designed to contain predominantely saturated and monounsaturated fats rather than polyunsaturated fats. We are not polyunsaturated creatures and, therefore, should not overeat these types of oils.

All Diseases are Cellular Disorders

All disease starts at the cellular level. An ailing colon, for example, doesn't all of the sudden become diseased. When enough cells in the colon become diseased or dysfunctional, the entire organ loses its ability to function properly; that in turn affects digestion and nutrient absorption. The result is illness and perhaps pain. The entire body is affected. Cellular degeneration throughout the body can cause a decrease in organ function, premature aging, aches, pains, fatigue, and any number of degenerative disease conditions.

If the cells in your body do not function correctly, what happens to you? What happens to your health? Let's look at the answer to these questions from the opposite direction. If all the cells in your body were healthy, what would you

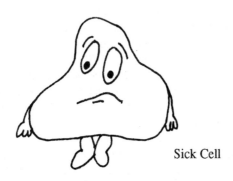

Sick Cell

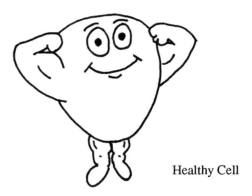

Healthy Cell

be? You would be healthy, right? If all your cells were functioning as they should, wouldn't that make the tissues and organs composed of those cells healthy? If all of your organs were functioning with health and vigor, then it stands to reason that you, too, would have good health and vigor.

The opposite is also true. If the cells in your body were weakened by deformed or injured molecules hampering proper function, then the organs composed of such cells will not function optimally and you, as well, will have a lesser degree of health. If your white blood cells, for instance, contained faulty materials such as trans fatty acids, do you believe they can effectively fight off infection? Is it any wonder why some people always get seasonal infections while others in the same environment do not, or why people develop degenerative diseases, even at young ages, while others remain relatively healthy through old age?

When you give your body clean, healthy foods, you supply it with the building blocks it needs to make healthy cells. Most of us live on diets composed of poor-quality building materials, so many of our cells, and consequently tissues and organs, are inferior to nature's intended design. When you eat good foods, in time, old cells made with inferior materials will be replaced by new healthier cells. There is profound truth in the saying, "You are what you eat." Are you made of the components of wholesome fruits and vegetables, or are you the product of soda pop, wieners, and Ding Dongs?

You Are What You Ate

You are what you eat, or more aptly, what you ate. Your body is actually the sum combination of not just the food you eat now, but all foods you have eaten. All the cells in your body have obtained their building blocks—the molecules, the proteins, fats, etc.—from the food you've been eating for years. You are the sum total of your diet. The chicken you ate for dinner last week has been broken down into amino acids (the building blocks for protein) and fats (cholesterol and fatty acids). Most of the nutrients in the foods we eat are burned up as a process of metabolism to generate energy. The rest is recycled and incorporated into your body tissues. Excess compounds and many harmful substances are discarded as waste.

The saying, "you are what you ate," is true more with fat than it is with carbohydrate and protein. Carbohydrate and protein, when digested and broken down, go directly to the liver. The liver, the manufacturing and processing plant of the body, converts them into glucose to be used as fuel to produce energy or makes compounds that will be incorporated into body tissues such as fat and enzymes.

The fat we eat does not go directly to the liver, but is absorbed through the intestinal wall into the blood stream (in the form of lipoproteins) where it is distributed throughout the body. The same fat you eat, is the same that is distributed to your cells. So if you eat a meal with a fat content of 80 percent polyunsaturated fat and 20 percent saturated fat, these very same fats will become your body tissues.

The liver also makes fat from the fat circulating in the blood (lipoproteins) and the proteins and carbohydrates in your food. The liver makes all types of fats, including, to some extent, the essential fatty acids.[1]

Approximately 95 percent of the fat in our bodies consists of a combination of saturated, monounsaturated, and polyunsaturated fats. The remaining 5 percent or so is composed of phospholipids (e.g., lecithin) and sterols (e.g., cholesterol). The fatty acids in the bodies of humans is about 45 percent saturated, 50 percent monounsaturated, and 5 percent polyunsaturated.[2, 3] At least these are the percentages for people who eat a relatively balanced diet devoid of junk foods—like we should. Note that our body fat should be only about 5 percent polyunsaturated. The predominante fat in the body is monounsaturated, followed closely by saturated fat. When our bodies synthesize their own fat from carbohydrates and proteins, it will make primarily saturated and monounsaturated fat. This is what the body prefers. The body ordinarily contains very little polyunsaturated fat. The polyunsaturated fat in our bodies comes directly from the foods we eat.

The fat which makes up our bodies is influenced directly by our diet. People who eat a lot of monounsaturated fat, such as olive oil, in place of the others, have as much

> "We are the sum total of the things we eat. If we use trashy building material (food) we will have a trashy body. This is law."
> —Dr. Eugene Christian

as 90 percent of their body fat of this type. Human tissues have been reported to contain up to 14 percent trans fatty acids from hydrogenated vegetable oil.[4] A person who eats more polyunsaturated fat in relation to monounsaturated and saturated fat will also have a different fat profile. The polyunsaturated percentage could be extraordinarily disproportioned—which it is for many people in Western cultures who eat a lot of polyunsaturated vegetable oils.

Competition for the enzymes in the body determines what type of fats body tissues are made of. For example, linoleic acid and alpha-linolenic acid both compete with each other for incorporation into the brain and heart tissues.[5] The fat that goes into the construction of our cells is determined by the fat that is available in the body. So the fat in our diet even affects the fat composition of our white blood cells and, therefore, their function and, consequently, the efficiency of the entire immune system.[6]

As you see, the fat in our foods is incorporated directly into our body's cells and tissues. The same is true for cattle, sheep, pigs, and other animals raised for food. Their diet influences their body fat composition. Farm animals given feed rich in polyunsaturated fatty acids also become more polyunsaturated themselves.[7] Animals are now being bred and raised to have more polyunsaturated fat, unlike the animals in past generations. This, in a sense, has given rise to the polyunsaturated cow—Western civilization's new farm product. Corn, soybeans, fish meal, flaxseed, as well as additives fed to cattle are all very high in polyunsaturated oils. So the meat we buy at the store has a higher percentage of polyunsaturated fat.

Scientists can engineer the tissue content in animals used for food. Cattle fed flaxseed contain more alpha-linolenic acid in both their meat and milk.[8] Chickens fed flaxseed meal produce eggs containing as much omega-3 fatty acids as a typical dietary supplement.[9] High omega-3 fatty acid eggs are available to those who want to get more of this fat but don't want to eat fish or take dietary supplements. Along with the polyunsaturated cow we now have the omega-3 chicken egg.

Eating meat, milk and eggs that are higher in polyunsaturated fats may sound good because it displaces the so-called "bad" saturated fat. Animals raised a century ago and those raised on free range ranches now, feed almost entirely on grass. The content of their bodies are more how nature intended it, with very little polyunsaturated fat. Nowadays, cattle are fed foods high in polyunsaturated fats so they can add weight faster and be prepared for market quicker.

Most of the meat we eat nowadays have a higher polyunsaturated fat content. Combine that with vegetable oils hidden in processed foods and used in cooking, and we consume more polyunsaturated fat than we realize. We eat

THE OMEGA-3 CHICKEN EGG
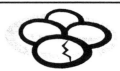

Anybody that knows anything about diet and nutrition has heard about omega-3 fatty acids. They are looked upon as rising stars in the world of nutrition. As a consequence, people have flocked to the store to buy more fish and oil supplements—the main sources for these essential fatty acids. But many people don't like fish or don't like to take supplements. So scientists have been working on ways to increase the omega-3 fatty acid content in foods which are more commonly eaten. The product with the most promise appears to be the chicken egg.

Once considered a heart disease patient's worst nightmare, because of its high cholesterol content, the egg is making a comeback. It's now gaining a status as a health food. Eggs have long been noted for their protein con-

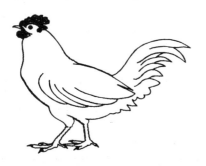

tent, providing the best balance of amino acids of any food. But now eggs can offer another nutrient—omega-3 fatty acids.

Normally, we think of eggs as high in cholesterol, not omega-3 fatty acids. But scientists have done the improbable. You can now go to your grocery store and buy eggs packed with omega-3 essential fatty acids. Eating a poached egg or an omelet sounds a lot more appetizing than a spoonful of raunchy-tasting cod liver or flaxseed oil.

How did they do it? It was accomplished by selective feeding. It's well known that in animals and humans body tissues resemble the fat content found in the diet. Even breast milk is influenced by diet, so why not eggs?

Researchers found that hens given flaxseed produced eggs with a substantial amount of omega-3 fatty acids. In one study, three diets containing 0%, 10%, and 20% of ground flaxseed were fed to hens and the omega-3 fatty acid content of their eggs determined. These diets resulted in a marked progressive increase in omega-3 fatty acids content with alpha-lino-

lenic acid measuring 28, 261, and 527 mg/egg and docosahexaenoic acid (DHA) measuring 51, 81, and 878 mg/egg. No alterations in the cholesterol concentration of the egg yolk were noted. Could humans benefit from the fatty acids in the eggs? To answer this question, the eggs were then fed to human volunteers. The subjects ate four eggs per day for two weeks. When the volunteers were tested there was no statistically significant changes observed in blood cholesterol, but there was a significant increase in omega-3 fatty acids.

The amount of omega-3 fatty acids from a single egg can supply all that's needed for the day. The author of the study suggested that regularly eating eggs from hens fed flaxseed may be a good way to reduce risk of heart disease. Eggs, a food that at one time were shunned as bad for the heart, are now recommended as a means to reduce heart disease.

Source: Ferrier, L.K. et al., 1995. Alpha-linolenic Acid- and Docosahexaenoic Acid-Enriched Eggs from Hens Fed Flaxseed: Influence on Blood Lipids and Platelet Phospholipid Fatty Acids in Humans. *Am J. Clin. Nutr.* 62:81

more polyunsaturated fat than our grandparents did. Our bodies, as a consequence, have a disproportionate amount of polyunsaturated fat as compared to other types of fat.

Nature's Design

Nature has designed our bodies to have more saturated and monounsaturated fat than polyunsaturated fat in our tissues. This is what the body prefers. We fight against nature's perfect design by eating refined vegetable oil.

International committees, namely the Food and Agriculture Organization (FAO) and the World Health Organization (WHO), along with those of many individual nations,

including the United States, Australia, the Scandinavian countries and others, have issued recommendations on fat intake. These recommendations state that we need a balance between polyunsaturated fat and saturated fat so as to achieve a polyunsaturated to saturated ratio of 0.6:1.0.[10] These organizations and governments recommend a ratio of almost twice as much saturated fat to polyunsaturated fat in our diet. This agrees more with nature's design than a diet with little saturated fat and more polyunsaturated fat.

The recommendation we hear in the United States most often comes from the American Heart Association (AHA) which states limiting fat intake to 30 percent of total calories. Out of this 30 percent, 10 percent should be from saturated fat, 10 percent from monounsaturated fat, and 10 percent from polyunsaturated fat. The AHA recommendation for saturated fat is lower than those noted above because of their belief that it contributes to heart disease. If saturated fat contributes to heart disease, why don't they cut their recommendation down even more? The reason is because they know our bodies need saturated fat. Reducing it too much may cause other health problems.

The saturated, monounsaturated, and polyunsaturated fatty acids we get from our foods all compete with each other for incorporation into the structure of our cells. The structure and function of the cell membrane is greatly influenced by the type of fatty acids from which it is composed. When all fatty acids are readily available, our bodies preferentially choose saturated and monounsaturated fats over polyunsaturated fat. The body knows what materials work best.

Restricting saturated and monounsaturated fats in the diet in favor of polyunsaturated fats causes our cells to use inferior materials in its construction. Food scientists are concerned, because the more polyunsaturated oils in food, the more likely lipid peroxidation is to occur.[11] The consequence is a greater number dysfunctional and damaged cells.

OILS AND DEGENERATIVE DISEASE

There is a strong correlation between the use of vegetable oils and the increasing incidence of degenerative disease. Researchers have already shown that free radicals are involved in at least 60 different types of degenerative diseases. Polyunsaturated fats are extremely susceptible to free-radical destruction. The more polyunsaturated fat in the body, the more chance of free-radical damage and, consequently, disease.

If our bodies have a high polyunsaturated fat content it is more susceptible to oxidative damage even when the fat is incorporated inside cells. You don't want your body made up of too much polyunsaturated fat. A polyunsaturated body is more prone to aging and disease than a more saturated or monounsaturated one.

Researchers have long debated why people who are overweight suffer with more health problems and die sooner than those of normal weight. The answer, at least in part, may be due to their body fat content. Most overweight people get that way by eating more calories than their body needs and the excess is stored as fat. Overweight people have more polyunsaturated fat as well as trans fatty acids in their body tissues. This may explain why being overweight is associated with many health risks.

Polyunsaturated fat when it oxidizes can affect other molecules, like cholesterol, causing it to become oxidized. Our brains are about 60 percent fat, mostly cholesterol. If the cholesterol in our brain is oxidized, the cells composed of the damaged cholesterol will not function properly. If the tissues in our brain cells become damaged by free radicals, what do you think will happen?

Oxidized cholesterol is the only type of cholesterol found in arterial plaque associated with atherosclerosis and heart disease. How did it become oxidized? It was either eaten that way in the food or became oxidized after being ingested into the body. The most likely culprit responsible for causing it to become oxidized after we have eaten it is polyunsaturated fat. Researchers know that the more polyunsaturated fatty acids in your cells, the greater the level of oxidation your body tissues experience.[12]

Lung Cancer

One look at the blackened diseased lung of a smoker would be enough to keep most people from considering smoking. Pictures of diseased organs from those who have died of lung cancer have often been displayed in schools to educate kids on the dangers of smoking. Smoking is known to greatly increase the risk of developing lung cancer, emphysema, heart disease and other health problems.

Cigarette smoke is filled with noxious gases and toxic chemicals, some of which are carcinogenic. The smoke is also a rich source of free radicals. In fact, most of the damage done by cigarette smoke is a result of free radicals. Free radicals contribute to the destruction of elastic fibers in the lungs (causing emphysema), and to lung cancer.[13] Smoke damages lung cells releasing substances that intensify free-radical activity causing further injury. Lung tissues in smokers are characteristically scarred as a result of free-radical injury.

Antioxidants that protect all our cells are quickly used up in their fight with smoke, leaving the cells in the lungs defenseless. This is why smokers are encouraged to take vitamin C and other antioxidants in doses nearly twice the RDA.

More people die from lung cancer than from any other form of cancer. As the facts on smoking have become publicized and as people have become more health-conscious, the percentage of those who smoke has steadily declined. While *less* people are smoking, cancer deaths are *increasing*. Over the past 30 years adults who smoke declined from 42 to 25 percent. During this same time period deaths from lung cancer have doubled. Not only are more smokers getting lung cancer but nonsmokers are dying from it as well. Yet not all smokers get lung cancer. If smoking causes cancer, why do nonsmokers get cancer while some smokers do not?

Undoubtedly there are many factors involved, but one of the biggest is diet. A person who eats lots of fruits and vegetables, rich in antioxidant vitamins and minerals, will unquestionably be much better off than one who doesn't. Another big factor is the amount of polyunsaturated fats consumed. A diet high in polyunsaturated fats predisposes people to lung and other types of cancer. These fats are incorporated into all the tissues of the body, including the lungs. Being highly susceptible to the oxidative chemicals in cigarette smoke, they readily transform into destructive free radicals. After many years of such abuse, it is no wonder cancer is often the end result.

A person who eats a lot of polyunsaturated oils will be much more sensitive to cigarette smoke and more likely to develop cancer. A nonsmoker who has a high amount of polyunsaturated fats in his body and low antioxidant reserves will be more vulnerable to lung cancer than a smoker with less polyunsaturated fats and higher antioxidant reserves. Lung cancer is increasing in part because people are eating too much polyunsaturated fat.

Skin Cancer and Sunlight

We've all been warned about the dangers of sunlight exposure on our skin. Too much ultraviolet (UV) light from the sun is considered a major risk factor in the development of skin cancer. Ultraviolet light does not necessarily cause skin cancer, but it is a risk factor. That means that a great deal of exposure to the ultraviolet radiation from sunlight is correlated with an increased risk or chance of developing skin cancer. The actual cause is still debated, but ultraviolet light seems to be one of the triggers that promotes it.

To say sunlight or overexposure to sunlight causes cancer is totally inaccurate. If sunlight or the ultraviolet component of sunlight were the cause of skin cancer, there would be a worldwide epidemic, an epidemic that would have extended back thousands of years. Skin cancer is primarily a modern disease, like other degenerative conditions common in Western countries. People in Third World countries and in ages past are not and were not troubled by skin cancer even though the vast majority of them are and were farmers who spent most of their lives working directly under the hot sun. Why all of the sudden in the latter half of the 20th century has skin cancer become a problem, especially since most of us spend almost the entire day indoors out of the sun?

The problem is in our diet. Skin cancer is a product of the overconsumption of polyunsaturated oils. When we eat foods rich in these types of oils, they become a part of the cells and tissues of our bodies, including our skin. The skin becomes susceptible to cancer when it become overly polyunsaturated. Researchers have found that the fat con-

tent of the skin is profoundly affected by the type of fats in the diet.[14] The more polyunsaturated fat in the diet, the more in the skin.

One of the primary causes of dry, wrinkled skin associated with aging is free-radical damage. Dry skin is associated with unsaturated fatty acids. One study showed dry skin contained a higher content of unsaturated fatty acids (60%) than normal skin (49%).[15] The more unsaturated fat in the skin, the greater the degree of free-radical damage.

Polyunsaturated oils, whether they are in a bottle on a store shelf or incorporated in the tissues of the skin, are easily oxidized by exposure to sunlight. The polyunsaturated fats in the tissues of our skin are bombarded by ultraviolet radiation from the sun and form free radicals. These free-radical chain reactions destroy molecules and cells and lead to the development of cancerous cells. The result is skin cancer.

People in past ages or in less developed regions of the world who eat more saturated fat and less polyunsaturated fat are not affected by ultraviolet radiation. They work 12 to 14 hours a day under the hot sun and experience no skin cancer. Saturated fat isn't easily oxidized, so body tissues made from saturated and monounsaturated fats are protected from the ultraviolet light.

Scientists know that free-radical damage to fats are involved in the development of many cancers. Antioxidants have been found to be useful in protecting polyunsaturated fats from free-radical damage and thus preventing the development of cancer. In one study melanoma (skin cancer) cells treated with the antioxidant vitamin E showed significant decrease in cell proliferation, accompanied by a significant decrease of free-radical levels and lipid peroxidation.[16]

Antioxidants don't necessarily need to be taken orally to be effective. Topical applications of antioxidants have been shown to be effective in reducing risk of tumors in test animals.[17]

Karen Burke, M.D., Ph.D. of the Cabrini Medical Center in New York City reported that 240 skin cancer patients demonstrated significantly lower blood selenium (an antioxidant mineral) concentrations than control volunteers without skin cancer. To determine the protective quality of selenium, she ran tests on several groups of mice. One group was fed a selenium supplement, on another group a selenium compound was applied to the skin, and a third group received no treatment. All the groups were then subjected to ultraviolet radiation. Both groups of the treated groups showed far less damage than those that were not given selenium. Also, none of the animals given either oral or topical selenium developed any blistering sunburn, but the nontreated animals did. This showed that selenium protected the fatty acids in the skin from UV radiation and reduced risk of skin cancer.[18, 19]

Scientists discovered that chlorophyll could undergo free-radical formation within plant tissues. Carotenoids, a group of plant pigments that act as antioxidants, were found to protect them against free-radical damage. When researchers gave animals extra beta-carotene, they discovered that it also had a major protective effect against free radicals.[20] In human volunteers carotenoids protected the skin against the harmful effects of ultraviolet radiation. Volunteers significantly reduced their erythema (skin reddening) upon exposure to UV radiation after taking a supplement of mixed carotenoids.[21]

Putting gobs of chemicals designed to block out UV light is not the answer to skin cancer. A much better solution is to make the body resistant to excessive exposure to sunlight, and that can be done by reducing polyunsaturated fat consumption and increasing the intake of fruits and vegetables rich in antioxidant vitamins and minerals.

Autoimmune and Inflammatory Diseases

Some of the most perplexing illnesses to plague modern society are known collectively as the autoimmune diseases. There is no known cause for these illnesses and no cure.

The medical explanation is that the immune system, which protects us from invading microorganisms and diseased cells, goes ballistic and, for no known reason, starts attacking itself. Doctors don't know why some people's bodies react in this way; they attribute it to genetics. Genetics is always a safe answer when medical science cannot explain why something happens.

The body, however, doesn't suddenly just make mistakes, it's not programmed that way. What happens is a normal and natural response in a toxic or diseased body.

Autoimmune processes can cause slow destruction of a particular type of cell or tissue, stimulation of an organ into excessive growth, or interference in its function. Organs and tissues frequently affected include the thyroid, pancreas, and adrenal glands, blood, connective tissues, skin, muscles, and joints.[22]

One of the characteristics of autoimmune disease is inflammation. Inflammation is a defensive healing response often considered a "symptom" to be suppressed. The body initiates inflammation to bring about healing. When there is an injury or infection, the inflammation response automatically kicks in. When it does, circulation of the blood increases into the infected area. This can cause swelling, generate heat, and increase pain. This process brings in an increased number of white blood cells to fight the infection and speed healing. Even the pain is beneficial because it

gives us a warning that something is wrong and to be careful. For example, if we sprained an ankle and there was little or no pain, most of us would continue to walk and use it as we normally do, quite possibly resulting in further damage. Pain tells us to ease off and let it heal.

Injury can occur anywhere and everywhere. It may even be self-inflected over a long time period like when you continually abuse your body with toxic food—particularly vegetable oils. Oxidized fat promotes inflammatory reactions encouraging autoimmune disease.[23]

Our bodies have billions of cells, and each cell is made of thousands of molecules. A few free-radical damaged molecules (or trans fatty acids) will probably have a relatively minor effect on the cell's ability to function (unless its DNA is damaged). A few hundred damaged molecules may begin to show signs of cellular degeneration as the cell loses its ability to function properly. The more damaged molecules the cell has, the more cellular function degenerates.

As these cells degenerate, they come to a point where the immune system identifies them as being a problem and attacks them just like a pathogenic microbe. That's exactly what happens with cancer. If a cell becomes cancerous or diseased, a healthy immune system will remove it as quickly as possible.

If the body is continually subjected to free-radical destruction, all of the cells will be affected to some degree. At some point, degenerative cells become so numerous that the immune system seems to be attacking the entire body. What we have is the onset of autoimmune disease. It appears as if the immune system is attacking itself and, in a sense, it is because so many of the cells have become degraded by damaged polyunsaturated fats.

Free radicals occur throughout the body. As a result, degenerative and autoimmune diseases can develop anywhere. The most likely place is where free radicals are most prevalent, like the sensitive skin of a sun bather, or the lungs of a smoker. Any organ that is abused or overstressed will feel the effects of degeneration first. A liver burdened with the job of continually detoxifying alcohol or other toxins will suffer free-radical damage and become diseased long before other organs begin to lose their functional capacity. The same is true for the kidneys, pancreas, or any other organ. If it is put under unusual stress for an extended amount of time, it will be the first to suffer.

The most common autoimmune disease is arthritis. Osteoarthritis is a noninflammatory condition where cartilage in joints degenerate. Rheumatoid arthritis is characterized by deterioration of soft tissues around the joints and is accompanied by chronic inflammation. These tissues become so degenerative that the immune system attempts to clean them out. Inflammation results, causing swelling and

Common Autoimmune Diseases

Addison's disease. Hyposecretion of adrenal hormones results in weakness, reduced blood sugar, nausea, loss of appetite, and weight loss.

Anemia. Abnormally low number of red blood cells lowers oxygen delivery to body which is necessary for proper metabolic processes.

Cardiomyopathy. Loss of pumping efficiency of heart and heart failure.

Crohn's disease. Chronic inflammatory disease that can affect any part of the gastrointestinal tract from the mouth to the rectum.

Diabetes mellitus. Hyposecretion of insulin by the pancreas results in extremely elevated blood glucose levels resulting in causing a host of metabolic problems and even death.

Glomerulonephritis. Disease of the filtration apparatus of the kidney results in fluid and electrolyte imbalance and possibly total kidney failure and death.

Graves' disease. Hypersecretion of thyroid hormone results in increase in metabolic rate.

Lupus. Chronic inflammatory disease has widespread effects and is characterized by arthritis, red rash on the face.

Multiple sclerosis. Progressive degeneration of myelin sheaths results in widespread impairment of nerve function and especially muscle control.

Myasthenia gravis. Muscle disorder is characterized by progressive weakness and chronic fatigue.

Myxedema. Hyposecretion of thyroid hormone in adulthood causes decreased metabolic rate; it is characterized by reduced mental and physical vigor, weight gain, hair loss, and edema.

Reproductive infertility. An inability to produce offspring resulting from destruction of reproductive cells.

Rheumatoid arthritis. Inflammatory joint disease is characterized by synovial inflammation that spreads to other fibrous tissues.

Ulcerative colitis. Chronic inflammatory disease of the colon is characterized by watery diarrhea containing blood, mucus, and pus.

Source: Thibodeau, G.A., and Patton, K.T.,1992, *The Human Body in Health and Disease*, Mosby-Year Book

pain. There is no recognized cure for arthritis. The standard treatment is to reduce pain and inflammation with anti-inflammatory and immunosuppressant drugs such as cortisone and ibuprofen.

Inflammation is a common symptom with many diseases, and chronic inflammation is often mistaken as a "disease" to be cured. Conditions involving chronic inflammation are classified as inflammatory diseases. Autoimmune diseases fit into this class. Inflammatory conditions such as allergy, arthritis, asthma, eczema, and chronic bronchitis are among the most common chronic diseases in the Western world. As we saw in the previous two chapters, all these symptoms have been linked to the consumption of polyunsaturated oils.

Allergy is an overactive response of the immune system to a relatively harmless environmental substance. These substances are called antigens. When we come into contact with an antigen, the immune system mistakenly interprets it as harmful and begins producing antibodies in self-defense. Antibody production triggers the release of histamine and other inflammatory substances. These responses may cause typical allergy symptoms such as runny nose, watery eyes, fever, and hives. But they also cause constriction of the airways, relaxation of blood vessels, and irregular heart rhythms.

Allergies may be triggered by pollutants in the air such as tobacco smoke or pollen, by components of food, or even by physical contact and absorption through the skin. The symptoms can vary greatly. Over one hundred symptoms have been medically recognized as being caused by allergic reactions to food and environmental chemicals; some of them include: depression, fatigue, irritability, hyperactivity, back pain, gallbladder pain, and indigestion.[24]

A healthy, properly functioning white blood cell will not overreact, but ignore harmless antigens. If the white blood cells aren't functioning properly, they can respond erratically to stimuli. Why would a white blood cell lose its ability to tell friend from foe? One easy answer is because it becomes degraded by too many trans fatty acids or free-radical damaged polyunsaturated fats. Taking antihistamines and pain killers may stop the symptoms, but that doesn't solve the problem.

Alpha-linolenic acid (flaxseed oil) has been recommended as a "natural" medication to reduce inflammation. Its anti-inflammatory effects come, not by the production of prostaglandins as we would expect, but through destructive free-radical reactions. [25, 26]

In this process, the immune system and inflammation response are suppressed.[27, 28, 29, 30, 31, 32] Using alpha-linolenic acid to reduce inflammation is no different than using anti-inflammatory drugs. Reducing inflammation does not solve the problem, it only masks the symptoms. In this process, it also suppresses the immune system, making healing more difficult. Can something that suppresses the body's natural system of healing be good? Discomfort may be temporarily lessened, but the disease will grow worse unless something is done to treat the cause.

Vegetable oils are known to *cause* inflammation and are suspect in numerous degenerative conditions including the autoimmune and inflammatory diseases.[33, 34, 35, 36, 37, 38]

A logical step in solving the problem is not to suppress the immune system with more polyunsaturated oil (in the form of alpha-linolenic acid), but to eliminate them from your diet.

Breast Milk

A pregnant or nursing mother can influence the development and future health of her baby by the type of fats she eats. Breast milk can be enriched with excessive omega-6 fatty acids as a result of too much vegetable oil in the mother's diet. A British study showed that nursing mothers with the most linoleic acid (omega-6) in their milk were more likely to have children with allergies. They found no correlation with saturated and monounsaturated fats.[39]

It has been observed that babies who are given infant formula are more likely to develop allergies than those who are breast fed. Dry infant formula contains oxidized fatty acids. It's no wonder that those who are bottle-fed experience more health problems as they get older. Polyunsaturated fatty acids are incorporated in the nerve tissues and brain. Free-radical damaged or oxidized oils can affect mental ability, behavior, and visual function.[40]

A child's health can be directly affected by its mother's diet. Breast feeding is able to provide protection against the development of allergies.[41, 42] This is particularly true when

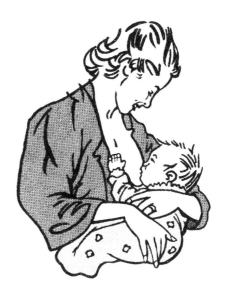

the mother eats a wholesome, balanced diet, low in polyunsaturated oils.

This doesn't mean all those people who were not breast fed or those breast fed by mothers who consumed lots of convenience foods (high in vegetable oil) are hopelessly doomed. Cells in the body are continually being replaced. What you ate while growing up and as you got older will have greater influence over your level of health now. A child born with allergies or an autoimmune disease of some type will continue to have problems the rest of his life if he continues to eat poor-quality foods. A person who changes his eating habits may overcome problems he inherited at birth. Likewise, a person who was healthy as a child may experience health problems later in life if the foods he eats don't supply the proper nutrients.

Chapter 7

THE CHOLESTEROL CONTROVERSY

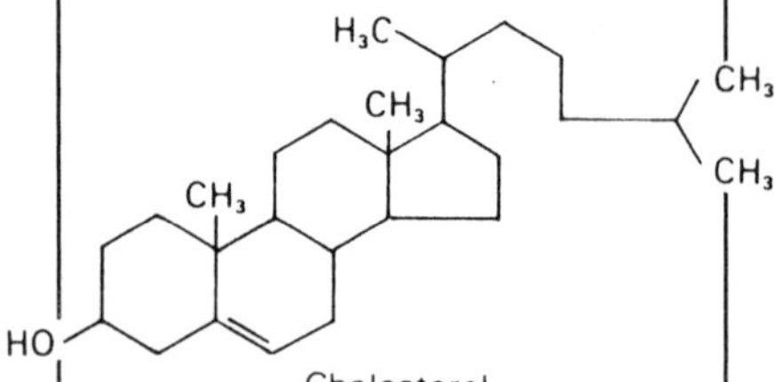

Cholesterol

"I think this low cholesterol business is pretty much nonsense."
—Linus Pauling, Ph.D., Two-Time Nobel Prize Winner

"The diet-heart hypotheses has been repeatedly shown to be wrong, and yet, for complicated reasons of pride, profit, and prejudice, the hypothesis continues to be exploited by scientists, fund-raising enterprises, food companies, and even governmental agencies. The public is being deceived by the greatest health scam of the century."
—Dr. George V. Mann, Vanderbilt University

THE CHOLESTEROL MYTH

When we hear the word "cholesterol," the first thought that comes to most people's minds is clogged arteries and heart disease. Cholesterol has almost become synonymous with heart disease. Everyone "knows" that cholesterol causes heart disease. You see it in the paper. You read about it in books. You hear it on television and the radio. They all loudly proclaim "High cholesterol causes heart disease." We hear it so much that it must be true. So many "experts" can't be wrong. Right?

We also know that saturated fat causes heart disease, don't we? That is what we read and that is what everyone says. Saturated fat has been labeled a villain because it can raise blood cholesterol levels too. And since saturated fat is much more abundant in our foods than cholesterol, it is considered by far the greater threat.

For years we have been told that cholesterol and saturated fat raise blood cholesterol and, therefore, cause cardiovascular disease. But actually, there never has been a study that demonstrated that high blood cholesterol *causes* heart disease. Not a single one! In fact, the opposite is true. There are numerous studies that demonstrate that blood cholesterol does not cause clogged arteries or heart disease. People die of heart disease without having high blood cholesterol. Others with high blood cholesterol show no signs of cardiovascular disease—no plaque in arteries, no abnormal clotting, and blood pressure within normal ranges. If high blood cholesterol causes cardiovascular disease, then it would *have to be present in all people who die from it*. But it's not. This fact is clearly recognized.

Most cholesterol researchers will admit that high blood cholesterol does not cause heart disease. The drug industry has had a lot to do with creating a false impression because they sell billions of dollars worth of cholesterol-lowering drugs. Their cry that high blood cholesterol leads to cardiovascular disease has been so loud and so popular we've been brainwashed into believing it. Throughout history, dubious political leaders have held to the philosophy that if you tell a lie often enough and loud enough, eventually everyone will accept it as truth, no matter how preposterous it may be. That is the situation we have with cholesterol.

"The cholesterol theory is not compatible with the history of coronary artery disease," says Charles T. McGee, M.D. in his book *Heart Frauds*. "Dietary consumption of fats and cholesterol does not effect blood levels of cholesterol significantly in the vast majority of people. Many people with high blood cholesterol never experience coronary artery disease. People with low blood cholesterol can and do develop coronary artery disease. About one-third of the people who have a heart

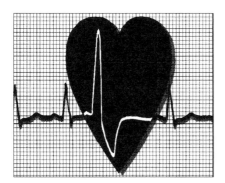

attack have a blood cholesterol level that is well within the range accepted as normal. Attempts to lower death rates from coronary artery disease with the American Heart Association diet have consistently failed. In addition, when drugs are given to try to lower blood cholesterol, overall death rates have gone *up*, not down, as anticipated."[1]

In an attempt to prove the cholesterol hypothesis, researchers have worked for over fifty years trying to demonstrate that cholesterol and saturated fat cause heart disease. No study has been able to do this. Science has not gotten any closer to a solution. The Framingham Heart Study which has monitored the health of some 5,000 people for several decades has shown that people who eat more saturated fat do not develop heart disease any more than anyone else.[2]

Michael DeBakey, a heart surgeon, performed a study using a large number of patients at Baylor University. He found that out of 1,700 patients who had atherosclerosis, which leads to heart disease, severe enough to require hospitalization, only 1 patient out of 5 had high blood cholesterol.[3] Dr. Harlan M. Krumholz reported in the *Journal of the American Medical Association* that people with higher cholesterol are not necessarily the most likely to have heart problems or die from heart disease. In a study, he monitored 997 people 65 years of age and older. Those with high cholesterol had about the same rates of heart attack and death as those with normal levels. You would expect that as we age, more cholesterol will build up in the arteries and thus increase the risk of heart disease. Indeed, risk of heart attack does increases with age. However, research doesn't show any correlation between age and cholesterol. For example, in one study of a mean age of 79, there was found "no evidence that an elevated level of cholesterol increased the risk of death or heart disease among this group."[4] Paul Addis and Gregory Warner, professors in the Department of Food Science and Nutrition at the University of Minnesota state: "The prevailing opinion, that atherosclerosis is simply an accumulation of cholesterol on arteries, has clearly shown to be erroneous. Therefore, the 'lipid hypothesis' has

become less well accepted by serious researchers and has been replaced by a competing hypothesis, i.e. 'response-to-injury hypothesis.'"[5] Because of the many inconsistencies with the cholesterol hypothesis, it has often been called the cholesterol myth.

In 1950, coronary artery disease became our leading cause of death, and it still is today. Avoidance of cholesterol and saturated fat, the availability of cholesterol-lowering drugs, and eating foods low in cholesterol and saturated fats have not stopped the heart-disease epidemic. It should be obvious that something else, that is generally overlooked, yet much more sinister than these two fats, is at the root of the problem.

CHOLESTEROL REGULATION

According to the cholesterol hypothesis, a diet high in cholesterol and saturated fat leads to high blood cholesterol. Saturated fat is included because it can be converted into cholesterol by the liver. The fat we eat, according to this theory, is directly responsible for the amount of cholesterol in our blood. The problem with this argument is that dietary consumption of fat has only a minor affect on cholesterol levels. Why? Because the vast majority of the cholesterol in our blood does not come from the diet, but comes from our liver. More than 80 percent of the cholesterol in our blood is manufactured in our own bodies.

To account for this fact, it is claimed, by those who believe in the cholesterol hypothesis, that the saturated fat in our diet is automatically converted into cholesterol and the more saturated fat we eat, the more cholesterol we have floating around in our bloodstream. The liver is depicted as a machine that blindly cranks out as much cholesterol as it possibly can. The more saturated fat we eat, the more cholesterol it cranks out.

Such a scenario is inconsistent with human physiology. The liver produces and carefully regulates a balance of hundreds of compounds essential for growth, digestion, and protection. Blood cholesterol is not an accident that is easily influenced by diet. The liver doesn't just crank out chemicals, like cholesterol, for the fun of it. It does it for a specific reason. And the amounts are carefully controlled and monitored so as to achieve and maintain homeostasis or chemical equilibrium. The liver carefully regulates the amount of cholesterol in our bodies, so it doesn't really matter how much saturated fat we eat, the liver will only manufacture the amount we need to maintain homeostasis. Everyone's bodies are different so everyone has a different level of cholesterol that the body is happy with. This level is consistent regardless of our diet and lifestyle within about 5 percent.

The liver doesn't need saturated fat to make cholesterol. It can make it from other fats and even from sugar or carbohydrates.[6] So, the claim that saturated fat raises blood cholesterol, while ignoring other fats and sugar, is illogical and inaccurate. If not enough cholesterol is eaten, the liver will make it from other dietary sources. This is why even drastic decreases in dietary cholesterol intake often produce only small drops in blood cholesterol levels.[7]

Kilmer S. McCully, M.D. is a pathologist and medical researcher who has investigated the connection between diet and heart disease and cancer for over 30 years. He states: "The amount of cholesterol that is formed in the liver is carefully controlled and adjusted according to the needs of the different organs of the body. If the amount of cholesterol is increased in the diet, a healthy, well-functioning liver makes less cholesterol for the needs of the body. If the amount of cholesterol in the diet is decreased, the liver makes more cholesterol. In this way the body regulates very precisely how much cholesterol is produced for its needs."[8]

Each day the body churns out approximately 1,000 mg of cholesterol; in comparison, an average American man's daily cholesterol intake is only 327 mg and a woman's is 221 mg. Of the cholesterol we eat, only about one-third is absorbed through the intestines; the rest is excreted.

Theoretically, the dietary cholesterol that is absorbed by the body in a day would raise a man's blood cholesterol by some 163 mg/dl. However, this doesn't happen. Here's why. Instead of responding in a set way to a high-fat meal, the body has several options: the intestine can absorb large or small amounts of cholesterol; the liver can turn down its own cholesterol production; and the liver can also convert

---

Cholesterol Content in Vegetable Oils

While it is generally believed that vegetable oils do not contain any cholesterol, they actually do contain very small amounts. The amount of cholesterol found in a few common oils are tabulated below. Measurements are in parts per million (ppm). As you can see by comparison, vegetable oils contain far less cholesterol than fats of animal origin.

Coconut oil: 0-14 ppm	Whole milk: 140 ppm
Palm oil: 16 ppm	Cheese: 1,100 ppm
Palm kernel oil: 17 ppm	Butter: 3,150 ppm
Sunflower oil: 17 ppm	Lard: 3,500 ppm
Corn oil: 50 ppm	Eggs: 5,000 ppm

Source: Thampan, P.K. 1994. *Facts and Fallacies About Coconut Oil*. Jakarta: Asian and Pacific Coconut Community.

---

some of this cholesterol into bile acids ready for excretion. The degree to which these responses occur depends both on the cholesterol content of the meal and the genetic makeup of the person. Some people absorb more than others, but some excrete more.[9]

For most people the blood cholesterol level is determined more by heredity than it is by diet. However, drastic diets, toxins, or drugs can upset normal cholesterol balance. Lowering cholesterol will have little, if any, effect on your overall health. Lowering it too much may even be detrimental.

HDL AND LDL

Blood cholesterol, the amount of cholesterol present in the bloodstream, is measured in terms of milligrams per deciliter of blood, expressed as mg/dl. In regards to health, serum cholesterol levels below 200 mg/dl are considered desirable. Levels between 200 and 239 mg/dl are borderline high. Above 240 mg/dl, risk of heart disease is said to be high. This scale has proven to be inadequate in determining risk of heart disease because *most* people who have heart attacks don't fit into the high-risk category. And as much as 40 percent of those people who do have heart attacks have cholesterol levels below 200 mg/dl.

In an attempt to reconcile the discrepancy between the heart disease rate and the cholesterol hypothesis, a new scheme was developed. Cholesterol was divided into subcatagories with some being classified as good (HDL cholesterol) and the others as bad (LDL cholesterol). Total cholesterol (both HDL and LDL) became less important and the ratio of the bad to good was viewed as what really determined risk. Under this new concept, a person can theoretically have a total cholesterol level above 240 mg/dl (high risk), yet be at low risk for heart disease; likewise, a person can have a total cholesterol level below 200 mg/dl and be at high risk. While this attempts to account for the observed discrepancies in cholesterol level, it doesn't adequately solve the problem. People who have high blood cholesterol usually have a high LDL to HDL ratio (also bad). And people who have low blood cholesterol often have a low LDL to HDL ratio (presumably good). So little has actually changed. Even high LDL (bad) cholesterol shows little correlation to the actual occurrence of heart disease, but it is often used as a standard to judge risk.

Since HDL (good) isn't considered a contributing factor in plaque formation, LDL is used as the major determinant in estimating risk. When people speak of high blood cholesterol, they are usually referring to LDL. The HDL level is really unimportant. Many people have speculated that HDL protects against coronary artery disease and the ratio of HDL to LDL would give a more accurate indication of risk. In recent studies, however, this has proven to be false. In one study, for example, published by *The American Journal of Cardiology* (Vol. 79, p. 705), HDL levels did not correlate with a healthy heart in an 82-year-old women. Despite elevated HDL and normal LDL cholesterol, the woman still had heart disease.[10] The conclusion is that even the ratio of HDL and LDL is no better of an indicator of heart disease risk than LDL alone.

We hear a lot nowadays about high-density lipoproteins or HDL (the good cholesterol) and low-density lipoproteins or LDL (the bad cholesterol). Both together constitute total cholesterol measured in our blood. The HDLs are considered good because they carry cholesterol from the tissues back to the liver, where it can be processed into other substances or removed from the body. LDL comes from the cholesterol we eat and from our liver. This cholesterol is packaged into compounds called lipoproteins along with saturated and polyunsaturated fatty acids and released into the bloodstream. As the lipoproteins circulate in the bloodstream, fat and cholesterol are extracted by tissues to be used as building blocks for new cells and to make hormones and other compounds. Fat is also pulled out of the lipoproteins and stored in adipose cells (the body's fat cells). This is how our body stores fat. When we need energy beyond what we get from the calories we eat, this fat is withdrawn from storage and used as fuel. HDLs are sent out by the liver to gather up fat from storage cells and bring it back to the liver to be converted into energy. HDL does *not* take fat out of the plaque in arteries. The cholesterol and fatty acids in HDL are taken from our fat cells. It does not reduce blood fat concentration because, again, it is taking fat from storage and not from the blood.

Because HDL (good) is removing fat from our bodies, it is considered a good thing. The advantage of HDL is that it reduces our body fat. When you go on a calorie-restricted diet, your HDL level increases because you are burning up more stored fat to compensate for the reduced calories you eat. The result is a reduction in fat and body weight. You can affect your HDL blood concentration by your diet and lifestyle. The fewer calories you eat and the more exercise you get, the higher your HDL level will be. The opposite is also true. The more calories you eat and the less exercise you get, the lower you HDL level. These two parameters are the only two that matter in regards to HDL levels. Eating a certain food like broccoli may raise HDL, but it does it because broccoli is a low-calorie food, so it reduces your calorie intake thus promoting HDL. Exercise may also raise HDL because it burns up calories.

WHERE DID WE GET HEART DISEASE?

Heart disease is an affliction of modern society. In primitive cultures, both ancient and modern, it is extremely rare. There were no recorded cases of this illness until the latter half of the 19th century. The first proven case of a patient suffering a heart attack was documented in Britain in 1878. Dr. Adam Hammer reported the unusual case of a patient that experienced crushing chest pain, then collapsed and died. An autopsy found that muscle tissue in the patient's heart had died resulting in heart failure and death. Nowadays, the signs of heart attack are well known and common. Thousands of people die every day. But a century ago it was almost unheard of.

The advancement of medicine took a giant leap forward during the 19th century. From 1830 to 1880 most of the diseases that plagued mankind at the time were identified and named. In Europe autopsies became routine. Tens of thousands of autopsies were performed during this time to accelerate the advance the science of medicine. Much of our current knowledge of anatomy, physiology, and pathology developed at this time. During this period, not a single case of heart disease was recorded until 1878. Nowadays, almost one out of every two deaths is heart related.

Some people might claim that heart disease wasn't recorded before that time because the doctors of that period didn't know what the disease looked like. In other words, the doctors were too ignorant to know what they were looking at. This argument isn't valid because these "old time" doctors were the ones who identified the signs of the disease that are used today. Also, there were many doctors who lived during the era of transition into modern medicine who saw first-hand the changes that occurred in the human body over time.

Dr. Paul Dudley White is known as the founder of cardiology—the study of the heart and its diseases. He graduated from medical school in 1910 and served as President Dwight D. Eisenhower's personal physician during his terms in office. As a young man, he wrote that he had an interest in a rare new disease that he had read about in the European medical literature. It was 1921, 11 years after he began his practice, when he saw his first heart attack patient. At that time, heart attacks were extremely rare.[11] Later in his career, and as the foremost authority in the world on cardiology and, consequently, heart disease, he was asked for his opinion about the cholesterol theory. He stated that he couldn't support the theory because he knew it didn't fit the history of the disease.

Europeans began to record heart attacks as a separate and distinct cause of death in 1930. Some localities in the United States began recording them as early as 1910, but

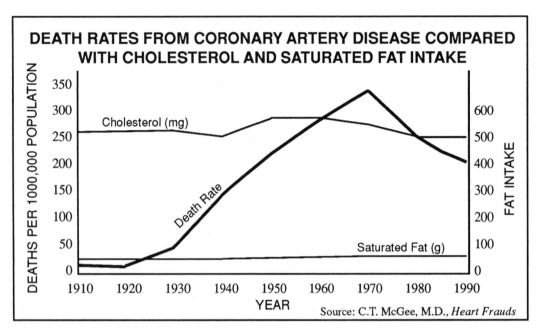

DEATH RATES FROM CORONARY ARTERY DISEASE COMPARED WITH CHOLESTEROL AND SATURATED FAT INTAKE

Source: C.T. McGee, M.D., *Heart Frauds*

Consumption of cholesterol and saturated fat have remained fairly constant since 1910. From 1910 to 1970 deaths form coronary artery disease increased an incredible 3,010 percent! By 1970 heart disease deaths began to decline but cholesterol and saturated fat intake remained the same. This clearly shows that there is little correlation between cholesterol or saturated fat with heart disease.

the country as a whole didn't record them separately until 1950. Although heart attacks could be clearly identified, they were usually lumped with deaths from other diseases. Before this time, heart attack deaths weren't recorded because they were uncommon.

The graph above shows the number of heart attack deaths per 100,000 people plotted over time in comparison to cholesterol intake. Note that cholesterol and saturated fat levels have remained essentially constant, but heart attack deaths have skyrocketed. There is clearly no correlation between heart disease and cholesterol/saturated fat consumption.[12]

From 1910 to 1920 heart disease deaths were fairly low, affecting only about 10 out of every 100,000 people per year. By 1930 the death rate jumped to 46 per 100,000 and by 1970 the rate reached 331 per 100,000. It is interesting to note that vegetable oil consumption started to become more common at the begining of the century and has steadily increased, almost mimicking the rise in heart-disease rate. There is a correlation between vegetable oil consumption and heart disease, but no correlation with cholesterol or saturated fat.

This information may surprise you, but it's not hidden or secret. The facts are here. You probably haven't heard them because there is no industry that can profit by spending advertising dollars publicizing this information. Even the meat industry which you might think would love to show that fat in their products as not so bad after all, doesn't want this information to be known. Why? Because meat, not fat, is a bigger factor in the development of heart disease and

many other diseases of modern society. If the meat industry can point an accusing finger at fat, it directs the focus away from them. After all, we can always buy leaner (more expensive) cuts of meat or cut the "horrible, disease-causing" fat off the "healthy, protein-packed" meat, right?

In 1968 the death rate from heart attacks fell for the first time in over 40 years and has continued to slowly decline ever since. By 1990 the death rate had fallen to 194 per 100,000 people. Those who support the cholesterol hypothesis have not attempted to take credit for this decline because fat consumption has remained relatively constant the entire time. The reason why the death rate has fallen since the 1970s and why meat may be worst for you than either cholesterol or saturated fat, is explained in Chapter 12 and 13.

WHAT DOES THE RESEARCH SAY?

We are led to believe the theory that animal fat consumption causes coronary heart disease is backed by abundant evidence. Most people would be surprised to learn that there is, in fact, very little evidence to support the belief that a diet low in cholesterol and saturated fat actually reduces death from heart disease or in any way increases one's life span.

The cholesterol hypothesis implies that animal fat consumption must have increased significantly since 1920 to correlate with the rise in heart disease, but in fact the consumption of saturated animal fats in America declined steadily during that period, while use of vegetable fats increased dramatically. During the 60-year period form 1910 to 1970, the proportion of traditional animal fat in the American diet declined from 83 percent to 62 percent, and butter consumption plummeted from 17 pounds per person per year to about four pounds. During the past 80 years, dietary cholesterol intake has increased only one percent. During the same period the percentage of dietary vegetable fat in the form of margarine, shortening, and processed oils increased about 400 percent, and the consumption of sugar and processed foods increased about 60 percent. When you look objectively at all the facts, the lipid or cholesterol hypothesis doesn't hold up.

A look at the development of the cholesterol hypothesis starting from the first studies that supported it nearly a century ago until the present provides a perspective as to its prevalence today. Professors Addis and Warner have stated in this regard: "A historical view of the cholesterol-atherosclerosis connection provides a fascinating account of how a single flawed experiment and equally flawed sequels can mislead medical science and the public. The relationship of these events to the popularity of the lipid hypothesis of atherosclerosis over the past 50 years is also interesting."[13] The development of science, like most everything else, is strongly influence by profit. Facts and theories that can be used for financial gain receive much more emphasis and funding than those that show little potential for profit. The cholesterol hypothesis is a classic example.

Before the beginning of the 20th century, heart disease and atherosclerosis were extremely rare. At that time, only the wealthy seemed afflicted by it. In the late 1800s and early 1900s nutrition was becoming recognized as an important factor in health and the first vitamins were identified. Because atherosclerosis appeared to be a disease of affluence, physicians suspected a dietary cause. The wealthy class consumed much more meat, milk, and eggs than poorer classes. Could meat or protein be the culprit, they wondered? Researchers began investigating this possibility.

The first connection between cardiovascular disease and diet came from studies performed by M.A. Ignatovsky, a young teacher in a military medical school in St. Petersburg, Russia in 1908 and 1909.[14, 15] Ignatovsky fed a high animal-protein diet to rabbits and observed the changes in the arteries. He purposely chose rabbits because they are strictly vegetarian, obtaining all the protein they need entirely from plants. If animal protein were a factor in the development of atherosclerosis and cardiovascular disease, then it should be quickly evident in the rabbits.

After feeding a protein-based diet to rabbits for several months, Ignatovsky found that the animals had developed hardened arteries and plaque similar to those found in humans. He suggested that it was the high *protein* diet that

was responsible for the hardening of the rabbits' arteries.

At another medical school in St. Petersburg, Nikolai Anitschkov became interested in Ignatovsky's findings. Anitschkov, however, believed that the cholesterol in the meat and dairy products Ignatovsky fed his rabbits might have produced the atherosclerotic plaques rather than the protein.

Anitschkov, repeated Ignatovsky's experiments using cholesterol rather than animal protein. Anitschkov fed cholesterol to rabbits either mixed *dry* with rabbit chow or dissolved in *vegetable oil*.* After several months, Anitschkov and fellow researcher, S. Chalatow, found that the arteries of the animals developed plaque-like deposits. This plaque contained a great deal of fat (triglycerides) and cholesterol. They proposed that atherosclerotic plaque is produced by cholesterol in meat and eggs and that cholesterol is what caused the plaque in Ignatovsky's experiments rather than protein.[16] This study was published in a German medical journal in 1913. From this beginning the cholesterol hypothesis was born.

Since cholesterol was the primary fat identified in human arterial plaque, it was assumed that cholesterol was the villain. Scientists, although they did not understand how, theorized that cholesterol, accumulated in the arterial walls, gives rise to the plaque deposits characteristic of atherosclerosis and, consequently, leads to heart disease. It was reasoned, the more cholesterol there is in the blood, the more that will be deposited in the arteries. This led to the assumption that a diet high in cholesterol and saturated fat (which the body can convert into cholesterol) *caused* cardiovascular disease. This process has been labeled the lipid or cholesterol hypothesis. This theory provided a simple answer to a perplexing problem.

Over the next several decades researchers performed study after study to prove this theory, but none of them seemed to turn out as well as the researchers had anticipated. The proof they had hoped to uncover, demonstrating the cause and effect relationship between cholesterol and heart disease, couldn't be found. Maybe the population sample used in the past wasn't big enough some reasoned. Bigger studies involving more than one country were conducted to find the missing proof.

A major international study conducted in the early sixties called the International Atherosclerotic Project put the theory to the most extensive test up to that time. This study involved examining arteries of over 20,000 autopsied bodies from the United States, Finland, Greece, Italy, Japan, the

---

*The fact that Anitschkov used dried cholesterol as well as vegetable oil in his experiments completely invalidated his findings. This is discussed in more detail later in this chapter.

Netherlands, and Yugoslavia. The results of this study revealed a high incidence of atherosclerosis, coronary heart disease, and stroke in those countries where the people ate large quantities of meat and animal fat. The United States and Finland, both of which consume a lot of meat, had the highest incidence. Japan, where relatively little meat or animal fat is eaten, the rate was the lowest. The correlation seemed unmistakable. The conclusion many drew from this is that high-fat diets are accompanied by a high rate of cardiovascular disease.[17] This was all the proof many needed to declare that cholesterol and saturated fat leads to heart disease. But it still didn't prove that cholesterol caused heart disease. The study results implicated meat as much as fat, but researchers in their zeal to prove the cholesterol theory somehow ignored this fact. Meat was considered simply the medium through which most saturated fat and cholesterol is eaten, but meat itself was overlooked as a cause.

More evidence came from a landmark study which was begun in 1948 called the Framingham Heart Study. This study was set up to continue throughout the lifetime of the volunteers, monitoring all parameters believed to be associated with the risk of coronary artery disease at the time. The study included a large portion of the population of Framingham, Massachusetts (population 5,127). Subjects were monitored every two years. After several decades, this study still could not provide proof for the cholesterol theory, and the real cause of coronary artery disease remained unknown. The researchers, however, were able to identify a few things that occurred more often with those that died of heart attacks from those that didn't. These were called risk factors, and the more of these a person had, the higher his or her risk of getting coronary artery disease. High blood cholesterol was one of these factors, but it was one of the weakest, being barely measurable. The researchers had to be greatly disappointed.

The investigators, perhaps unwittingly, ignored data that went contrary to the cholesterol theory. Information they didn't publicize was the fact that dietary intake of cholesterol and fats did *not* influence blood cholesterol levels to any significant degree. Although blood fat levels increase slightly immediately after eating, the body maintains a fairly constant blood fat level which changes only slightly regardless of the diet.[18] The Framingham study showed that some people who ate a lot of saturated fat and cholesterol had low blood cholesterol levels. Some people who ate only a little saturated fat and cholesterol had high blood cholesterol levels. These findings seemed to support the idea that normal cholesterol level is determined more by genetics than by diet.[19]

After 40 years of research, the director of the Framingham study, Dr. William Castelli, admitted: "In Framingham, Mass., the more saturated fat one ate, the more cholesterol one ate, the more calories one ate, the lower the person's serum cholesterol...we found that the people who ate the most cholesterol, ate the most saturated fat, ate the most calories, weighed the least, and were the most physically active."[20]

We now know that about 80 percent of cholesterol in our blood does *not* come directly from our food but is manufactured by our liver. Dietary fat intake has little effect on blood cholesterol levels in most people because of an internal feedback mechanism. The body, for whatever reason, sets a blood cholesterol level it likes, then tries to keep it constant. If you eat more cholesterol, the body makes less. If you eat less, the body makes more. Diet can affect blood cholesterol levels, but not nearly as much as we are led to believe. Reducing fat intake from a typical 40 percent of daily calories to the American Heart Association's recommendation of 30 percent may drop cholesterol level by a mere five percent, if at all. Hardly enough to make much of a difference according to the cholesterol hypothesis.

A study similar to the Framingham Heart Study was published in 1976 that involved 4,057 volunteers from Tecumseh, Michigan. The findings were the same. Blood cholesterol had a very weak association with heart attacks. And, like with the Framingham group, dietary intake of cholesterol was not related to blood cholesterol levels the way researchers hoped.[21]

The cholesterol theory provided a logical connection between dietary fat and cardiovascular disease. It is the story often told by countless newspaper articles and diet books. Today everyone "knows" that saturated fat and cholesterol *cause* heart disease. The connection between high blood cholesterol and fatty plaque deposits in the arteries seem obvious. There is only one problem. It isn't true. If fat slowly builds up in the arteries, why doesn't everyone develop atherosclerosis? Older people should have many years of accumulation if this theory were true, but people as old 100 have been found to be completely free from the disease.[22]

Most scientists agree that high blood cholesterol does not *cause* atherosclerosis. If it did, *all* people who died of cardiovascular disease would have high blood cholesterol. Likewise, *all* people who have high blood cholesterol should have cardiovascular disease. But they don't. All people who eat a high-cholesterol and high-saturated-fat diet should be expected to get cardiovascular disease. But they don't.

If cholesterol and saturated fat caused heart disease, numerous peoples around the world who live on high-fat diets would all be dropping dead from heart failure. But they don't. The traditional Eskimo diet is one of the highest in meat and saturated fat in the world, yet heart disease has been rare—until they began eating the same types of food we do. The same is true with other cultures that have high-saturated-fat diets like certain Pacific Islanders, Filipinos, and others in Southeast Asia. Many of the American Indian cultures survived for hundreds of years on a diet consisting almost entirely of the buffalo and other game that roamed the great plains.[23]

Some of these people even today consume diets with 60 percent of their total calories coming primarily from fat, and have cholesterol readings as high as 245 mg/dl (the high-risk range), yet have absolutely no arterial plaquing and show no signs of cardiovascular disease, even in old age.[24]

One argument for the reason that Eskimos have had such a low heart disease rate is because their diet includes lots of fish, which is high in omega-3 fatty acids. These fish oils are believed to offset some of the effects of cholesterol and saturated fat. That may have some bearing with the Eskimos, but it doesn't figure in with many of the other populations in the world that have a high-fat diet but low heart disease rate. Two notable examples are the Pukapukans and Tokelauans, both Pacific Island peoples who eat relatively little fish but consume huge quantities of saturated fat, primarily from coconuts. Some of them have moderately high blood cholesterol levels but suffer no cardiovascular disease. The cholesterol theory doesn't hold up.

Yet people in America, Western Europe, and other industrialized countries who eat far less saturated fat and cholesterol are dying in mass numbers from heart disease and other related cardiovascular conditions.

Dr. Alfred E. Harper, professor of biochemistry and nutritional sciences at the University of Wisconsin, and past president of the Food and Nutrition Board, pointed out exceptions to the theory in several countries. In Israel, Chile and a few other low-cholesterol-consumption countries, the incidence of coronary artery disease was high. In Scandinavian countries, fat consumption dropped while the incidence of the disease went up. As the consumption of animal fat in Switzerland *increased*, its rate of coronary artery disease went *down*.[25]

More studies, with more test subjects over longer periods of time were conducted. In 1982 the results from the MRFIT (Multiple Risk Factor Intervention Trial) study were released. This study recruited 12,866 high-risk men between the ages of 35 and 57. The volunteers were randomly divided into two groups. One group started a program involving the reduction of the commonly accepted risk factors. This included eliminating smoking, reducing fat consumption, and treating high blood pressure with drugs. The other group made no dietary changes and received routine medical care. Those who smoked in this second group continued to do so. The study ran for seven years.

When the investigation was completed, the results were not as anticipated. The researchers had expected to find a

significant improvement in the cardiovascular health of the treatment group as compared to the control group. The heart attack death rate was only *slightly* lower (less than .1%) in the treatment group. The big shocker discovered by the researchers was that the treatment group had a *higher* overall death rate because of an increase in cancer deaths. *The control group continued to smoke and eat all the saturated fat they wanted, yet had fewer deaths.*[26] It is of interest to note that the researchers only publicized the favorable results and ignored the increased death rate. Reporting studies in an honest manner has become a growing problem. It's a known fact of life, with few exceptions, that researchers report only the results that support their preconceived beliefs or the views of the organization funding their studies. If this is the case, we need to be careful about accepting too quickly the results of any study.

One of the most glaring shortcomings of the cholesterol hypothesis is its failure to demonstrate a correlation between the cholesterol and fat composition of the diet and the level of LDL (bad cholesterol) in susceptible populations as demonstrated by the 50-year-old Framingham Heart Study. Experiments with animals all fail to demonstrate a correlation between dietary cholesterol and the level of cholesterol in the LDL in the blood.[27]

Every doctor sees patients who have highly elevated cholesterol yet are not troubled with any form of cardiovascular disease, and others who have low cholesterol and are considered at low risk, yet still suffer heart attacks. Charles T. McGee, M.D. reports in his book, *Heart Frauds,* that he has seen patients with blood cholesterol over 400 mg/dl and family members with levels up to 600 mg/dl that have no cardiovascular problems and lived to ripe old ages. Keep in mind that cholesterol readings above 240 mg/dl are classified as high risk. So 400 mg/dl is extremely high and, therefore, should be at extremely high risk. Levels below 200 mg/dl are considered normal. He has also treated patients with cholesterol levels as low as 115 mg/dl which were considered to be at very low risk, yet still suffered from heart disease.[28] If cholesterol were the villain it was supposed to be, this type of thing just shouldn't happen, but does happen. And it happens all the time.

Physicians know that the majority of their patients with coronary heart disease, stroke, and other forms of atherosclerotic disease have no evidence of elevated cholesterol or LDL levels. In a study of 194 consecutive autopsies of mostly male veterans, for example, Dr. Kilmer McCully found that only 8 percent of cases with severe atherosclerosis had total cholesterol levels greater than 250 mg/dl, and the mean blood cholesterol level in the group with the severest disease was only 186.7 mg/dl, well within the normal or safe range.[29] The large majority—two-thirds of the patients with severe atherosclerosis—had no evidence of elevated blood cholesterol or hypertension (high blood pressure).

Herbert Naito, Ph.D. and Henry Hoff, Ph.D. agree with Dr. McCully. They report in *Medical Applications of Clinical Nutrition* that the mean blood cholesterol level in coronary heart disease patients is only 190 mg/dl. This is below the optimal level of 200.[30]

The International Atherosclerosis Project, which analyzed 31,000 autopsies from 15 countries, found no correlation between animal fat intake and degree of atherosclerosis of blood cholesterol. Michael DeBakey, the famous heart surgeon, surveyed 1,700 patients with atherosclerosis and found no relation between levels of blood cholesterol and degree of hardening of the arteries. Other studies like the Veterans Clinical Trial, the Minnesota State Hospital Trial, the Honolulu Heart Program, and the Puerto Rico Heart Health Study, found no significant relation between a diet high in cholesterol and saturated fats with coronary heart disease.[31]

Blood cholesterol is not affected much by the type of fat in the diet. Because the body can make cholesterol, for most people with normal blood cholesterol levels, restriction of dietary cholesterol and saturated fat has only small effects on the blood level. In patients with elevated blood cholesterol, drugs are usually recommended to decrease it. Clinical trials have shown some effects of such drugs in decreasing mortality from heart disease, but the results are not very striking and may actually cause more serious problems. Hence, many experts are now skeptical about whether changes in diet or the taking of drugs to decrease cholesterol levels are really justified.[32]

Faced with these facts, some experts have spoken up against the cholesterol hypothesis. Dr. H. Kaunitz of Columbia University has pointed out that autopsies show that some of the most severely diseased arteries are found in people who have low blood levels of cholesterol.

Eminent researcher, Dr. George V. Mann, a nutritional biochemist and physician long associated with Vanderbilt University, tried to lay the cholesterol theory to rest as far back as 1977. Mann wrote an article in the *New England Journal of Medicine*. He pointed out that the Framingham and Tecumseh studies did not show a cause-effect relationship between cholesterol intake, blood cholesterol levels, and coronary artery disease. He was one of the first to publicize the finding that "risk factors for coronary artery disease don't count after the age of 55." He also warned about the dangers from abnormal trans fatty acids produced in the processing of hydrogenated vegetable oils.[33]

In a later article Mann referred to supporters of the cholesterol dogma as the "Heart Mafia" because they received all available research funds aimed at coronary artery disease.

The funding comes from pharmaceutical companies who have a heavy financial interest in the cholesterol hypothesis. Dr. Mann stated that the cholesterol hypothesis was valid when it was first proposed, but after thorough testing was found to be false. Rather than abandon the theory, researchers were encouraged by financial backers to continue their studies. In an effort to prove the theory, researchers unwittingly manipulate the facts to make them fit their beliefs and to satisfy their financial backers—the pharmaceutical industry.[34]

Dr. Mann has stated: "The diet-heart hypothesis has been repeatedly shown to be wrong, and yet, for complicated reasons of pride, profit, and prejudice, the hypothesis continues to be exploited by scientists, fund-raising enterprises, food companies, and even governmental agencies. The public is being deceived by the greatest health scam of the century."[35]

Criticism by Dr. Mann and others motivated the pharmaceutical industry to take more aggressive measures to promote their products. Convincing government agencies to support their cause, they hoped this would overpower much of the opposition. Under the prodding of the drug and medical industries, in 1987 the U.S. government launched the National Cholesterol Education Program, an aggressive campaign to convince people and physicians about the dangers of high blood cholesterol. Those with cholesterol levels between 200 to 240 mg/dl were advised to get medical counseling. For those who had levels above this, the recommendation was to get immediate treatment with cholesterol-lowering drugs. This sudden push to fight cholesterol was obviously an industry-sponsored campaign motivated purely by profit. Many physicians, knowing cholesterol was not the cause of heart disease, opposed this national campaign and in 1989 it erupted into a national debate. This was precipitated by an article published in the September issue of *Atlantic Monthly* written by Thomas J. Moore titled *The Cholesterol Myth*. Moore reviewed all of the scientific data concerning cholesterol up to that time and concluded, "It is irresponsible to force the public into a costly cholesterol-reducing program without firm scientific evidence of the effectiveness of the intervention."[36]

Michael Gurr, Ph.D., renowned expert on lipids and author of an authoritative textbook on lipid biochemistry, recently stated that, "whatever causes coronary heart disease, it is not primarily a high intake of saturated fat." He criticized "...the degree of self-delusion in research workers wedded to a particular hypothesis despite the contrary evidence!"[37]

Authorities from around the world spoke up on the issue. Peter Skrabanek, Professor of Community Health at Trinity College, Dublin, told a conference, "Lowering blood cholesterol does not lower overall mortality. None of these studies have shown people live any longer. It is a fascinating sociological phenomenon that some experts, in the face of massive evidence to the contrary, have come up with recommendations based on wishful thinking and dogmatic beliefs. They are guilty of unethical behavior."

William E. Stehbens, professor of pathology at New Zealand's Wellington School of Medicine, claims, "There is no scientific evidence that dietary fat and cholesterol, or even elevated blood cholesterol, causes atherosclerosis. Researchers who fed rats increased amounts of cholesterol did cause fat to accumulate on the walls of their arteries, but these pathological changes are not true atherosclerosis."

Germain J. Brisson, professor of nutrition at Universite Laval, Quebec, Canada, was equally blunt in his 1982 book, *Lipids in Human Nutrition*. Brisson stated, "Those who take action and make recommendations as if the lipid hypothesis has been verified are in danger of making a serious mistake. Increasing the consumption of fats rich in polyunsaturated fatty acids and decreasing the intake of cholesterol and fats of animal origin is ineffective in prevention programs designed to reduce the incidence of coronary heart disease."[38]

Dr. U. Ravaskov evaluated 22 studies in which lower blood cholesterol levels were studied to see if heart attack death rates would fall. In about half of the studies the death rates fell, in the other half the death rates increased. Dr. Ravaskov found statistical errors in most of the articles that were supportive of the cholesterol theory. His article points out that there is so much bias on this subject that since 1970 only articles supportive of the cholesterol theory are cited as references in other medical articles. Studies that provide evidence contrary to the cholesterol theory are ignored.

The author concluded that, "Lowering serum (blood) cholesterol concentrations does not reduce mortality and is unlikely to prevent coronary heart disease. Claims of the opposite are based on preferential citation of supportive trials."[39]

Despite 50 years of research, the theory has not been proven and, in fact, cholesterol appears to have little effect on heart disease. While most researchers acknowledge that cholesterol does not have as strong an effect as once believed, most of them agree that high blood cholesterol can at least *slightly* increase a person's chances of developing heart disease. High blood cholesterol is, therefore, considered a *risk factor* for heart disease, but not the cause. This is a far different cry from their position a few decades ago.

High blood cholesterol is just one of several risk factors. The more risk factors a person has, the greater his chance of dying from a heart attack. Other risk factors include glucose intolerance (diabetes), hypertension (high blood pressure), lack of exercise, being overweight, smoking, stress, and being male. Being a male is a risk factor, just as high blood cholesterol is, but because someone is a male doesn't mean he will develop heart disease or that being a male causes the disease. None of these risk factors cause heart disease. In fact, about 50 percent of those who die of heart disease don't have any of the standard risk fac-

Cholesterol A Risk Factor?

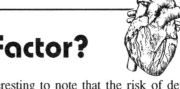

Statistically, a very *small* correlation exists between some groups of people who have high blood cholesterol and those with cardiovascular disease. That is to say, people who have cardiovascular disease sometimes also have high blood cholesterol levels. This correlation is only found with middle-aged men—those between tha ages of about 35 and 57. The correlation of high blood cholesterol with the younger and older men and women of all ages is essentially nonexistent. Not everyone who has cardiovascular disease has high cholesterol levels, nor does everyone with high cholesterol have cardiovascular problems. For this reason, we know that high blood cholesterol does not *cause* cardiovascular disease. High blood cholesterol has been used as a sign that a problem may exist and, therefore, is considered a *risk factor*. It is, however, only a risk factor for middle-aged men.

It's interesting to note that the risk of developing heart disease increases with age (age is also a risk factor and a much stronger one than blood cholesterol), yet the correlation between cholesterol and heart disease *diminishes* with age.

A woman or elderly man with high blood cholesterol is at no greater risk of heart disease than someone with optimal blood cholesterol levels. Unfortunately, such people are often put on cholesterol-lowering drugs which will do nothing to prevent them from developing heart disease but will subject them to serious side effects such as liver failure and cancer.

The real risk associated with high blood cholesterol is not from heart disease but from cholesterol-lowering drugs. These drugs can pose a far greater risk to your health than high blood cholesterol.

tors. It is apparent there are other, more important, yet un-discovered, factors involved.

Professors Paul Addis and Gregory Warner of the University of Minnesota state: "Most major blood epidemiological studies reveal an *extremely weak* relationship between blood cholesterol and coronary heart disease (CHD), often showing an increase in annual CHD rate of *less than 1% across most, or all, of the blood cholesterol range*."[40] This is saying that there is less than 1% difference in CHD from the lowest blood cholesterol levels to the highest. From this very tiny and insignificant correlation rests the whole basis of the cholesterol-heart disease connection. The correlation with most all other risk factors show a much stronger correlation than blood cholesterol. If it weren't for certain groups with financial interests at stake, who are actively campaigning for the cholesterol hypothesis, it would have died long ago.

You are at greater risk of getting heart disease by being a male than you do by having high cholesterol. Being a male is a much higher risk factor than high cholesterol, so is smoking and high blood pressure. Cholesterol is a very minor risk factor, yet it is the one we always hear about. Why? Mostly because of money. Cholesterol-lowering drugs outsell all other prescription drugs. They are the financial backbone for many drug companies. Obviously, these companies will promote them aggressively. This is the main reason why the cholesterol hypothesis continues to be broadcast loudly and frequently even when most all the evidence is against it.

FOOD AND DRUG COMPANIES

As the cholesterol hypothesis gained acceptance, pharmaceutical companies quickly jumped on the bandwagon and began searching for new drugs that could lower cholesterol. The concept was fairly simple. Since 80 percent of the cholesterol in our blood is manufactured by the liver, the easiest solution would be to develop a drug that could block the liver's ability to produce cholesterol.

MER-29, the first cholesterol lowering drug to come on the market, made its appearance in the early 1960s. MER-29, however, didn't stay around long. The drug caused cataract and was withdrawn from the market after a couple of years. Other cholesterol-lowering drugs soon followed. Today, there are several available from different companies. All of them have side effects, both known and unknown. Most of them work by interfering with normal liver function.

Drug companies aggressively advertised their new products along with their research demonstrating that the drugs can lower cholesterol and, therefore, must also reduce the risk of heart attack. Advertising literature sent to doctors and the media were so bold that the statements conveyed the idea that by taking these drugs lives would be saved. The cholesterol hypothesis found a powerful ally to fight for its cause.

Cholesterol-lowering drugs are the most profitable drugs on the market today, costing as much as $2,000 to $3,000 per person per year. And these drugs must be taken for life in order to keep blood cholesterol down. It is estimated that some 100 million Americans have elevated blood cholesterol and, therefore, are candidates for these medications. If 100 million people, in the United States alone spent a couple thousand dollars a year, you can easily see the enormous profit potential for drug companies. Cholesterol-screening tests and cholesterol-lowering drugs already constitute a 20 billion (that's *billion* with a "B") dollar a year industry. The word billion is used with such frequency today that it tends to lose its meaning. A billion is one thousand million! We are taking about 20 billion every year—now that's BIG business. With this kind of money at stake, the pharmaceutical companies have been aggressively marketing and educating the medical profession and the general public. Is it any wonder why cholesterol's role in health is so misunderstood?

The power and influence that drug companies have over our lives is incredible. They finance the majority of the research done in the medical field. If a researcher publishes results of a study that is unfavorable to a drug company's interests, these companies can literally destroy the researcher's career. Since they are the ones who give the grants to universities and research institutions to fund the studies, they can refuse to fund research for any particular researcher who will not report findings favorable to the industry. That person cannot do research if funds are not available. The "publish or perish" philosophy reigns in the academic and research world. If you can't get funds to do research, you can't publish, and if you can't publish, you can't make a living as a researcher. It's that simple.

The food industry wields a power similar to that of the drug industry. Jane Heimlich described in her book, *What Your Doctor Won't Tell You*, what happened to one researcher who was working on vegetable oils and the harm they can do. After publishing results which were detrimental to the vegetable oil industry, the researcher found she could no longer get funding to continue her work.[41]

Even if a researcher did get the funds for a study that may be contradictory to the food or drug industry's interests, it would be very difficult to get it published. None of the leading medical publications would dare publish it. Why? Because all of their revenue comes from the drug companies in the form of advertisements. When articles that were even slightly negative to a drug product have been published, the drug companies have threatened to pull all advertising. This is enough of a threat for editors to carefully screen all potential articles so nothing that is obviously detrimental to any drug company's interests gets into print.

Some years ago a medical journal published a study demonstrating the beneficial effects of a particular herb. One drug company that viewed this herb as competition for its own products contacted the editors and threatened to never advertise in the journal again if they ever published a similar article. Since advertising is the life blood of these publications, the editors complied. We don't hear about this type of thing often. As you might expect, such occurrences are keep under wraps. In this case, however, the story leaked out and became public.[42]

Most medical journals nowadays devote about a third of their space to advertisements for drugs. According to *The Wall Street Journal*, drug companies spend over $330,000,000 on advertising directed toward doctors. Medical journals quite literally rely on drug money for their survival.

There are about 3,000 different medical journals that are published. Out of this number, only about 10 percent are included in the medical indexes, such as Medline. Articles on controversial topics must be published in relatively obscure journals that are not cross-indexed in computer databanks. Most people, including physicians, don't even know these other publications exist. So studies that are not funded by food and drug companies, or conform to popular opinion, are extremely difficult to find.

Because of the power wielded by food and drug companies, researchers pick parameters in their research in such a way as to make results favorable to their sponsors. If the results aren't in agreement with the sponsor's interests, the study is left unpublished or manipulated to give positive results. For example, studies have been ignored that showed when animals ate less saturated fats and more polyunsaturated oils cancer rates went up. Also ignored are human studies that showed that as consumption of vegetable oil increased, blood cholesterol levels fell, but the heart attack death rate *increased*.[43] In some cases, the researchers may even proclaim that because cholesterol was lowered, *risk* of heart disease was reduced—even though cancer and heart attack deaths actually increased.

You can't trust the result of any single study because of author prejudice or errors that may affect the results. The World Health Organization (WHO) conducted a multi-country survey spanning 10 years. The survey focused on diet and fat consumption with the assumption being that it is primarily the saturated fat in our diet that leads to heart and other diseases. Their conclusion was that there is a "prob-

able" relationship between a high saturated fat intake and a high incidence of coronary atherosclerosis. The results of this study were widely accepted as "proof" between the relationship between saturated fat and heart disease. In the researchers zeal to find proof of the lipid hypothesis, data was preferentially selected to give the results desired and calculations skewed.

A couple of years after publication, statisticians from the Rockefeller Research Institute discovered errors in the data and reanalyzed the entire study. The results of the re-evaluation were published in the *New York State Medical Journal*.[44] While WHO researchers studied 27 countries, they included only six in their final analysis. Why choose only six? Perhaps they were the only ones that would provide data that was in agreement with the researchers' preconceived viewpoint. Furthermore, they utilized figures for

❓ QUESTIONABLE RESEARCH

Manipulating data to arrive at conclusions supporting the researcher's or sponsor's beliefs is common. Some researchers take too much liberty in their handling of the data and their research is openly questioned. A recent example that drew some notoriety was a 1992 study linking high-voltage power lines to cancer. Dr. R. Liburdy, a cellular biologist, claimed to have found a link between the electromagnetic fields around power lines and certain cellular changes in the body.

The possibility that electromagnetic fields can cause childhood leukemia and other illnesses has raised fears among people living near high-tension power lines. The theory had been raised before Liburdy's study, but he found what was thought to be the first plausible biological explanation for such a connection.

Seven years after the study was published independent investigators concluded that Liburdy deleted data that did not support his conclusions producing inaccurate and misleading results. "The evidence demonstrates Liburdy knew his data manipulations were significant to the conclusions of the paper," they reported.

When confronted, Liburdy didn't argue about the fact that he deleted important information, yet he denied doing anything wrong other than failing to explain his graphing procedures. It appears that he felt justified in what he did because data manipulation is a common practice.

This is also why no single study can be taken as absolute proof of any theory and why several studies by different researchers are necessary before new ideas are accepted.

saturated fat "available" rather than estimating the actual amount ingested. Correction for these two factors showed that death rates from coronary heart disease were more closely related to increased intake of *animal protein* in the diet than to saturated fat content.

Manipulating data to achieve results that correspond to researchers' preconceived ideas or that support the sponsor's viewpoint isn't anything new, it's been going on for years. Every researcher is aware of it. A few who have tried to publish what they considered to be the truth which went contrary to drug company propaganda, have found themselves blackballed by the ones who control research funding. Without funds, they cannot do any further research. It's a very strong incentive to conform to industry's pressure.

The scientific community has been harsh on anyone who would dare rock the foundations of the cholesterol hypothesis. Those who have questioned this theory and backed it up with hard scientific evidence have been ostracized and even persecuted.

John Yudkin, a professor of nutrition at the University of London, studied the relationship between refined sugar consumption and coronary artery disease for many years. He found the association with sugar was stronger than between cholesterol and fats and coronary artery disease.[45]

No one in the medical community would listen to him even though he had hard scientific evidence. Yudkin's findings created friction with both the pharmaceutical companies and the food industry. Sugar production and use is a major element within the food industry. These companies provide the financial support for nutritional education and research. Yudkin was singled out as a risk to their financial interests and every effort was exerted to keep him quiet. Yudkin became frustrated in his attempts to inform colleagues and the public of his findings. He wrote that it became common for the food industry to arrange to have entire conferences canceled when his name was listed as a speaker. As a consequence, few people know that overconsumption of refined sugar is a greater risk factor in the development of atherosclerosis than saturated fat.

In the late 1960s and early 1970s, Kilmer McCully, a professor at Harvard Medical School, proposed the idea that amino acids from protein, rather than fat or cholesterol, were the real cause of atherosclerotic diseases. His ideas were completely contrary to the cholesterol dogma. Consequently, his research was viciously criticized and completely ignored. He was persistent in his belief that cholesterol was not the cause of heart disease and eventually was dismissed by Harvard. Because of his unorthodox beliefs, no university or research institution was willing to hire him. It took him two years before he found a job at a veterans hospital and there, under less than ideal conditions, he was able to continue his research. McCully's story is described in more detail in Chapter 12.

Because contrary views are ignored by the food and drug industries, the information readily available to the media and the public, as well as the information doctors receive, is highly biased. Doctors depend on research and drug company educational materials and seminars to keep them abreast of what is happening in the medical field.

Dean Ornish, M.D., the author of *Dr. Dean Ornish's Program for Reversing Heart Disease* and other books states: "The influence of drug companies is so pervasive that, from the first day of medical school, it affects and in many ways determines how medicine is practiced and how disease is viewed.

"Drug companies spend millions of dollars educating physicians. Drug companies are the major advertisers in all medical journals. They fund clinical trials to determine the effectiveness of their drugs and they pay these researchers to speak at hospitals and medical schools. And if a drug company that makes a cholesterol-lowering drug provides most of the funds to conduct research on the effectiveness of that drug, then there is a potential for bias, even if unwittingly, despite independent monitoring committees that sometimes oversee these studies. Drug companies provide sandwiches and doughnuts at hospital conferences and for the doctors' lounges. They provide free samples of their products. Drug companies also sponsor scientific meetings on the importance of lowering cholesterol, often emphasizing the importance of cholesterol-lowering drugs. These meetings are sometimes held in resorts, and doctors who attend may even be given free transportation and expenses in addition to their food and entertainment."[46]

There is nothing wrong with corporations providing seminars and educational materials. Many businesses do it, not just pharmaceutical companies. But the continuing education doctors get often come solely from drug companies, so that's the only view they understand. They are easily brainwashed into thinking drugs are the only way to solve a problem. That's what the companies are hoping to accomplish. And they do a very good job of it.

The result is the mistaken belief that cholesterol is an important risk factor. There is too much evidence against the cholesterol hypothesis to say that high cholesterol alone leads to heart disease. But that is the impression we still get from many doctors and the media.

CHOLESTEROL-LOWERING DRUGS

Cholesterol-lowering drugs are based on the presumption that cholesterol is the primary determinant of atherosclerosis and coronary heart disease. If cholesterol were the problem it is made out to be, than a reduction in blood levels should have a direct influence on coronary health. Only problem is, that it doesn't work. Since cholesterol isn't the cause or even a very strong risk factor, lowering cholesterol level does little good. The fact is, taking cholesterol-lowering drugs actually *increases* your chances of death rather than reduces it.

Dean Ornish, M.D. is widely known for his studies in reducing risk of coronary artery disease using diet and lifestyle modifications. He found that cholesterol-lowering drugs, while they reduced blood cholesterol, do not reduce incidence of heart attack deaths.

For example, "One of the patients in the comparison (control) group of our study," explains Dr. Ornish, "took lovastatin (Mevacor), a powerful cholesterol-lowering drug, for one year, and he stopped smoking. His cholesterol level decreased from 248 to 172 during the year, yet his coronary artery blockages worsened substantially and he had a heart attack at the end of the year."[47]

Similar results were reported by Dr. David Blankenhorn in a study published in 1987. Patients with a history of elevated cholesterol were divided into two groups. One group received very high doses of two cholesterol-lowering drugs in combination—30 grams per day of colestipol (a fat-lowering drug) plus 8 to 12 grams per day of Niacin (vitamin B-3)—the other group received no medication. Both groups were placed on a 30 percent fat diet in accordance with the American Heart Association guidelines. A 30 percent fat diet includes vegetable oils for cooking and salads, lean red meats, chicken with the skin removed, fish, and no more than three eggs per week. Only patients whose blood cholesterol levels were substantially lowered by drugs were included in this study.

Coronary angiograms were performed at the beginning of the study and two years later for comparison. It was found that only 16 percent of the participants who took the cholesterol-lowering drugs showed any measurable reversal of their coronary artery blockages, 44 percent of the subjects had no change in their blockages, and almost 40 percent actually got *worse* despite intensive drug treatment. Also, the participants reported no overall reduction in the frequency of their chest pains.[48]

Another important study was conducted by F. Greg Brown, M.D. at the University of Washington Medical School in 1990. In this study men with heart disease and elevated cholesterol levels were divided into three groups. Group A was given high doses of niacin plus colestipol; Group B was given high doses of lovastatin plus colestipol; Group C was put on a 30 percent low-fat diet. After two and one-half years, patients in Group A showed a slight amount of overall reversal (less than 1%) of their coronary blockages and patients in Group B showed even less reversal (0.3%). The majority of patients in both groups became

worse, that is, their coronary arteries became more blocked despite drug treatment. Group C patients also become worse, showing a 1.7% worsening of the coronary artery blockages.[49]

If lowering cholesterol were the primary factor in causing reversal of heart disease, then the blockages of most of the patients in the studies by Dr. Blankenhorn and Dr. Brown who were taking cholesterol-lowering drugs should have shown improvement. Almost all of the patients, however, either stayed the same or worsened despite treatment with cholesterol-lowering drugs.

Other studies, including the $170 million dollar National Heart, Lung, and Blood Institute "Type II" study, have also found that cholesterol-lowering drugs do not reverse coronary heart disease.[50] To date, no study has shown that medication to lower cholesterol to be of any value in reversing heart disease.

Dean Ornish points out in his studies that "While there was a direct correlation between adherence to each part of our program (diet, stress management, exercise, and giving up smoking) and the degree of improvement, there was very little correlation between blood cholesterol levels and degree of change in their arteries. In particular, reversal did not correlate with blood levels of total cholesterol, HDL, LDL, total cholesterol/HDL, LDL/HDL, or changes in any of these."[51] Dr. Blankenhorn's study also found that there was little correlation between changes in any of these blood cholesterol levels and arterial blockages."

Despite the decades-long effort by thousands of medical researchers and the availability of cholesterol-lowering drugs since the 1960s, coronary heart disease still remains the leading cause of death in most Western countries. In the face of severe criticism, the American Heart Association (AHA) and the National Heart, Lung, and Blood Institute (HHLBI) have steadfastly supported the lipid hypothesis and have, in terms of funding, studiously ignored other promising areas of research.[52] In America, more money is spent on treating heart disease than any other illness—*$78 billion* an-

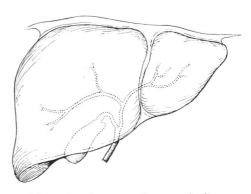

Cholesterol-lowering drugs can damage the liver.

nually. I wonder if this has anything to do with their reluctance to abandon the cholesterol hypothesis?

Cholesterol-lowering drugs are expensive, costing as much as $3,000 a year. And the drugs must be taken for life to keep cholesterol levels down. If blood cholesterol really isn't as important as we are led to believe and cholesterol-lowering drugs aren't useful in reducing risk of heart attack, they are at best a waste of money. Even more important is the fact that they can actually do harm.

Most cholesterol-lowering drugs interfere with the normal function of the liver. This can cause serious liver damage. For this reason, those people who use these drugs are required to get liver function tests every two to three months. Since cholesterol-lowering drugs do not reduce the risk of heart attack, but do increase the risk of liver disease, it seems senseless to use them.

Liver damage isn't the only problem caused by these drugs. In the four largest studies published to date in which cholesterol-lowering drugs were used, along with reducing other risk factors, heart attack deaths fell by 7 percent. However, deaths from other causes *increased* by 20 percent. The net result was an *increase* in overall death rate.[53]

The Lipid Research Clinics Coronary Primary Prevention Trial received intense media attention and was cited as proof that a low-fat diet combined with cholesterol-lowering drugs works. All subjects in the trial were put on a low-cholesterol, low-saturated-fat diet. One group received a cholesterol-lowering drug, the other a placebo. Statistical analysis of the results indicated a 24 percent reduction in the rate of coronary heart disease in the group taking drugs compared with the placebo group. Both the popular press and medical journals touted the survey as the long-sought proof that animal fats are the cause of heart disease and that lowering blood cholesterol can prevent heart disease. Many researchers questioned the results because it didn't fit previous studies nor did it match clinical observations. Independent researchers retabulated the results of this study and found *no significant statistical difference* in the coronary heart disease death rate between the two groups. In addition, a rarely publicized finding of this study was the fact that there was an *increase* in deaths from cancer, intestinal disease, stroke, violence, and suicide in the group taking the cholesterol-lowering drug.[54]

One of the newest groups of cholesterol-lowering medications that have shown some success in lowering blood cholesterol and reducing risk of heart disease are the statin drugs. It is believed that their effectiveness is due primarily to their antioxidant effects rather than their cholesterol-lowering ability. The same benefit can be obtained from antioxidant vitamins at a fraction of the cost and without the side effects. These drugs are toxic to the muscles and liver and promote cancer![55] You may lower your risk

of heart disease, but at the same time increase your risk of liver disease and cancer.

Keep in mind that the body makes cholesterol only when it is needed. So if your body is turning saturated fat into cholesterol, there is a reason for it. Likewise, if you take cholesterol-lowering drugs and your liver isn't damaged in the process, your body will become cholesterol poor. This could lead to a cholesterol deficiency. Also, if you stop taking the drugs, your body will try to make up for this deficiency by producing even more cholesterol than before and your blood cholesterol level will soar. For this reason, once you are put on cholesterol drugs you are told to stay on them for the rest of your life. Remember, cholesterol is used to make hormones, bile, and vitamin D (which helps us absorb calcium for healthy bones), and is an important building block for every cell, especially nerve and brain cells. I wouldn't want to stifle the production of such an important chemical if my body says it needs it.

GENETICS AND CARDIOVASCULAR DISEASE

In studying populations from around the world, the cholesterol hypothesis just doesn't hold up. Studies have shown certain populations from such diverse places as South and Central Africa, South America, Europe, the Middle East, and Western Asia to be free of heart disease and high cholesterol despite the fact that their diets are very high in saturated fat.[56, 57, 58, 59, 60, 61, 62, 63, 64]

A typical example of this is the Masai. The Masai are a nomadic people who live in East Kenya and Northern Tanzania. They herd cattle, goats, and sheep. Most of their diet consists of fresh, raw cow's milk. Adults consume up to five liters of milk a day. This is whole milk, not skim or 2%, so it's loaded with saturated fat and cholesterol.

About 66 percent of calories in their diet come in the from of saturated fat. Even with a diet high in animal fat, the blood cholesterol of the Masai runs only 135 mg/dl and they don't have heart attacks as long as they eat their traditional diet.

Cholesterol researchers traveled to Kenya to study the Masai. During the study, cholesterol in their diet was manipulated in volunteers. When fed 2,000 mg day of cholesterol (one egg yolk contains about 300 mg) blood cholesterol averaged 135 mg/dl. When fed no cholesterol at all, blood cholesterol levels stayed the same. These people did not fit the parameters of the cholesterol hypothesis at all. In order to explain the apparent discrepancy, the researchers simply concluded that the Masai must have some genetic trait that protects them from getting high cholesterol and heart disease.[65]

Genetics has been the favorite answer in defense when those who champion the cholesterol hypothesis are faced with facts that go contrary to their beliefs. Several studies testing the genetic hypothesis have been performed and all have given similar results much to the dismay of the cholesterol promoters.

Japanese Study

To explain the difference why some people are affected by cardiovascular disease and why others are not, even when both have high blood cholesterol levels, people have pointed to genetic differences. It's all in the genes they say. Some people are more susceptible to heart disease than others. Perhaps those people whose ancestry were predominantely meat eaters have a higher tolerance for animal fats than those who descended from agrarian societies. We know that carnivorous animals, such as dogs and cats, can consume huge quantities of saturated fat and cholesterol without any ill effect; maybe the human population varies in its ability to handle such fats.

A study to verify this hypothesis was undertaken. Men of Japanese descent were chosen for the study because the Japanese have one of the lowest rates of cardiovascular disease and many have migrated to various parts of the world. The study analyzed the rate of heart disease and stroke of Japanese men in different countries who ate according to the local diets. The results showed that the death rate from heart disease and stroke of the Japanese men matched those of their adopted countries.[66]

This study clearly showed that heredity was not a factor. Diet and lifestyle were the essential ingredients to cardiovascular health.

Pedigree Studies

Despite the Japanese and other studies, heredity is still often considered a risk factor, thus giving the idea that genetics is an important factor in the development of the disease. If you have a close relative who has suffered a heart attack, you are considered to be at a higher risk. If heart disease is hereditary, then those who are at risk now should have a family history of heart disease.

The University of Utah School of Medicine screened 1,134 high-cholesterol men from eighteen families. In four of the families, cholesterol levels averaged 352 mg/dl. Men with the disease averaged having their first heart attack at 42 and dying at 45.

Pedigrees were traced back to four males who were born before 1880 who must have carried the assumed "abnormal" gene. These men survived to ages 62, 68, 72, and 81. The authors concluded that some unknown healthy lifestyle factors must have protected them against this hereditary defect.

What lifestyle factors could these have been? If they ate the same types of foods most Americans did at the time, they were not eating vegetable oil or flaxseed oil, but cooked their food in lard, ate bacon and eggs, fried chicken and beef, and whole milk, butter, and cream.

Heart disease is our number one killer and has been so for nearly 50 years. Our ancestors, from which we supposedly inherited the genetic defect to have heart attacks, should also have had a high death rate from this illness, but they didn't. Before the late 1800s, heart attacks were so rare they were not even recorded. It was only after the 1930s that heart disease became a major problem.

Irish Study

In a classic study begun in 1963, researchers at the Harvard School of Public Health joined with scientists at Trinity College in Dublin, Ireland. At the time of the study, the heart disease rate in the United States was four times greater than in Ireland. The goal of the study was to determine why Irish immigrants who had lived in the United States for ten or more years experienced the same rate of heart disease as native-born Americans.

To eliminate genetic differences, the subjects chosen in the United States had brothers living in Ireland who also participated in the study. By comparing electrocardiograms, blood pressure readings, and cholesterol levels, the researchers discovered that the cardiovascular condition of the subjects in Ireland was far superior to that of their American brothers. Autopsies performed on subjects who died during the course of the study revealed that the hearts and arteries of the American brothers had "aged from fifteen to twenty-eight years more rapidly."[67]

Most astonishing of all, the Irish participants consumed a diet *much richer in saturated fat and cholesterol* than that of the Americans! If cholesterol and saturated fat were the major factors affecting coronary health, the Irish brothers would have been less healthy. Why the difference? Several answers have been suggested. The American brothers took on the dietary habits of their adopted country which included more polyunsaturated oil and more sugar, both of which we now know to contribute to the deterioration of cardiovascular health. Another factor is that the Irish brothers generally worked at more physically demanding jobs, giving them more exercise. Both diet and physical activity probably made the difference. Exercise does help, but the biggest factor was probably diet. It is of interest to note that now in areas of the world where people still work hard physically, since they have adopted diets more like those of affluent countries, like the United States, by eating more polyunsaturated oils and sugar, their rates of cardiovascular disease has skyrocketed.[68]

BUTTER IS BETTER

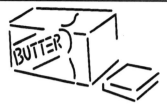

When I was growing up in the 1950s and 1960s, butter was considered an unhealthy food because it was high in saturated fat and cholesterol. Margarine made from polyunsaturated vegetable oil was considered a much healthier alternative.

Before the use of margarine in the 1930s, everyone ate butter—and lots of it. They used it as a spread and in cooking and baking. Heart disease and cancer were rare back then. From 1935-1939 the consumption of butter averaged 17 pounds per person per year. No one was concerned about eating too much fat and ate as much as they liked. With the growing concern that saturated fat and cholesterol may contribute to heart disease, people started switching from butter to margarine. By 1977 butter consumption dropped to only 4.4 pounds per person and that's about where it is today.

During the same time period, margarine rose from 2.9 pounds to 11.6 pounds per person. In 1957 margarine consumption exceeded butter. Our current consumption of margarine is still around 11-12 pounds per person each year.

Butter is making a comeback. While margarine has been promoted as a healthy alternative to butter because it is made from polyunsaturated vegetable oil, the discovery of the toxic nature of trans fatty acids has turned the tables. Margarine rich in trans fatty acids is now considered by most nutritionists to be less healthy than butter. And besides, butter tastes better.

Claims that butter causes chronic high-cholesterol values have not been substantiated by research, although some studies do show that butter consumption can cause a minor increase. Butter, unlike margarine and other vegetable oils, contains fat-soluble vitamins A, D, and E and other naturally occurring nutrients. These vitamins are necessary for the proper utilization of many minerals. Lecithin is a natural component of butter. It is known to assist in the proper assimilation and metabolization of cholesterol and other fats and is an important component of brain tissue.

Butter contains glycosphingolipids. This special category of fat protects against gastrointestinal infections, especially in the very young and the elderly. For this reason, children who drink skim milk have diarrhea at rates three to five times greater than children who drink whole milk.[70]

Many trace minerals are incorporated into the fat globule membrane of butterfat, including selenium, manganese, zinc, chromium, and iodine. Selenium is particularly important because it acts as an antioxidant. Butter contains more selenium per gram than herring or wheat germ, two other sources of this important mineral.

Nutritionists don't argue about the nutrient value of butter. Their concern has been with the saturated fat and cholesterol content. In this chapter you've seen that eating cholesterol does not contribute significantly to blood cholesterol or heart disease. So saturated fat is the only remaining issue. There are different types of saturated fat and not all of them promote blood cholesterol. Stearic, butyric, and caproic acids are three that don't.[71] These make up the bulk of the saturated-fat content of butter.

Monounsaturates such as oleic acid (like that found in olive oil) seem to decrease blood cholesterol. Stearic acid, which is a saturated fat, is easily converted into oleic acid in humans, which perhaps explains reports that stearic acid might actually lower blood cholesterol. Thus, butter fat, which contains about 30 percent of its total fatty acids as monounsaturates and most of its saturated fat from stearic acid (which is converted into monounsaturated fat), butyric acid, and caproic acid* may not be as bad as nutritionists have suggested.[72] Blood cholesterol does not accurately predict heart disease nor does it contribute to it in any significant way.

Another advantage of butter is that it is 66 percent saturated fat. Being saturated it is not easily affected by free radicals and does not have the detrimental effects polyunsaturated oils have.

Margarine is void of all vitamins, minerals, and other nutrients. It is full of toxic trans fatty acids and free-radical forming polyunsaturated fats. Butter, on the other hand, is a good source of many essential vitamins, minerals and other nutrients. It is composed predominantely of monounsaturated fatty acids and other beneficial saturated fatty acids. Studies, such as those conducted in India discussed on page 95, show people are much healthier eating butter in comparison to vegetable oils. When compared to margarine, butter is a health food. Butter truly is better.

---

*Butyric acid is a short-chain fatty acid and caproic acid is a medium-chain fatty acid. The health benefits of short- and medium-chain saturated fatty acids are discussed in detail in Chapter 8.

Butter Study

When we think of butter, we often associate it with cholesterol and saturated fat. Many health-conscious people have switched from butter to margarine with the belief that vegetable oils are healthier. Butter is nearly 100 percent fat, with traces of protein and some vitamins and minerals, most notably vitamins A and D.

People have been eating butter for thousands of years. Greeks and Romans used butter as a hair dressing, ointment, and medicine, as well as for food. Butter has been used in India for more than 3,500 years. In India a type of butter called ghee is popular. Ghee is made by heating butter until protein precipitates to the bottom and the clear liquid (ghee) remaining at the top is skimmed off. Ghee, therefore, has a higher concentration of fat than ordinary butter.

Margarine has been in use for over 60 years. It was not popular at first, but because it costs less than butter and because it was made from vegetable oil instead of saturated fat, its popularity grew. By 1957 more people were using margarine than butter. Today we consume more than twice as much margarine as we do butter.

An interesting study was undertaken in India that compared the health effects of people who use butter with those who use vegetable oils. The study was first reported in *the American Journal of Clinical Nutrition* in 1967.[69]

The director of the study was Dr. Malhotra, medical doctor for the Indian National Rail System. Dr. Malhotra compared two population groups in India, one in the north, the other in the south. The main source of fat in the northerners' diets was from ghee. Ghee was commonly used in all their cooking.

The southerners did not use ghee or any other type of animal fat. As researchers anticipated, their cholesterol levels on the whole were lower than their ghee-loving neighbors. However, even though their cholesterol levels were lower and they ate no cholesterol and consumed very little saturated fat, they had a heart disease rate that was *fifteen times greater* than their northern neighbors. The diets of the two populations were very similar. The major difference, Dr. Malhotra found, was in the kind of fat the southerners used. They had abandoned the traditional use of ghee in favor of margarine and polyunsaturated vegetable oils.

A follow-up study done twenty years later found that heart attack deaths in north India had greatly increased essentially matching those in the south. The British medical journal, *Lancet* on November 14, 1987, contained a letter from Bihari S. Raheja of the Jaslok Hospital in Bombay. He wrote that heart attack deaths in India have greatly increased as the polyunsaturated liquid vegetable fats and the margarine made from them have largely replaced ghee in the Indian diet.

There were two reasons why the Indians abandoned ghee for vegetable oils: one was that margarine and vegetable oils were cheaper than ghee; the other was that doctors had been telling people that they would be healthier if they replaced the "bad" saturated fat of ghee with the "good" polyunsaturated fat of refined vegetable oil. This is the same lie that has been told to us and we've been suffering the consequences of it for years. As inexpensive vegetable oils slowly replace the natural animal fats characteristic of traditional diets throughout the world, we will see a steady rise in heart disease. In fact, it was reported that, for the first time in history, heart disease has now become the number one cause of death worldwide, surpassing infectious diseases. The number one disease of the industrialized world has now spread like a raging plague into less developed countries. Replacing natural, highly saturated fats with processed vegetable oils has proved to be a worldwide health disaster.

You Have Control Over Your Health

The role of genetics in heart disease, cancer, and other degenerative illnesses is greatly overstressed. Genetics provides a convenient excuse when conventional medical science doesn't have an answer. Studies, such as the ones described above, have dispelled the belief that heredity is a major factor in the most prevalent degenerative diseases. The Centers for Disease Control and Prevention recognize this fact and label heart disease and most cancers as primarily lifestyle-caused illnesses. This means that lifestyle choices and not genetics have the greatest influence over our health.

Despite numerous studies to the contrary, drug companies continue to teach physicians that genetics is an important indicator for heart disease. This keeps the idea alive among physicians, and the general public, that cholesterol is the primary villain, that dietary changes won't be enough to overcome hereditary factors, and the only way to reduce risk of heart attack is by using cholesterol-lowering drugs.

You may know a family, perhaps even your own, where two or three members have suffered from a heart attack or other cardiovascular disease. In other families, few suffer with these illnesses. This may seem like there is a genetic relationship. But, according to statistics, about half of us will develop some type of cardiovascular disease. That means you should expect half of your family members to be affected regardless of genetics. Not only that, but families learn to eat the same types of foods—the foods that contribute to heart disease. Kids grow up eating basically the same types of foods they were taught to eat as children, they in turn, teach their children to eat the same way. So a family that uses a lot of vegetable oil or margarine, processed foods, etc. will be more susceptible to disease. Families that eat more healthfully will experience less illness and disease.

This is why the Indians who ate ghee instead of vegetable oil were healthier. This is why Irishmen who ate more saturated fat but less vegetable oil than their American brothers lived longer. This is why the Japanese who live in Japan have a much lower heart disease rate than their relatives who migrate to the United States, Canada, and other Western countries. Among industrialized nations, the Japanese have the longest life expectancy. This is primarily due to the fact that heart disease, cancer, and other degenerative disease are not as common among them.

When Susan Shinagawa, an American of Japanese decent, visited her doctor, he told her not to worry about the lump in her breast because, "Asian women don't get breast cancer." And at 34, she was much too young, especially since she had no family history of cancer, her doctor said.

Shinagawa's doctor made his conclusion based on National Cancer Institute data that showed a low incidence of breast cancer among females of Asian and Pacific islander extraction. But the data lumped all Asian-Americans and Pacific islanders into one group and ignored the fact that the more Americanized these people become, the higher the incidence of cancer. People living in Japan have one of the lowest rates of cancer, but by the time Asians become a second- or third-generation Americans, their risk of cancer is actually higher.

The lumps in Shinagawa's breast didn't go away and she grew concerned. Eventually she went to another doctor. Tests verified the presence of cancer. By this time it had spread to her spine. She has undergone a mastectomy, chemotherapy, and radiation therapy. Two years ago doctors thought she had only a few months to live. Although she has survived beyond those predictions, the cancer is still present and she is dying. Her health frail, she can stand with the aid of a cane but needs a wheelchair to get around. She is a dramatic example of how the health care system has failed many patients simply because of fatal misconceptions about heredity.

We are not helplessly under the control or destiny of genetics. For the most part we have control over our current level of health and our future health. By wisely choosing the foods we eat and avoiding those that may cause the most harm, we can greatly improve our health and avoid many of the degenerative diseases that have swept over industrialized countries during the past century.

ANIMAL STUDIES

One question you might have asked after reading this far is: What about the animal studies mentioned earlier? Rabbits given diets high in saturated fat and cholesterol de-velop a form of atherosclerosis that may plug up their coronary arteries within three months. Doesn't this prove that eating saturated fat/cholesterol causes atherosclerosis? The answer to this question is a simple "no." The early studies on animals have since been shown to be seriously flawed.

What happens in an animal that is strictly a herbivore (vegetarian) by nature may not be the same that happens in a carnivore or omnivore (consumes both meat and plants) like us. We cannot take the results from any animal study and blindly state that the same thing happens in humans. The processes that operate in an animal's body are not the same as those in humans. All researchers know this, but when a study yields results supporting a prevailing dogma, people are quick to extrapolate the results to humans. Extrapolating the results of these animal studies to humans is grossly misleading. Further studies have demonstrated that carnivores and omnivores handle fat differently than rabbits and other vegetarian animals. When researchers fed high-fat diets to dogs and cats, which by nature are carnivores, no plaque was found in their arteries.

The fatty deposits that develop in rabbits are distinctly different from the type of plaque that is found in humans. In rabbits the fatty deposits build up on the inner surface of the arterial wall. In humans the plaque doesn't attach itself to the artery wall, but grows *inside* of it. Researchers looking for proof for their theory ignored this important fact and equated the fatty deposits in rabbits with the plaque found in humans.

Feeding experiments have been repeated using a variety of animals. High-fat diets, which included as much vegetable oil as saturated fat or cholesterol, produced similar fatty obstructions in several herbivorous animals, but did not work with carnivores. Obstructions did not form in dogs unless their thyroid glands were removed before conducting the experiment. This demonstrated that carnivores and omnivores, including humans, are born with the chemistry to handle saturated fat and cholesterol in the diet.

It is interesting to note that researchers included just as much vegetable oil as saturated fat or cholesterol. Why they found it necessary to add vegetable oil when they were testing the effects of cholesterol and saturated fat is not revealed. Could it be that the vegetable oil enhances the development of atherosclerosis? It certainly wasn't used to retard its development, for this would make their studies meaningless. Keep in mind that vegetable oil is highly susceptible to free-radical formation and will cause free-radical degeneration (oxidation) of cholesterol. It is only this form of cholesterol that is found in arterial plaque.

Another problem with the cholesterol-feeding experiments of Anitschkov and other scientists is that the arterial plaques contained too much fat and cholesterol in comparison with plaque found in humans. Typical human lesions are fibrous, have a lot of calcification, and contain a relatively small percent of cholesterol deposits. But over the years the emphasis has been so heavily on the fat deposition that the connective tissue changes have been overlooked.

Atherosclerosis in humans is characterized by tough fibrous tissue and calcium deposits. That is why it is referred to as "hardening" of the arteries. Arteries become so tough and brittle that they are very difficult to cut with scissors or even a surgical knife. Only in the aorta and some large arteries do the excessive deposits of fat and proteins cause soft plaques to become prominent. The idea that arteries in human atherosclerosis are narrowed only by greasy fatty deposits is simply not true for most arteries.

OXIDIZED CHOLESTEROL

Both animal studies and human autopsies show cholesterol in atherosclerotic arteries. Regardless of the amount found, doesn't this suggest that cholesterol plays an important role in the development of the disease? Not necessarily. Cholesterol has unjustly been accused as the primary instigator of arterial plaque. Normal cholesterol, the type used to make hormones, vitamin D, and brain tissue is guilty only by association. It's like a group of school children playing baseball and the batter hits the ball through a neighbor's window. All the kids involved in the game run for cover. The only kid that sticks around was one who was sitting watching the game and minding his own business. When the owner of the house comes out and sees only that boy, he is automatically accused as the guilty party. Cholesterol is that innocent bystander. The real troublemakers have hidden out of sight and until recently have escaped detection.

It was in the 1970s that researchers discovered that dietary cholesterol existed in two forms, oxidized and reduced. In fresh, natural foods, cholesterol and other fats occur only in the harmless reduced form. This is the normal cholesterol, the innocent bystander, the type that makes up the majority of our brain tissue or that is used as a component of cell membranes; it is *not* found in human arterial plaque. The type of cholesterol that builds up in the arteries is *oxidized* cholesterol and oxidized fatty acids. These are the *only* types of fats found in plaque.[73, 74]

Only the oxidized form is toxic to arteries. Dr. Ishwarlal Jialal of the University of Texas Southwestern Medical Center in Dallas states, "Fats in the bloodstream become lodged in artery walls and begin to clog arteries *only* when their transporters, the lipoproteins, have chemically combined with oxygen to turn rancid."[75] Lipoproteins are tiny bundles of protein packed with cholesterol and fatty acids (including polyunsaturated fats). The polyunsaturated

fats are highly susceptible to oxidization which causes free radical formation. When polyunsaturated oils turn rancid, they produce free radicals that attack the cholesterol, causing it to become oxidized as well. The result is that both the cholesterol and polyunsaturated fats in the lipoprotein become oxidized. (Could this be why cholesterol, when added to vegetable oil in the animal studies mentioned above, was found in plaque deposits?)

In a series of studies of oxidized cholesterol, medical scientists at Albany Medical College showed that highly purified cholesterol, without contamination from polyunsaturated oils, chemically free of all traces of oxidized cholesterol, and protected from the oxygen in air, does *not* produce atherosclerosis.[76, 77] Pure unadulterated cholesterol is not harmful to the arteries and cannot initiate or promote heart disease.[78] Cholesterol *must* be oxidized before the artery cells will trap it.[79]

A very large number of research publications support the fact that oxidized fats (both cholesterol and polyunsaturated fats) are far more harmful to arterial health than native or ordinary fats. Therefore, cholesterol is now viewed as harmless unless it becomes oxidized.[80]

It is very important to understand the difference between normal (reduced) and oxidized cholesterol. Cholesterol doesn't simply come strolling freely down the artery and suddenly decide to stick somewhere. The process begins with an injury to the inner lining of the arterial wall. The injury can be caused by a virus, excessive blood pressure, or other factors, even free-radical damage. Because of a process which is still not fully understood, cells in the artery wall attract oxidized cholesterol and oxidized triglycerides (e.g., fatty acids such as those found in vegetable oil) from the blood. Only oxidized fats are involved. Other materials such as calcium and fibrous tissue also combine with fat to form plaque. As the plaque builds up within the wall of the artery, the wall bulges inward, slowly closing off the arterial opening. Over many years, the process gradually obstructs the artery, blocking the flow of blood.

When it was discovered that only oxidized fat is involved in the generation of arterial plaque, researchers became curious enough to repeat the original rabbit-feeding studies. They suspected that early researchers put the fat-rich food into cages and left it for the rabbits to eat throughout the day. This allowed the fat on the surface of the food to react with the oxygen in the air and become oxidized. As you recall oxygen, sunlight, and heat (even room temperature) can initiate free-radical reactions.

When researchers repeating these experiments made efforts to protect the fat in the food from oxidizing, the animals' arteries remained healthy. The fat content of the food was increased and the rabbits' blood cholesterol went as high as 1,500 to 2,000 mg/dl—ten times the upper limit currently considered acceptable for humans—but no fatty deposits formed! So even in vegetarian animals cholesterol is harmless.

Some researchers questioned that the small amount of fat that would be oxidized on the surface of the food in the original studies would make any significant impact. So researchers designed experiments using very small quantities of oxidized fat. Rabbits fed a diet containing a mere 1% oxidized cholesterol developed extensive obstructions in their coronary arteries. In another group, rabbits ate the same amount of fat and cholesterol which was protected from oxidation, and their arteries remained disease-free. So even a tiny amount of oxidized oil can have a very significant impact on health.[81]

Several factors affected the cholesterol in early studies to give erroneous results. If the cholesterol was mixed with vegetable oil, the oxidation process was accelerated. Vegetable oil was routinely added in many studies. Because eggs contain a high percentage of cholesterol, they were often used as the source in many studies. However, the type of eggs they used were always in dried, powdered form. Drying the eggs *oxidizes* the cholesterol in them. So the researchers were conducting tests using highly oxidized cholesterol and not the type typically found in ordinary foods.

Most of the older scientific articles don't specify the type of cholesterol and other oils used. So there is no way of telling if the fats were oxidized or not. If not specified, it is assumed that steps were *not* taken to protect fats from oxidation, usually because researchers did not recognize the difference at the time. Because of this, most feeding studies reported over the past 80 years are worthless. The results of these flawed studies were then applied to humans in making dietary recommendations. This is why in real life doctors and researchers have failed to find a correlation between people who eat a high-cholesterol diet and heart disease.

All oxidized fats, whether they are cholesterol or polyunsaturated fatty acids, because they involve free radicals can damage arterial walls. Studies on rabbits showed those fed oxidized cholesterol had damage, while those fed normal cholesterol didn't.[82] What we know now is that it's not the total level of fat or the LDL (bad cholesterol) in the blood that's important, but the amount of *oxidized* fat that is the issue. Many people with relatively low blood fat levels develop cardiovascular disease because a large amount of this fat is oxidized. Others who have high cholesterol readings do not experience cardiovascular disease because the fat in their blood is normal or not oxidized.

How does the body accumulate oxidized fat? That is a very important question in regards to cardiovascular health, and knowing the answer may save your life.

Oxidation can occur in food either before or after it's eaten. Rancid or heat-damaged oils become oxidized before eating. Once these damaged oils are consumed, through free-radical chain reactions, they can cause other oils inside the body to become oxidized. The best defense against free-radical destruction is to eat oils that are not oxidized and those that are not susceptible to oxidization. As noted above in the rabbit studies, even a very small amount of oxidized fat can have a dramatic effect on cardiovascular health.

Probably the biggest contributor to fat oxidation and free-radical formation in the body comes from eating polyunsaturated vegetable oils. Saturated fats are not a problem because they are not vulnerable to oxidation like unsaturated fats or even cholesterol. Cholesterol is an unsaturated fat, meaning it can accommodate more hydrogen atoms in its structure and, therefore, is more susceptible to oxidation than saturated fat. Cholesterol can be oxidized within the body, so a higher level of cholesterol in the blood can theoretically increase the risk of developing oxidized cholesterol which has been shown to be involved in atherosclerosis. This is why there is a risk, howbeit very small, with elevated cholesterol levels. The vast majority of the cholesterol in our blood is made by the liver and is pure and natural, thus harmless, unless it comes in contact with rancid polyunsaturated fatty acids or other free-radical-causing substances like homocysteine, xanthine oxidase, or iron, each of which is described fully in later chapters.

Heat is a major factor in free-radical formation, and cooking with vegetable oils causes massive free-radical generation. When you eat anything that is cooked in vegetable oil, you are quite literally damaging your heart, your brain, and all other organs and tissues in your body. Any unsaturated oil that has been heated contains free radicals. Almost all vegetable oils, often including those labeled "cold" or "expeller" pressed, are subjected to high temperatures in processing. The cold-pressed oils undergo lower temperatures, but still are damaged. Extra virgin olive oil, long known to be one of the healthiest oils, is the least contaminated because it is extracted under low-temperature conditions.

Cooking meat causes some fat oxidation particularly on the surface where it is exposed to oxygen. Currently, however, there is little evidence to show that cooked meat causes any significant problems from oxidized fats. The reason is probably because meat contains primarily saturated and monounsaturated fat, both of which are fairly stable under heat. The oils in the meat that are oxidized first are the unsaturated fatty acids. Cholesterol may also be affected to some degree but is present in very small amounts. You don't need to worry about the saturated fat in the meat because it is not vulnerable to oxidation and free-radical formation like unsaturated fats are. This is why our ancestors could cook all their meals in lard and butter without experiencing any signs of cardiovascular disease.

Eggs have frequently been condemned because they are high in cholesterol and saturated fat. A much bigger health hazard is the vegetable oils commonly used in cooking eggs. It's safer to cook them in lard than in vegetable oil. Hard boiled eggs are cooked at temperatures below 212° F (100° C)—the boiling point—and are not exposed to oxygen during cooking, so the cholesterol they contain is not oxidized. Despite the fact that eggs are high in cholesterol and saturated fat, when hard boiled they do not contribute to heart disease.

Charles McGee, M.D., tells in his book, *Heart Frauds,* about an experience with one of his patients who participated in an animal-feeding study. This patient worked in a regional primate center, one of several research centers funded by the federal government. "One old baboon named George was selected to participate in the study because he had a mean disposition and none of the animal keepers liked him," relates Dr. McGee.

"The staff dreamed up an experiment in which George was given the opportunity to give his life for science and not be around to bother them any more. They fed the old baboon nothing but hard boiled eggs for one year, then put him down (killed him) and performed an autopsy.

"Because of the propaganda about the cholesterol theory, the staff confidently expected to find massive obstructions in the old baboon's arteries. They dreamed of seeing their names in large print on the top of a published scientific paper supporting the widely accepted and popular cholesterol theory.

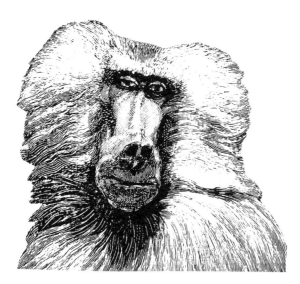

George gave his life for science but no one ever knew.

"But it was the old baboon who had the last laugh. Because no evidence of atherosclerosis was found in George's arteries, no paper was written. This feeding study demonstrated once again the fats and cholesterol in fresh eggs are harmless because they do not become oxidized. It also demonstrated that studies that do not support an accepted theory usually don't get published."[83]

Dr. Kilmer McCully states: "The entire history of the cholesterol/fat hypothesis explaining the cause of atherosclerosis is based on the unproved assumption that the disease is produced by overconsumption of the normal dietary constituents—cholesterol and fat. Only in the case of the oxycholesterols (oxidized cholesterol) is there compelling evidence to suggest that a trace or contaminant constituent associated with fat and cholesterol in the diet is actually injurious and capable of initiating atherosclerotic plaques."[84]

All cells in our bodies need cholesterol. It forms an integral part of the cell's membrane. It has an important structural role in the brain and in the conduction of nerve impulses. "Because cholesterol is so important physiologically," states Nicholas Sampsidis, M.S., "it is a rather foolhardy assumption that, since the dawn of mankind, the human system has been performing the suicidal experiment of becoming dependent on a biochemical which can trigger its self-destruction. The human system takes very good care of itself and it does not manufacture cholesterol in order to clog up its own arteries and start heart disease."[85]

VEGETABLE OILS AND CARDIOVASCULAR DISEASE

Vegetable oils are recommended in place of saturated fat and cholesterol because they do not raise blood cholesterol levels. For this reason, they are often said to reduce the risk of heart disease. But we have seen that blood cholesterol level really isn't important. What is important is the amount of oxidized fat in the blood from both cholesterol and polyunsaturated fatty acids. Polyunsaturated fats are the primary source of oxidized oils in our bodies and a major catalyst in the oxidation of cholesterol.

Mary G. Enig, Ph.D., a Fellow of the American College of Nutrition and an internationally recognized expert in lipid chemistry, along with Sally Fallon, a nutritional journalist, reported that a recent study found that excess consumption of omega-6 fatty acids, the kind found in most vegetable oils, increases the amount of oxidized cholesterol in the arterial plaque. They go on to say that it is the polyunsaturated omega-6 fatty acids—not saturated fat—that forms the major fat component of arterial plaque, yet for many years the American Heart Association and many health and nutrition writers advocated the consumption of polyunsaturated oils.[86] But these oils should be the last things you would ever want to eat.

Let's take a look at the oils and see what happens to them physically, then you be the judge if you want to put them inside your body or not.

Many oils and fats have a tendency to "dry" or solidify when exposed to air. The drying is caused not by evaporation, but by oxidation or chemical combination with oxygen. The rate of drying or oxidation varies depending primarily on the degree of unsaturation. In the oil industry oils are grouped into three classifications:

- *Nondrying*—coconut oil, tallow, palm oil, and lard (saturated fats)

- *Semidrying*— olive, peanut, rapeseed (canola), cottonseed, corn, soybean, sunflower, and sesame (moderately unsaturated fats)

- *Drying*—fish oils, tung, linseed (flax), perilla, and oitcica (very highly polyunsaturated fats)

Both semidrying and drying oils are used in paints, varnishes, linoleum, and printing ink. These oils quickly oxidize and harden, making good mediums for industrial use. Linseed oil, which is also known as flaxseed oil, is particularly useful in the paint industry because it readily oxidizes and becomes hard. It is used to make linoleum, paint, putty, enamel, and varnish. It was the primary source for linoleum until the late 1940s before the use of cheaper synthetic petroleum-based oils became popular. In fact, linoleum derives its name from linseed oil. When oil producers began marketing linseed oil as a food and dietary supplement, they didn't want people to associate it with the toxic industrial products it had been used for, so they began to call it flaxseed oil. It's ironic that a toxic substance used to make turpentine and varnish is now used as a dietary supplement!

When unsaturated oils go rancid, they oxidize and become hardened. It is this property that makes the oil useful for industrial purposes. Oxidation of the oil in oil-based paints is what causes them to dry or harden on canvas. When oil molecules inside our bodies become oxidized, they harden just like the paint on a canvas or the lacquer on a tabletop. This process has been suggested as a contributing factor in the development of arterial plaquing and vascular disease.[87]

Atherosclerosis or hardening of the arteries occurs when plaque builds up in the wall of blood vessels. If the cells in a person's arteries contain a lot of polyunsaturated fatty acids from vegetable oils, what do you suppose will happen when these cells are bombarded with free radicals or free-radical catalysts (substances that initiate free-radical reactions)? Oxidation hardens the polyunsaturated oils in the lining of the arteries just as it does in the paint on an artist's canvas. The oils used in the making of paints and varnishes are the very same ones we put in our food and eat as dietary supplements. Think about it. If linseed (flaxseed) and other polyunsaturated oils harden when they oxidize, what are they going to do inside your body—inside your arteries, your skin, your kidneys, and other tissues?

Saturated fat does not harden; it is classified as a nondrying oil. If your tissues are filled with polyunsaturated fats when they are subjected to the oxidizing effects of free radicals, they harden. It's no wonder why studies have shown that people develop heart disease at a faster rate when they switch from using butter to vegetable oil.[88] Draw your own conclusions, but I would much rather have my tissues made up of flexible saturated fat than potentially dangerous and brittle polyunsaturated fat.

The American Heart Association recommends that people lower their total fat intake from the typical 35-40 percent of total calories to 30 percent. When we hear about lowering fat consumption, we all assume that means lowering saturated fat and cholesterol and not vegetable oil. So when people reduce their total fat intake, they are primarily reducing these two fats, but continuing to eat just as much vegetable oil. Besides, many people have the mistaken notion that vegetable oil helps protect them from heart disease. To reduce to 30 percent fat, the typical guidelines include eating fewer eggs, trim fat off meat, remove skin from chicken, replace red meats with fish or chicken, and drink nonfat milk. Notice that these recommendations lower primarily saturated fat and cholesterol consumption. Nothing is usually said or done about lowering vegetable oil consumption. Consequently, people continue to eat just about as much vegetable oil as they always have. Even with these guidelines heart disease continues to kill more people than any other disease.

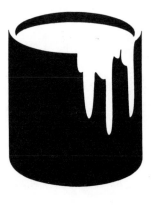

Linseed (flax) oil, soybean oil, and other polyunsaturated oils have long been used in the making of paint and varnish because they easily oxidize and harden.

When people reduce saturated fat and cholesterol to limit total fat intake to 30 percent or less, health does *not* improve. A study published in the *New England Journal of Medicine* reported that even a diet with only 20 percent fat did not reduce risk of heart disease any more than a diet containing 30 percent fat.[89]

Dean Ornish, M.D., has had success in helping people gain better health and overcome cardiovascular problems, but in order to do this they had to change their diets drastically. All processed and refined foods are eliminated and consumption of whole grains and fresh fruites and vegetables encouraged. Total fat intake is limited to only 10 percent of total calories. In order to reduce it this much, a person must eliminate *all* fats from the diet. All meat (including fish and chicken), egg yolks, and milk is eliminated as well as all vegetable oils. Just about the only oils people get are those that are found naturally with the fresh fruits, vegetables, and grains they eat. Since all processed vegetable oils are eliminated, the people show dramatic improvement in cardiovascular health as well as all types of degenerative disease. Dr. Ornish showed for the first time that it was possible to reverse obstructions in coronary arteries.[90]

The primary reason why vegetable oils are considered good or at least better than other oils is because they have a tendency to lower blood cholesterol levels. Much is said about *blood* cholesterol, but cholesterol is in other parts of the body as well. High intakes of polyunsaturated fatty acids have been found to *increase* whole body cholesterol, especially liver cholesterol. Dietary changes in favor of polyunsaturated fatty acids usually lower both the so-called "bad" LDL cholesterol and the "good" HDL cholesterol. So there is no benefit. Similarly, excess polyunsaturates are known to enhance platelet aggregation and interfere with cell-wall permeability to various metabolites.[91]

Let me ask you a question. When polyunsaturated oils lower blood cholesterol what happens? Where does the cholesterol go? Vegetable oil does not magically make cholesterol disappear. And cholesterol is not excreted with the consumption of vegetable oil, so how does it lower blood cholesterol levels? I'll tell you. It causes the cholesterol to migrate out of the blood and into surrounding tissues. The cholesterol is still there, but now it is in the cells and tissues rather than floating in the blood. Where else is it going to go? Some of this cholesterol becomes oxidized by the polyunsaturated oils that are eaten. Where do oxidized fats end up? In the arteries. You get a lower blood cholesterol reading, but is it any healthier? No, because you'll likely have more oxidized cholesterol in your arteries.

The question one might ask is why does cholesterol migrate into the cells when polyunsaturated fat is eaten? The answer is that the membranes of the cells are made predominantely from fatty acids, both saturated and unsaturated. Cholesterol is also an important component of the cell membrane. Polyunsaturated fatty acids make the membrane fluid or flexible. Saturated fat and cholesterol act as stabilizers, providing support. A balance is needed in all of them for the cells to function optimally. When the diet is rich in polyunsaturated fatty acids, more of these fats are used as building blocks for the cell membranes. As a consequence, the cells become too fluid and become leaky, resulting in a loss of function. In order to maintain optimal function, more cholesterol is extracted from passing lipoproteins and incorporated into the cell membrane to strengthen it. Therefore, less cholesterol is left in the blood. Eating polyunsaturated oils to reduce blood cholesterol doesn't do a bit of good for your health. Actually it causes more harm and increases the chance of packing more oxidized cholesterol and triglycerides (fatty acids) into the arteries.

As far back as 1965, studies clearly showed vegetable oils contribute to cardiovascular disease. But because they could also lower cholesterol, and everyone believed that lowering cholesterol was good, the bad side effects were ignored. In one example, a study was conducted where volunteers ate either a diet high in saturated fat and cholesterol (the control group) or a low-fat diet supplemented with four teaspoons of corn oil per day. After two years, blood levels of cholesterol in the corn oil group went down, but the incidence of major cardiac events doubled![92] Vegetable oils also increase platelet stickiness, thus promoting blood clots. Even canola and olive oils which are considered relatively heart safe, increase platelet stickiness.[93]

From the evidence presented it appears that vegetable oils contribute far more to the development of atherosclerosis and heart disease than might either cholesterol or saturated fat. It's no wonder the recommendation to cut back on these two fats has not produced any improvement in cardiovascular health and why heart disease is still our number one killer. Perhaps if we cut out the vegetable oils and stopped worrying about how much saturated fat and cholesterol we ate, the heart disease rate would finally come back down to levels before the "age of vegetable oils."

DEATH RATES AND VEGETABLE OIL CONSUMPTION

In 1911 the two biggest killers in the United States and much of the Western world were tuberculosis and pneumonia. Today these infectious diseases have been overtaken by degenerative disease. Of the top 10 causes of death in this country, seven are due to degenerative disease—diseases that a century ago were relatively uncommon.

The Ten Leading Causes of Death in the United States

Rank	Cause of Death	% of Total Deaths
1	Heart disease	35.7
2	Cancers	22.4
3	Strokes	7.0
4	Accidents	4.4
5	Chronic obstructive lung disease	3.7
6	Pneumonia and influenza	3.2
7	Diabetes mellitus	1.8
8	Suicide	1.4
9	Chronic liver disease and cirrhosis	1.2
10	Atherosclerosis	1.1

Source: National Center for Health Statistics, *Monthly Vital Statistics Report*, vol. 37, no 1.

Vegetable oils promote the mechanisms that clog arteries, raise blood fat levels, and contribute to cardiovascular disease and cancer. Polyunsaturated oils contribute most to all degenerative disease.

Of the top ten causes of death, cardiovascular disease (heart disease, stroke, and atherosclerosis) make up 43.8 percent and cancer 22.4 percent. Either one is by far greater than any other cause of death.

A good percentage of these deaths are caused by dietary oils. Vegetable oils probably cause more deaths than tobacco and alcohol combined. But because the oil industry has propagated the idea that their products are "healthy" alternatives to saturated fat, the danger they cause is largely ignored. It's time we stop ignoring this threat to our health!

As the use of vegetable oils has gained popularity around the world, deaths from cardiovascular disease and cancer has risen. The number one killer in the world now is heart disease (6.3 million a year). Stroke is second (4.4 million). Cancer has risen to fifth (2.4 million)[94] behind lower respiratory infections and diarrheal disease. The striking thing about these figures are that up until recently, most deaths in Third World countries had been due to infectious diseases, but now since vegetable oils and other highly processed foods have made their way into these areas, the death rate from degenerative disease is soaring. When people abandon their native foods for cheaper mass-produced ones, like vegetable oil, their death rate from cardiovascular disease and cancer approaches those of more industrialized nations.

Over the past 50 years, margarine has nearly replaced butter in our diets. We currently eat some 12 pounds of it a year. Lard has dropped from 5 pounds per person in 1970 to about 1.5. Over the same time period, shortening has increased from 17 pounds per person to 23 pounds. Salad and cooking oils have increased from 15 pounds per person to 25 pounds. Total fat consumption from 1970 to 1995 has increased while saturated fats (lard and butter) have decreased. Vegetable oils have increased from almost nothing in 1900, to 43 pounds per person in 1970 to 58 pounds per person in 1995. We consume 58 pounds of vegetable oil every year. This is predominantely polyunsaturated oil. Much of it is hydrogenated.

In Puerto Rico, the breast and colon cancer rate is only 30-40 percent that of that in the United States in spite of the fact that Puerto Ricans eat considerably more animal fat than Americans use (88% versus 62% of the total fat intake). But Americans use much more vegetable oil.[95, 96]

When you put all these facts together, it should become crystal clear to you that saturated fat and cholesterol aren't the enemy. Vegetable oils are a much greater health hazard.

LOW CHOLESTEROL IS DANGEROUS TO YOUR HEALTH

Low cholesterol dangerous to health? How can that be? The low-cholesterol mantra has been forced down our throats for so long now that we tend to think of cholesterol as an evil villain equal to the eboli virus or small pox. But in truth, cholesterol is an essential component of our bodies. It is absolutely vital to life and to the life of every cell in our bodies. Believe it or not, we need to have cholesterol in our blood, and too little of it can be life threatening. So much interest has been placed on elevated levels of cholesterol in the blood that researchers have all but ignored the consequences of having too little. Evidence indicates that a cholesterol deficiency can lead to cardiovascular disease, cancer, and death.

As far back as 1974 researchers discovered that low cholesterol can lead to serious health problems. Since cholesterol and saturated fat were being blamed for heart disease, some researchers suggested that theses fats might also be responsible for other illness as well, so they began looking at cancer. Studies were conducted to compare the incidence of colon cancer with blood cholesterol levels. What they found was shocking. Instead of finding another deadly illness to blame on high cholesterol, they discovered just the opposite: cholesterol levels that were lower than average for the populations studied, correlated with an *increase* in cancer rate. The researchers were baffled. Other studies performed by researchers from many different nations showed the same trend.[97]

By the early 1980s so many investigators had found the association between low cholesterol and cancer that researchers Paul D. Sorlie and Manning Feinleib went back to the Framingham studies to evaluate the data. They found the same correlation between low blood-cholesterol levels and cancer. They also discovered that low cholesterol was evident as far back as 16-18 years before cancer was diagnosed. That made low cholesterol a powerful predictor of cancer. Their result was reported in the *Journal of the National Cancer Institute*.[98] Many still refused to accept it. How can something, namely cholesterol, that is believed to cause one disease, provide protection against another?

In 1987 researchers at the National Cancer Institute measured this relationship among 12,488 men and women who participated in the National Health Nutrition and Examination Survey. This was a bigger, more recent, and more representative sample of the American population than the Framingham group. They found that the men with the lowest cholesterol levels were more than twice as likely to be diagnosed with cancer as those with the highest cholesterol levels. Further, the longer the follow-up the stronger the relationship. These results were published a 1987 *Lancet* article.[99]

If the link between low cholesterol and cancer wasn't bad enough, researchers were also discovering other health risks. While low cholesterol has been viewed as good for the heart and cardiovascular system, evidence indicated otherwise. A study presented at the American Heart Association's annual stroke conference in February 1999 provides an example.[100] The study was conducted by Dr. David Tirschwell of Harborview Medical Center in Seattle, Washington. Tirschwell studied 587 victims of ischemic strokes (strokes that occur when a blood clot blocks an artery, choking off oxygen and nutrients to a section of the brain) and 137 victims of hemorrhagic strokes (those caused by excessive bleeding) and compared them with 3,743 healthy people. Among the findings, Tirschwell found people with cholesterol less than 180 mg/dl had double the risk of those at 230 mg/dl for a hemorrhagic stroke. While it isn't known exactly how low cholesterol contributes to hemorrhagic stroke, Tirschwell said one possibility is that cholesterol is needed to keep blood vessels strong to prevent rupture. Weak blood vessels are more apt to burst.

For many years, experts have been convinced that too much cholesterol, particularly low-density lipoproteins (LDL—the bad cholesterol), increases the risk of heart disease and stroke. There are two kinds of strokes, bleeding strokes (hemorrhagic stroke) and clot strokes (ischemic strokes). The above study attempted to look at the effects of cholesterol on each of these. It found that low cholesterol increases the hazard of the less common hemorrhagic strokes that result from leaky blood vessels in the brain.

The study calculated that the perfect cholesterol level for preventing strokes is about 200 mg/dl, which coincidentally is the target established by the U.S. Government's National Cholesterol Education Program. The current recommendation for cholesterol is less than 200 mg/dl as desirable, 200-239 mg/dl is borderline high, more than 240 is high risk. The belief has been that the lower the cholesterol level the better. So a cholesterol level of 140 mg/dl would be excellent. Now we know such a person is at a greater risk for experiencing a bleeding stroke.

The threat of stroke or hemorrhage occurring anywhere in the body is a real danger with omega-3 polyunsaturated fatty acids. Flaxseed and fish oils are the most common sources of these fatty acids. They are converted to prostaglandins (PGE3) which thin the blood and, in excess, can cause spontaneous bleeding, bruising, and hemorrhagic stroke. While the Eskimos are looked upon as prime examples of a people who have been free of heart disease because of the large amount of fish oil they consume, the biggest cause of death among Eskimos has always been hemorrhagic stroke—a cardiovascular disease. We always think of the Eskimos traditionally having very healthy cardiovascular systems because their rate of heart attacks was low, but they have an extraordinarily high incidence of stroke. Why? One reason is because they consume so much fish that they get too much of the essential fatty acids from fish oils, which produces too much PGE3, which weakens their cardiovascular system to such an extent that their blood vessels fall apart with the slightest stress.

One nutritionist discovered the dangers of omega-3 fatty acids by accident. In her studies, everything she ran across reported the benefits of omega-3 fatty acids, particularly from flaxseed oil. From the material she read it seemed to be an immensely healthful nutrient without any adverse side effects. So, like thousands of other health care professionals, she began recommending it to her clients. She took flaxseed oil herself because it was the "healthy" thing to do. After a few months, she noticed that areas on her arms and legs became darkened much like liver spots that so commonly affect the elderly. She also began to bruise easily. She didn't know the cause. When she began seeing the same symptoms occurring to all the clients whom she had recommended flaxseed oil, she began to suspect a connection. These people were developing large bruises almost spontaneously, a problem that did not exist before they were taking flaxseed oil. Fearing that it was caused by the oil, she had them discontinue its use. Their bruising subsided. She now feels it is extremely dangerous for people to use flaxseed oil or any omega-3 supplement because it can greatly increase the risk of not only weakening blood vessels in the arms and legs, but also in the brain, which could lead to a hemorrhagic stroke and possibly death. Stroke (both hemorrhagic and ischemic) is the third leading cause of death behind heart disease and cancer.

Too little cholesterol and too much omega-3 fatty acids can both increase the risk of suffering a stroke. Stroke is a cardiovascular disease. While lowering cholesterol and taking omega-3 fatty acids have been recommended as a means to fight cardiovascular disease, they can also contribute to it.

Another study published in May of 1999 has demonstrated further detrimental effects of low cholesterol.[101] This study, conducted by Edward Suarez, a psychologist at Duke University, recruited 121 women ages 18 to 27. Researchers took blood samples to determine cholesterol levels and administered a psychological test. Comparing the cholesterol levels with the test, they found that those women who had had blood cholesterol less than 160 mg/dl had a higher rate of depression and anxiety. Suarez states that when cholesterol dips too low, it can affect the brain. He says without enough cholesterol, brain cells don't get enough serotonin, a feel-good chemical made by the body, and depression may result.

THE CONTROVERSY RAGES

Campaigns have been launched by various groups advising us to consume less saturated fat and cholesterol. Radio and TV commercials echo the cry. Hundreds of cholesterol-free products are on the market. Drugs and medical diagnostics and treatments based around measuring or reducing blood cholesterol abound. Low-fat diets and health programs are religiously promoted by nearly every health guru. Even natural or herbal cholesterol-lowering products are aggressively marketed. Lowering cholesterol has become *big* business. As a consequence of the intense hype these prod-

ucts and enterprises generate, most of the public still believes cholesterol is the culprit responsible for heart disease.

The cholesterol controversy has been hotly debated, and an increasing number of honest investigators are seriously questioning the sketchy evidence upon which the theory is based.

The Food and Nutrition Board of the National Research Council challenged the view of the American Heart Association by stating that "there is no reason for the average healthy American to restrict consumption of cholesterol, nor should fat intake be reduced."[102] This group found no link between cholesterol in the diet and cholesterol levels in the bloodstream. Within a year, a report in the *New England Journal of Medicine* disputed the National Research Council's viewpoint.

The presumption that cholesterol may be the causative agent in heart disease has been disproven time and time again. The only connection cholesterol has with heart disease is when it is in an oxidized form, usually in association with polyunsaturated oils (oxidized triglycerides). Many new findings have come forth over the past few decades that explain the cause of heart disease and fit all the observed facts much better than the cholesterol hypothesis (as you will see in later chapters).

So what keeps the cholesterol hypothesis alive? Politics, greed, and money. The low-cholesterol push has been an enormous money maker for all sorts of industries from drug and food companies to the health and fitness industry. Even the media has joined in the fray. Have you ever noticed how many books, magazines, and tapes promote low cholesterol? With all these people getting rich off the cholesterol scare, they are not about to let their cash cow go easily. Many people will refute the facts presented here, but refuting a fact does not make it any less factual. The only way you can know the truth for yourself is to study the data and apply it in your life. Because this book isn't tied into the cholesterol profit machine, it is one of the few resources that presents the facts as they really are.

Chapter 8

SATURATED FAT

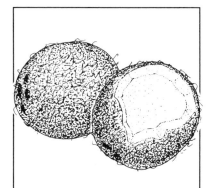

THE TRUTH ABOUT SATURATED FAT

Although we don't normally consider saturated fat as an essential nutrient, it is just as essential to good health as the essential polyunsaturated fatty acids. We need saturated fat for proper digestive function, growth, and a host of other processes. In fact, saturated fat is an essential component of every cell. It is so important to proper function and good health that nature has incorporated saturated fat into almost all of the foods we eat both of animal and plant origin. Even the so-called polyunsaturated oils like safflower oil, corn oil, and even flaxseed oil contain saturated fat. The World Health Organization and even the American Heart Association recommends that we get saturated fat in our diet to maintain optimal health. This type of information is usually ignored because saturated fat is considered a health hoodlum lurking in our food just to cause problems, and the less we eat the better. But this is simply not true. Why has nature considered saturated fat so important to include it in all our foods? Nature doesn't do things just for the fun of it. In nature there is always a reason for everything. Nature doesn't put saturated fat in vegetables, mother's milk, and other foods for kicks. It's there for a reason.

The Food and Agriculture Organization (FAO) and the World Health Organization (WHO), two international committees, recommend a polyunsaturated to saturated fat ratio (P:S) of 0.6:1.0. Or almost twice as much saturated fat as polyunsaturated fat in the diet. The membrane of our cells preferentially chooses saturated and monounsaturated fat for incorporation into its structure.[1] Only in a few specialized structures are the polyunsaturated fats preferentially selected over saturated and monounsaturated fatty acids.

Since the proposal of the cholesterol hypothesis, saturated fat has been tagged a dietary monster, sneaking into our foods to cause heart disease, cancer, and a host of other health problems that now plague Western civilization. Isn't it interesting that saturated fat has been a staple part of the human diet for thousands of years and yet only recently has it turned bad, or so they say. In reality, saturated fat isn't as bad as it has been portrayed; most of this negative publicity is profit motivated. Polyunsaturated vegetable oils, with few exceptions, are relatively new to the human diet. Their use corresponds precisely with the decline in human health in Western nations.

Cholesterol and saturated fat have been tagged as the biggest dietary villains of all time. As I have shown in the last chapter, cholesterol is not as bad as it is made out to be. It is, in fact, vital to good health, a necessary component of every cell and the basic building block for brain tissue.

"The greatest discovery of any generation is that human beings can alter their lives by altering the attitudes of their minds."
—Albert Schweitzer

"An old error is always more popular than a new truth."
—German Proverb

As knowledge of dietary cholesterol has increased, its status as a troublemaker has fallen somewhat. As a result, more heat has been placed on saturated fat, which is now considered a much more serious problem. According to the cholesterol theory, coronary artery disease is caused by cholesterol buildup in arteries, so why is saturated fat condemned? Saturated fat is attacked because our bodies can turn it into cholesterol. We get more cholesterol from saturated fat than we do from the cholesterol in our food. But this native cholesterol, which is made by our liver, is the material used to build healthy cells and is not the "oxidized" cholesterol that finds its way inside artery walls. So eating saturated fat contributes little, if anything, to the development of atherosclerosis and heart disease.

It is because of the cholesterol hypothesis that saturated fat is condemned. Since ordinary cholesterol is not a factor in the development of heart disease, saturated fat, likewise, is not as big a problem as it is made out to be.

Saturated fats, like the polyunsaturated fats, come in families consisting of several members. And like polyunsaturated fats, each individual saturated fat has a different effect on the body. A few saturated fats do increase the tendency of blood to clot (increasing platelet stickiness). But vegetable oil, particularly linoleic acid (omega-6), is more of a problem because it produces PGE2 which also stimulates platelet stickiness as well as constricting blood vessels and increasing blood pressure, all of which can contribute to cardiovascular disease. Saturated fat also doesn't produce harmful free radicals or become oxidized like polyunsaturated fats do and, therefore, is not nearly as destructive.

History has proven this fact. Our ancestors lived on a diet rich in grease, lard, and butter. Those were the only oils they ever used. It wasn't until the 20th century that vegetable oils became widely available. Use of oils rich in saturated fat have declined over time while vegetable oils have skyrocketed. Along with the greater use of vegetable oil and the decreased use of saturated fat has come a plague of degenerative diseases that the world has never known before. To blame cholesterol and saturated fat for the heart disease, cancer, and other degenerative diseases does not fit the facts and is inconsistent with the historical record.

There are many types of saturated fat that do not harm the cardiovascular system. Their primary purpose is to supply energy for the body and building materials for cellular components. Since saturated fat does not degenerate into destructive free radicals, they do not prematurely age the body or put a strain on the antioxidant and immune systems of the body. They provide nutrients and cellular building blocks necessary for metabolism and growth without causing any of the harm that polyunsaturated oils do. It's no wonder our ancestors could eat a meal of roasted beef fat, or

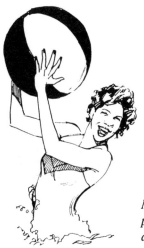

Many saturated fats promote better health and are good for you.

fry all their meals in lard, or make a sandwich by spreading a thick coat of bacon fat between two slices of bread. This type of fat did them no harm, at least not like the vegetable oils we use nowadays.

There have been many studies that demonstrate that saturated fat is not nearly as bad as it has been made out to be. If saturated-fat consumption caused heart disease then eliminating it from the diet would prevent the illness. The *Lancet* reported a study of 2,000 men who went on a low saturated-fat diet to see how that would affect cardiovascular health. The study found that those participants who went on diets low in saturated fat didn't experience any reduction in heart attack death risk over a two-year period.[2] If eliminating saturated fat didn't stop heart disease from developing, it is logical to assume there is another cause.

Researchers have shown in animal studies that saturated fatty acids actually help to prevent stroke rather than cause it. In particular, Dr. Yamori[3] reported decreased stroke incidence among rats fed a high-fat, high-cholesterol diet. In addition, Dr. Ikeda[4] demonstrated a decreased stroke risk among rats fed a diet high in milk fat.

Two ecological studies in the 1980s from Japan found correlations between increased fat intake and decreased death from ischemic stroke in humans.[5, 6] In another cohort study of Japanese men living in Hawaii, intake of both total fat and saturated fat was inversely associated with all stroke mortality, after adjustment for multiple risk factors.[7] These studies were generally ignored because they were contrary to the prevailing belief that saturated fat promotes ischemic stroke rather than protects us from it.

On December 24, 1997, headlines around the world proclaimed that saturated fat *lowers* rate of strokes. This pronouncement came after the publication of a 20-year study performed by Dr. Matthew Gillman and colleagues at Harvard Medical School and published in the *Journal of the American Medical Association*.[8] The study involved 832 men aged 45 through 65 years of age who were initially free of cardiovascular disease. The results of the study raised howls of protest from health experts who had spent years trying to teach (brainwash) us to eat less saturated fat. Yet many researchers familiar with fat metabolism and cardiovascular disease were not surprised at the results of this study.

The purpose of the Harvard study was to examine the association of stroke incidence with intake of fat and type of fat during 20 years of follow-up among middle-aged men participating in the Framingham Heart Study. In conformity with other studies performed in Japan, intakes of saturated fat were associated with *reduced* risk of ischemic stroke in men. The study also showed that the *highest* incidence of stroke was associated with the most *polyunsaturated fat* consumption.

Again, polyunsaturated oils were linked to cardiovascular disease more than saturated fat. It's ironic that the oils that are safest to eat are condemned the most, and those that cause the most problems are hailed as "healthy." Why are people ignoring these facts? It is sad that politics and money have such a great influence.

If all of this is true, why have there been so many studies reporting bad effects from eating saturated fat? There are four major reasons: (1) Many of the early studies used hydrogenated fat as their source of saturated fat. We now know that hydrogenated fats produce trans fatty acids which have a detrimental effect on health. (2) To some degree most studies either consciously or subconsciously reflect the bias of the researchers or funding organization. Data can be preferentially selected or manipulated to present results favorable to preconceived beliefs or financial interests. It's almost comical to read some of the reports and see the gymnastics the researches have taken to design studies that will give the results they desire. Unfortunately, when the results of these studies are reported in the media there is no mention of their validity, as long as they agree with the generally accepted belief at the time, they're accepted as true. (3) Many of the studies do not measure saturated fat intake directly but measure foods containing fat. The highest concentration of saturated fat is in meat and dairy products. In fact, there is much more protein in these foods than fat. So, these studies are not really measuring the effect of saturated fat on health, but rather the effects of meat or protein. The preconceived notion that fat is the culprit has shifted blame away from excess protein consumption, a much more likely cause of ill health. (4) The biggest criticism of saturated fat is that it can raise cholesterol levels and, therefore, it must cause heart disease and other health problems. As you have seen from the previous chapter, blood cholesterol is not a problem you need to be too much concerned about.

When you take in to account all the above facts saturated fat becomes a relatively harmless food if eaten in moderation. In some cases it can even promote better health.

A NEW HEALTH FOOD

There is a new health food sweeping the nation. This remarkable product can protect you from the effects of many degenerative diseases, aid you in losing unwanted weight, give your skin a more youthful appearance, and help you feel years younger. Technically, it really isn't new, it's been used for thousands of years in the Far East as a food and as a medicine. While not exactly new, its health benefits have only recently been revealed to the rest of the world. What is this amazing substance? This new health food is coconut oil. Yes, ordinary coconut oil, which by the way, is predominately a saturated fat.

As food, coconuts and coconut oil have been a staple in the diets for many Polynesian and Asian peoples for thousands of years. It still is a major food source in Malaysia, Polynesia, and parts of the Philippines and India. Among these people, coconut oil has served as their sole source of cooking fat. Interestingly, the people who use these products have a much lower incidence of heart decease, hypertension, atherosclerosis, stroke, and cancer than those of us who eat modern foods, in which vegetable oils, meat, and dairy are the predominante dietary sources for fat.

These people have been consuming coconut oil and other kernel products in their daily diet without any ill effects on their health. In fact, they have regarded coconut products as health foods with medicinal value. In the traditional medical systems such as Ayurveda in India, coconut products enjoy a place of importance and are essential components of some of the medicinal preparations.

In the Western world, coconut oil has been branded a villain because of its high saturated-fat content (as much as 92 percent). Despite the negative publicity coconut oil has received in recent years, it is only due to its association with the words "saturated fat." To date, there has been no study that can show that unadulterated coconut oil has any adverse health effects (some studies cleverly use hydrogenated and heat-damaged tropical and other oils in order to manipulate data). To the contrary, research has turned up many beneficial effects unique to the tropical oils.

THE MIRACLES OF COCONUT OIL

So much has been said against saturated fats over the years that the idea that all saturated fats are harmful is firmly entrenched in our minds. It may come as a surprise to you to learn that at least some saturated fats can promote better health. There is a group of saturated fats that are unlike any other fat. These unique fats have no known harmful effects, yet do provide many health benefits. This class of saturated fats are known as short- and medium-chain saturated fatty acids, also called short- and medium-chain triglycerides.

Short-chain fatty acids (SCFA) are those whose carbon chains contain 2 to 4 carbons and are relatively rare in nature. The most common sources are found in vinegar and butter. Medium-chain fatty acids (MCFA) are those that contain between 6 to 12 carbons. They are found in moderate amounts in certain tropical plants. Long-chain fatty acids (LCFA) are those that contain over 12 carbons. They are by far the most common fatty acids in nature. Long-chain fatty acids provide the most efficient or compact energy package and thus make the best storage fats in both plants and animals. Fat cells in our bodies and those of animals are almost entirely long-chained. Shorter chained fatty acids, being less effective as energy storage units, are therefore, not produced to any appreciable degree.

Both saturated and unsaturated fats in our foods are almost entirely long-chain fatty acids. Only a very few foods contain any appreciable amount of the short- or medium-chain fatty acids and all of them are saturated. Milk contains tiny amounts of the shorter chain saturated fatty acids. These fats are concentrated in the making of butter and comprise about 12 percent of the total fat content. Palm kernel oil contains 58 percent MCFA and coconut oil 64 percent.

The length of the carbon chain has a dramatic effect on the way our bodies utilize and metabolize these fats. Coconut oil, being predominately a medium-chain saturated fat, is characterized by the properties associated with these fats.

Researchers have discovered a multitude of health benefits associated with the shorter chain saturated fatty acids. Some of the main benefits of these fatty acids are described below.

Digestion

Many of the health advantages of medium-chain fatty acids (MCFA) over long-chain fatty acids (LCFA) are due to the differences in the way our bodies metabolize these fats. Because the MCFA molecules are smaller, they require less energy and fewer enzymes to break them down for digestion. They are digested and absorbed quickly and with minimal effort.

Because MCFA are broken down quickly during digestion, pancreatic fat-digesting enzymes are not even essential.[9] This puts less strain on our pancreas and our digestive system.

Unlike other fatty acids, MCFA are absorbed directly into the portal vein and sent straight to the liver where they are, for the most part, burned as fuel much like a carbohydrate. In this respect they act more like carbohydrates than they do fats.[10]

Other fats require pancreatic enzymes to break them up into smaller units. They are then absorbed into the intestinal wall and packaged into bundles of fat and protein called lipoproteins. These lipoproteins are carried by the lymphatic system, bypassing the liver, and dumped directly into the bloodstream. As they circulate in the blood, their fatty components are distributed to all the tissues of the body. The lipoproteins get smaller and smaller, until there is little left of them. At this time they are picked up by the liver, broken apart, and used for making hormones or repackaged into another lipoprotein and sent back into the bloodstream to distribute its fatty load. Cholesterol, saturated fat, monounsaturated fat, and polyunsaturated fat are all packaged together into lipoproteins and distributed throughout the body in this way. In contrast, MCFA are converted into energy rather than stored as body fat. MCFA produce energy. Other fats produce fat.

Inside each of our cells is an organ called the mitochondria. The energy needed by the cell to carry on its functions is generated by the mitochondria. Mitochondria are encased in two membranous sacs which normally require special enzymes to transport nutrients through them. MCFA are unique in that they can easily permeate both membranes of the mitochondria without the need of enzymes and thus provide the cell with a quick and efficient source of energy. Longer chain fatty acids demand special enzymes to pull them through the double membrane and the energy production process is much slower and uses up enzymes.

Because of the above advantages, coconut oil has been a lifesaver for many people. It is used medicinally in special food preparations for those who suffer digestive disorders and have trouble digesting fats. For the same reason, it is also used in infant formula for the treatment of malnutrition. Since it is rapidly absorbed, it can deliver quick nourishment without putting excessive strain on the digestive and enzyme systems, and helps conserve the body's energy that would normally be expended in digesting other fats. Coconut oil is one of the major ingredients in most infant formulas commonly used today.

MCFA can also improve the absorption of other nutrients. The absorption of calcium and magnesium and also amino acids has been found to increase when infants are fed a diet containing coconut oil.[11] Coconut oil has been used to enhance absorption and retention of calcium and magnesium when a deficiency of these minerals exist. This is especially true in the case of rickets which involves a vitamin D deficiency and the demineralization of the bones. For those who are concerned about developing osteoporosis as they get older, coconut oil may be useful in helping to slow down this degenerative process by improving mineral absorption.

Most anyone who suffers from a digestive disorder can benefit from using coconut oil. More people fit into this category than may realize. Anyone who has had their gallbladder removed would greatly benefit from using coconut oil in place of other oils.

The function of bile in the digestive process is often given little notice, but is essential. The liver produces bile at a relatively constant rate. As the bile is secreted, it drains into and is collected by the gallbladder. The gallbladder, being hollow, functions as a container to hold bile. Fats and oils in our foods stimulate the gallbladder to pump bile into the intestine. Bile is essential in the digestion of fats because it emulsifies or breaks the fat into small particles so digestive enzymes from the pancreas can break the fat down into individual fatty acids which can then be absorbed.

When the gallbladder is surgically removed, fat digestion is greatly hindered. Without the gallbladder, the bile which is continually being secreted by the liver, slowly drains into the small intestine. The tiny amount of bile that drains directly from the liver into the intestine is not enough to adequately function in fat digestion when even moderate amounts of fat are consumed. This leads to malabsorption of fat-soluble vitamins, and to digestive problems. Bile must be present in the intestine to properly absorb fat-soluble vitamins (vitamins A, D, E, K, and beta-carotene). The consequence of these problems may not be immediately noticeable, but over time will manifest themselves in a variety of ways. Metabolism of MCFA does not require bile or pancreatic enzymes, so people who have had their gallbladder removed or people who have trouble digesting fats would greatly benefit from the use of coconut oil.

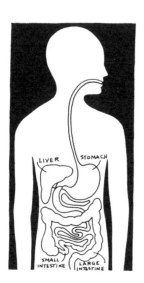

Medium-chain fatty acids (MCFA) are easily digested and quickly utilized for energy production.

Diabetics can also benefit from the use of coconut oil. As mentioned above, coconut oil puts less of a demand on the enzyme production of the pancreas. The pancreas produces insulin which pulls glucose (sugar) out of the blood and delivers it to the cells. In diabetes, the pancreas is not capable of producing adequate amounts of insulin, or the cells are not able to absorb glucose as they should. In either case, cells are deprived of glucose, the fuel they need for energy production. Coconut oil helps supply energy to cells (because it is easily absorbed without the need of enzymes) as well as improve insulin secretion and utilization of blood glucose.[12]

Weight Reduction

One of the remarkable things about coconut oil is that it can help you *lose* weight. Yes, there is a dietary fat that can actually help you take off unwanted pounds. That fat is coconut oil. Coconut oil can quite literally be called the world's only low-fat fat.

When people go on a diet to lose weight, the foods that are most restricted are those which contain the most fat. Why is fat singled out? Because it contributes the most to body fat. The fat we eat is the fat we wear—literally. When we eat fat, the fat is broken down into individual fatty acids and sent into the bloodstream where it is deposited directly into our fat cells. Other nutrients such as carbohydrate and protein are broken down and used immediately for energy. Only when we eat too much is the excess carbohydrate and protein converted into fat. As long as we eat enough to satisfy energy needs, fat in our food always ends up in our fat cells. Only between meals when physical activity outpaces energy reserves is fat removed from storage and burned for fuel.

MCFA are different. They do not circulate in the bloodstream like other fats, but are sent directly to the liver where they are immediately converted into energy—just like a carbohydrate. So when you eat coconut oil, the body uses it immediately to make energy rather than body fat. As a consequence, you can eat much more coconut oil than you can other oils before the excess is converted to body fat. The weight-loss effects of coconut oil have clearly been demonstrated by many researchers.[13, 14, 15]

Overeating any food will add additional pounds to our waistlines. But different foods affect us differently. Another reason fat is restricted on most weight loss diets is because gram for gram it contains more calories than either carbohydrate or protein. When completely broken down in the body, a gram of carbohydrate provides about 4 calories, a gram of protein also provides 4; but a gram of fat provides 9 calories—more than twice as much. So fat is twice as fattening as carbohydrate or protein.

All fats, whether they be saturated or unsaturated, from a cow or from corn, contain the same amount of calories. Coconut oil, however, contains a little less. As you recall from Chapter 1, all fats are made of triglycerides—three fatty acids attached to a glycerol molecule. Because medium-chain fatty acids are smaller than other fatty acids, coconut oil contains more glycerol per gram than other oils. This is important because glycerol is an alcohol and, as such, yields only 7 calories per gram. So coconut oil has *less* fat than other oils. Coconut oil has at least 2.56 percent fewer calories per gram of fat compared with that of long-chain fatty acids.[16] This means that by using coconut oil in place of other oils your calorie intake is less.

The reduction in calorie content and the fact that MCFA are burned as energy rather than stuffed away as body fat aren't the only reasons for coconut oil's status as a low-fat fat. Perhaps the best reason is its effect on our metabolism.

Often people have weight problems because their metabolism is slow. That is, they burn calories at a slower rate than someone who has a higher metabolism. If calories are used up slowly, less food is needed to fuel bodily functions. A person with a slow metabolism will put on more weight because the energy isn't needed. This is why one person can eat like a gorilla and look as skinny as a bird, while someone else can eat like a bird and still pack on weight.

If you could rev up your metabolism, you would burn up more calories and be able to eat more without adding excess pounds. MCFA can do that for you. In fact, they actually promote weight loss! MCFA shift the body's metabolism into a higher gear, so to speak, so that you burn off more calories. This happens every time you eat MCFA.

MCFA promote weight loss by *increasing* the metabolic rate. A dietary fat that takes off weight rather than putting it on is a strange concept indeed, but that is exactly what happens, so long as calories in excess of the body's needs are not consumed. The reason for this is due to the fact that they are easily absorbed and rapidly burned and used as energy for metabolism. This increase in metabolic activity even fuels the burning of the LCFA.[17] So not only are medium-chain fatty acids burned for energy production, but they encourage the consumption of long-chain fatty acids as well.

Dr. Julian Whitaker, a well-known authority on nutrition and health, makes this analogy between the long-chain triglycerides (LCT) and medium-chain triglycerides (MCT): "LCTs are like heavy wet logs that you put on a small campfire. Keep adding the logs, and soon you have more logs than fire. MCTs are like rolled up newspaper soaked in gasoline. They not only burn brightly, but will burn up the wet logs as well."[18]

Research supports Dr. Whitaker's view. In one study the thermogenic (fat burning) effect of a high-calorie diet

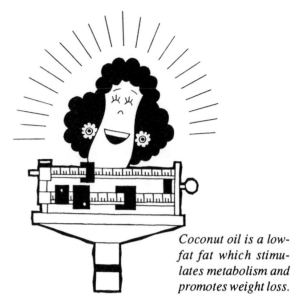

Coconut oil is a low-fat fat which stimulates metabolism and promotes weight loss.

containing 40% fat as MCFAs, was compared to one containing 40% fat as LCFAs. The thermogenic effect of the MCFAs was almost twice as high as the LCFAs, 120 calories versus 66 calories. The researchers concluded that the excess energy provided by fats in the form of MCFAs would not be efficiently stored as fat, but rather would be burned. A followup study demonstrated that MCFAs given over a six-day period can increase diet-induced thermogenesis by 50%.[19]

In another study, researchers compared single meals of 400 calories composed entirely of MCFAs and of LCFAs.[20] The thermogenic effect of MCFAs over six hours was three times greater than that of LCFAs. Researchers concluded that substituting MCFAs for LCFAs would produce weight loss as long as the calorie level remained the same.

Coconut oil contains the most concentrated source of MCFA available. Substituting coconut oil for other vegetable oils in your diet will help promote weight loss. The use of vegetable oils actually promotes weight gain, not just from its calorie content, but because of its harmful effects on the thyroid—the gland that controls our metabolism. Polyunsaturated vegetable oils depress thyroid activity, thus lowering metabolic rate—just the opposite of coconut oil. Eating vegetable oils will contribute more to weight gain than any other fat known even more than beef tallow and lard. According to Ray Peat, Ph.D., an endocrinologist who specializes in the study of hormones, unsaturated oils block thyroid hormone secretion, its movement in the circulation, and the response of tissues to the hormone. When thyroid hormones are deficient, metabolism becomes depressed.[21] Polyunsaturated vegetable oils are, in essence, a high-fat fat and encourage weight gain more than any other type of fat.

While controlling weight is desirable for appearances sake, it is also important for our health. Being overweight has become one of our biggest health problems. In the United States, as much as 25 percent of all teenagers and

50 percent of all adults are obese. A person is obese if he or she is more than 20 percent above ideal weight. This is easy to do on the typical Western diet loaded with sugary, polyunsaturated fat-filled foods. If you are overweight, losing some pounds could be one of the healthiest things you can do for yourself. Substituting coconut oil for polyunsaturated oils would be a smart step in that direction. Doing so will help you reduce your chances of developing the conditions listed in the table below.

Farmers are always looking for ways to fatten their livestock because big animals bring big bucks. Fats and oils have been used as an additive in animal feed as a means of quickly packing on weight in preparing them for market. Saturated fat would seem like a good choice to fatten up livestock and pig farmers tried to use coconut oil on their animals for this purpose, but when it was added to the animal feed, the pigs lost weight![22] Farmers found that the high polyunsaturated oil content of corn and soybeans were able to do what the coconut oil couldn't. Animals fed corn and soybeans packed on pounds quickly and easily. The reason these oils worked so well is that the polyunsaturated oils suppressed thyroid function decreasing the animal's metabolic rate. They could eat less food and gain more weight! Many people are in a similar situation. Every time we eat polyunsaturated oils our thyroid gland is assaulted and loses its ability to function normally. Weight gain is one of the consequences.

Common Health Problems Associated With Obesity

In General:
- Abdominal hernias
- Arthritis (especially in the knees, hips, and lower spine)
- Gout
- Coronary heart disease
- Hypertension
- Respiratory problems
- Varicose veins
- Atherosclerosis
- Diabetes
- Gastrointestinal disorders

For Men:
- Cancers of the colon, rectum, and prostate gland

For Women:
- Gynecological irregularities
- Pregnancy-induced hypertension
- Cancers of the breast, uterus, ovaries, gallbladder, and bile ducts

Cardiovascular Health

All of the criticism that has been aimed at coconut oil is based solely on the fact that it is a saturated fat and saturated fat is known to increase blood cholesterol. No legitimate research, however, has ever demonstrated any proof that coconut-oil consumption raises blood cholesterol levels.

The MCFA of coconut oil are burned almost immediately for energy production and so are not converted into cholesterol and do not affect blood cholesterol levels. Numerous studies have demonstrated that coconut oil has a *neutral* effect on cholesterol levels.[23, 24, 25, 26, 27, 28, 29]

Even the ratio of HDL (good) cholesterol to LDL (bad) cholesterol is not changed.[30] While coconut oil's direct effect on blood cholesterol may be neutral, it may in effect lower LDL (bad) cholesterol and increase HDL (good) cholesterol. This is because of its stimulatory effect on the metabolism. One of the factors that increases blood cholesterol is low metabolism. Because coconut oil stimulates metabolism it actually protects against high cholesterol.

In one study performed in the Philippines, for example, ten medical students tested diets consisting of different levels of animal fat and coconut oil. Animal fat is known to raise blood cholesterol. Total calories from dietary fat consisted of 20 percent, 30 percent, and 40 percent using different combinations of coconut oil and animal fat. At all three levels with a ratio of 1:1, 1:2, and 1:3, saturated fat to coconut oil, no significant change in cholesterol levels were observed. Only when the ratio was reversed so that animal fat consumption was greater than coconut oil and total fat calories reached 40 percent was a significant increase in blood cholesterol reported. This study demonstrated that not only did coconut oil have no effect on cholesterol levels, it even reduced the cholesterol-elevating effects of animal fat.[31] Anyone who says coconut oil contributes to high blood cholesterol is either ignorant of the facts regarding MCFA or has some financial interest at stake.

An even more important factor in relation to cardiovascular health is the blood's tendency to form clots. Special proteins in the blood called platelets cause clotting when they become sticky. Numerous studies have demonstrated that all fats—beef fat, lard, butter, vegetable oil, and even canola and olive oils—promote platelet stickiness. The more you eat, the stickier the blood gets, and the greater the risk of developing blood clots. The omega-3 fatty acids, like those found in fish oil, are an exception. They have the opposite effect on blood platelets. This is the main reason why they have been recommended for those at risk of heart disease. Too much, however, which is easy to do with dietary supplements, can interfere with normal blood clotting, and that can be just as dangerous. When this happens, blood vessels weaken and can rupture with the slightest degree of stress. Twenty-five percent of all strokes are caused by excessive bleeding within the brain.

Another group of fats that don't promote platelet stickiness are the MCFA. These fats are burned up immediately after consumption and, therefore, do not affect platelet stickiness either one way or the other. Of all the dietary fats, MCFA are the most benign.

People who traditionally consume large quantities of coconut oil as a part of their ordinary diet have a very low incidence of heart disease and have normal blood cholesterol levels. This has been well supported by epidemiological observations recorded in many studies. Those populations who consume large quantities of coconut oil have remarkably good cardiovascular health. Absent are the heart attacks and strokes characteristic in Western countries. After analyzing all available studies and reviewing epidemiological evidence, author and coconut researcher, P.K. Thampan, concludes that there is absolutely no correlation between coconut oil consumption and heart disease.[32] If anything, coconut oil consumption is heart healthy.

The native populations of the Polynesian Islands are high coconut consumers and derive most of their energy from coconut. In a study of the native populations of two islands Pukapuka and Tokelau it was observed that the male population of the two groups derive 35.2 percent and 55.7 per cent respectively of their energy requirements mostly from coconut. In both groups, the female population had a comparatively high intake of fat calories. The levels of blood cholesterol among the Pukapukans were low, ranging from 170 mg/dl to 176 mg/dl, despite a high fat intake. Among the Tokelauans, whose intake of fat was higher than that of the Pukapukans, the blood cholesterol levels were somewhat higher ranging between 208 mg/dl and 216 mg/dl. The prevalence of

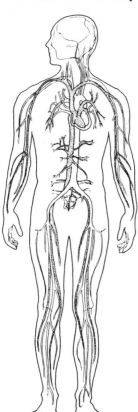

Coconut oil promotes cardiovascular health.

coronary heart disease among the two populations covered in the study was extremely low and has remained low.

In Sri Lanka coconut has been the chief source of fat in the diet for thousands of years. The average consumption in the island country has been reported to be 90 coconuts per capita annually. When the consumption of coconut oil is also taken into consideration, the total consumption in terms of coconut is 120 annually. Their heart disease rate is far lower than that of noncoconut-eating populations.

In the state of Kerala, in India, where large quantities of coconuts and coconut oil have traditionally been consumed, an average 2.3 out of 1,000 people suffered from coronary heart disease in 1979. A campaign against the use of coconut oils on the grounds that it is an "unhealthy" saturated fat decreased coconut oil consumption during the 1980s. Vegetables oils replaced it in household use. As a result, the heart disease rate shot up to 7 per 1,000 people by 1993. By substituting vegetable oils for coconut oil, the heart disease rate tripled! In Delhi where the consumption of coconut products is negligible, 10 out of 1,000 people had heart disease in the same time period.[33] In Western countries where vegetable oil is the main source of fat, heart disease accounts for nearly half of all deaths. It seems that if you want to protect yourself from heart disease, you should replace your polyunsaturated vegetable oils with coconut oil.

Antimicrobial

We live in an environment teaming with microorganisms. They are in the air we breath, the food we eat, the water we drink, and even live on our skin. Nature has provided plants and animals with a variety of defense mechanisms to protect themselves from attack by harmful pests.

One of the unique characteristics of coconut oil is its antimicrobial properties. Coconut oil is, in essence, a natural antibacterial, antiviral, and antifungal food.[34, 35] Coconuts grow in warm tropical climates where bacteria and other organisms live in abundance. Coconuts have developed a natural resistance to this swarm of potentially harmful microorganisms by using nature's own antimicrobial defense force—medium-chain fatty acids.

Coconut oil is composed of 48 percent lauric acid (a 12-chain saturated fat), 7 percent capric acid (a 10-chain saturated fat), 8 percent caprylic acid (an eight-chain saturated fat), and .5 percent caproic acid (a six-chain saturated fat). These medium-chain fatty acids, which make up the triglyceride molecules, form the antimicrobial properties of coconut oil. These are generally absent from all other vegetable and animal oils, with the exception of butter.

Human breast milk and the milk of other mammals all contain MCFA. This is why butter has a significant amount of MCFA. These fatty acids protect the newborn baby from harmful germs at its most vulnerable time in life while its immune system is still developing. Coconut oil is added to infant formula as protection and because it supplies easily digestible nutrients. Since our bodies mirror the food we eat, nursing mothers who avoid eating saturated fat, will produce less MCT for their babies. A mother who consumes coconut oil will have more MCFA in her milk to help protect and nourish her baby.

Our bodies have many ways of protecting us from microorganisms that can cause us harm. The strong acid excreted in our stomachs, for example, kills most organisms that we eat along with our foods. In our bloodstream, microorganisms are attacked and killed by our white blood cells. Our first line of defense against any harmful organism is our skin. In order to inflict harm, microorganisms must first penetrate the skin's protective barrier. While the skin is permeable to some degree, it is also equipped with chemical weapons to help it ward off attack. One of these weapons is the oil secreted by our sebaceous glands (oil glands). Sebaceous glands are found near the root of every one of our hairs. This oil is secreted along the hair shaft to lubricate the hair and skin. Some have described this oil as "natures's skin cream" because it prevents drying and cracking of the skin. It also contains medium-chain fatty acids to fight invading microorganisms.

A person who eats lots of vegetable oils will have less MCFA in their oil glands and thus dilute the germ-fighting capacity of the oil. Frequent washings will also remove this oil, exposing the skin to infectious organisms. This may be one of the reasons why acne is common among those in the Western countries, but rare in cultures that eat traditional diets void of processed vegetable oils. Eating less vegetable oil and more coconut oil will help replenish the body's MCFA reserves and help fight acne.

Another common skin problem that plagues mankind is fungal infections. Skin fungus afflicts many people in form of ringworm, jock itch, and athlete's foot. Skin fungus can afflict any part of the body from the head to the toe. Many people have fungal infections without even realizing it. Dry flaky skin that persists despite the use of hand lotion and skin creams could very well be a fungal infection. Often what people call psoriasis is really a fungal infection. Dandruff is caused, in part, by skin fungus.

Preadolescent children are the primary victims of scalp ringworm (tinea capitis), a skin fungus similar to athlete's foot. Not until puberty do glands secrete oil containing fatty acids that protect the scalp from skin fungus.

One of the most widespread health problems in Western society is candidiasis. Candidiasis is an infection caused by the fungus *Candida albacans*. Many women are familiar with this troublesome pest because it is a common cause of vaginal yeast infections. It is also the same organism that causes oral thrush and diaper rash in babies. Systemic candida infections can cause a myriad of symptoms ranging from headaches to intestinal pain. Candida is a single-celled fungus or yeast cell that inhabits the intestinal tract of every living person on the earth. Within days after birth, newborns are infected and have a budding colony living in their digestive tract. Normally, competition from friendly bacteria and the cleansing action of our immune system keeps candida numbers low and prevents them from causing any adverse health problems. But when the immune system is compromised or friendly bacteria in our gut are killed by taking antibiotics, a candida infection can quickly flair up. A single course of antibiotics (which does not harm yeast) can lead to a candida infection.

The most potent non-drug or natural yeast-fighting substance is caprylic acid, a medium-chain fatty acid derived from coconut oil. Polynesian women who live their native lifestyles rarely ever get yeast infections. Caprylic acid is commonly sold as a dietary supplement in health food stores. It is very effective against candida and other forms of fungi. It is even effective mixed with a little coconut oil or vitamin E oil as a topical application for fungal skin infections. I've seen fungal infections that have lasted for months clear up in a matter of days using caprylic acid and a little coconut oil. It works just as effectively inside the body killing fungi without the least bit of harm. Eating coconut oil on a regular basis, like the Polynesians do, would help to keep candida and other harmful microorganisms at bay.

It is interesting that people who eat a lot of coconuts live in areas where bacteria and fungi are extremely plentiful, yet they are rarely troubled by infections. Only in more temperate climates where vegetable oils are the main source of dietary fat, are skin fungus, acne, and other skin infections big problems.

Immune System Support

Polyunsaturated oils put a heavy strain on the immune system. They act as toxins overburdening the white blood cells and draining the body's antioxidant reserves. Polyunsaturated oils cause the immune system to shift into feverish activity while at the same time interfering with its ability to form protective compounds. Antioxidants are quickly used up fighting free radicals produced by the unsaturated oils. When antioxidants such as vitamins A, C, and E become depleted, the immune system slows down and becomes less effective. Vegetable oils produce an overall depressive effect on the immune system.

Coconut oil, on the other hand, supports the immune system. It causes no stress. Coconut oil is not toxic to the body so does not burden the immune system. Saturated fats are very stable and do not oxidize easily, so antioxidants are not used up.

The antimicrobial and anitparasitic properties of the MCFA also aid in reducing the stress that would otherwise be placed on the immune system. The immune system wages a constant battle with disease-causing microorganisms. Coconut oil provides artillery to help fight these invading organisms, thus reducing stress on the immune system which allows the immune system to function more efficiently. Studies with coconut oil have shown it to improve immune response to pathogenic bacteria.[36]

Sixty-three percent of coconut oil is composed of antimicrobial medium-chain fatty acids, and therefore, can be a powerful ally with the immune system in its fight against microscopic invaders. Coconut oil is ideal for immune-suppressed individuals. Oil researcher, Dr. Mary Enig, has proposed giving coconut and palm kernel oils to AIDS patients to help protect them against infections.

Next time you're sick with a viral or bacterial infection, do you want to depress your immune system even more and lengthen the duration of your sickness by eating foods containing polyunsaturated vegetable oils? Or would you like to boost your germ fighting ability with coconut oil?

Food Preservation

Coconut oil makes an ideal dietary oil not only for its health benefits, but because it doesn't spoil like other oils do. Polyunsaturated oils begin to go rancid before they leave the factory and long before you buy them at the grocery store. The extraction and processing operations cause oxidation and free-radical formation from the very start. And the longer they sit, the more free radicals they form. You have no idea how long these oils have been on the grocery shelf or in the distributor's warehouse or what conditions they were shipped in. Were they shipped in a hot truck or kept refrigerated? Since they are almost always on the grocery shelf without refrigeration, you can bet they were shipped in a hot truck. Heat, as well as light, accelerates oxidation. When the oils are on the store shelf, are they exposed to light? Yes, they are put in clear plastic bottles and placed in the store aisles were they are fully exposed to light.

After you bring them home, do you store them in the refrigerator where it is dark and cool? Probably not. The older they get, the more oxidized they become and the more dangerous they are to your health.

Coconut oil is made up of 92 percent saturated fat with only 2 percent polyunsaturated. Saturated fats aren't oxidized easily and, therefore, don't spoil as quickly as polyunsaturated vegetable oils. According to Leigh Broadhurst, Ph.D., a scientist at the USDA Human Nutrition Research Center in Beltville, Maryland, saturated fatty acids are 300

or more times more resistant to oxidation than alpha-linolenic acid (flaxseed oil). In other words, coconut oil will remain fresh 300 times longer than flaxseed oil. For instance, to equal the amount of oxidative damage that occurs in flaxseed oil in just 30 minutes of processing, coconut oil would have to be subjected to the same conditions for 150 continuous hours—that's over six days!

Because of coconut oil's antimicrobial properties, it isn't affected easily by microorganisms either. Oxidation, bacteria, and fungi are a food's worst enemies. Coconut oil, being resistant to all of these, is a safe product with a long shelf life. Manufacturers have known this for decades. Coconut oil has long been used for this purpose. Coconut oil can be safely stored, unrefrigerated, for two years or more without it going rancid. No other oil can do that and still remain even marginally edible.

When used in cooking, coconut oil is much more stable than unsaturated vegetable oils. It can be heated and reheated without producing damaging free radicals.[37] Coconut oil has a very mild flavor that is unnoticeable in foods. For cooking, it is the best oil you can use. Because it has a texture like butter, it can be used in recipes wherever butter, margarine, or shortening is called for.

Protection Against Disease

Coconut oil may be useful in preventing a wide assortment of diseases. Because of its unique metabolic properties, it can help shed unwanted weight, thus reducing the risk of many health problems associated with obesity. Since the 1950s it has been used to treat malabsorption problems in adults and infants. People who eat coconut oil on a daily basis have little or no cardiovascular disease, so it may provide protection against heart disease and atherosclerosis. Dr. Robert L. Wickremasinghe, head of the serology division at the Medical Research Institute in Sri Lanka, reports that coconut oil may even possess anti-carcinogenic properties. Studies have shown that coconut oil inhibits the induction of carcinogenic agents of colon as well as mammary tumors in test animals.[38]

Probably the biggest advantage to using coconut oil is that it can displace the use of unsaturated vegetable oils that are known to be involved in the development of numerous diseases as well as premature aging. While coconut oil may not prevent or cure all these conditions directly, it can limit the amount of potentially toxic polyunsaturated oil in our bodies and thus reduce our chances of suffering prematurely

> Coconut oil improves the texture of foods and helps keep them fresh and safe to eat.

from degenerative disease. It is an oil that is relatively benign in its effects as compared to unsaturated oils. In that respect it protects from many diseases that are encouraged by vegetable oils.

Body Lotion

For thousands of years coconut oil has been use to make the skin soft and smooth. Polynesian women are famed for their beautiful skin, even though they are exposed every day to the hot blistering sun and the chafing of the ocean breeze. As a skin lotion, no other oil can compare.

Because coconut oil has a natural creamy texture, comes from a vegetable source, and is almost always free from pesticides and other chemicals and contaminants, it has been used for years in soaps, creams, and other body care products. Its small molecular structure allows for easy absorption, giving the skin a soft smooth texture. It makes an ideal ointment for the relief of dry, rough, and wrinkled skin. It can be used in its natural form without adulteration by chemicals and other additives. For this purpose, it has been for many years, and still is, commonly used as a body cream.

Coconut oil makes the perfect body lotion. Antiseptic fatty acids in coconut oil help to prevent fungal and bacterial infections on skin. The Polynesians who use it regularly are never troubled by skin infections or acne.

Most other hand and body lotions promote dry skin. Commercial creams are predominantely water. This moisture is quickly absorbed into dry wrinkled skin. As the water enters the skin, it expands the tissues, like filling a balloon with water, so that wrinkles fade away and skin feels smoother. But this is only temporary. As soon as the blood can carry this excess water away, the dry wrinkled skin returns. Have you ever permanently cured dry wrinkled skin with any body lotion? It can't be done. Another ingredient in most lotions is oil or some type. It may be jojoba, almond, apricot kernel, lavender, or a host of others. Unless they use coconut oil, they all have one thing in common. They all contain unsaturated oils. What consequence does this have in a skin lotion? Lots!

All oils are absorbed easily through skin. Polyunsaturated oils in body lotions and creams penetrate the skin and are absorbed into the tissues and bloodstream. They may produce a temporary improvement against dry skin, but polyunsaturated oils will make your skin even worse over time. Free-radical deterioration of these oils ages skin, making it dry, leathery, and wrinkled. As the skin becomes dryer and more wrinkled, more lotion is used. The more lotion that is used the worse the skin becomes. It's a vicious cycle. Studies show that dry skin contains a higher content of unsaturated fatty acids (60%) compared to normal skin (49%).[39] The best oil to use is one that doesn't create free

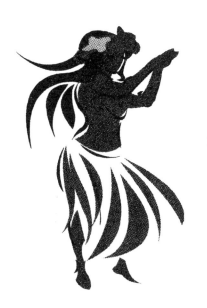

radicals. Saturated fats fit that requirement. The ideal skin lotion is pure coconut oil with a little bit of vitamin E oil. This combination will protect your skin from germs and free radicals as well as soften skin and strengthen the underlying connective tissues.

With all the advantages listed above, coconut oil can be considered the health food of the future. It has been the health food of many people for thousands of years. We can all benefit.

THE PUKAPUKA AND TOKELAU ISLAND STUDIES

If coconut oil is as good as it appears to be from laboratory studies, you would think that there might be some real life examples confirming what the studies show. And you're right, there is. It has long been noted that people in Polynesia and Asia whose diets are high in saturated fat from coconuts are surprisingly free from cardiovascular disease, cancer, and other degenerative diseases. Since saturated fat has been tagged as a major culprit in the development of these diseases, it seems an enigma that people who have diets higher in saturated fat than those in North America and Europe are much less prone to degenerative disease. Coconuts are used extensively in the diet in many different parts of the world. In these populations coronary heart disease is rare.

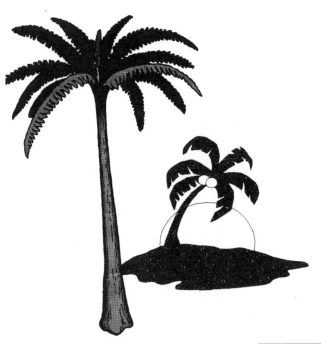

Pukapuka and Tokelau are part of the Cook Islands located in the South Pacific.

Some of the most thorough research conducted on people who have a high-fat diet derived primarily from coconuts are the Pukapuka and Tokelau Island studies. These studies involved many researchers and extended for over a decade.

The Islands of Pukapuka and Tokelau lie near the equator in the South Pacific. Pukapuka is an atoll in the Northern Cooks Islands and Tokelau, another atoll, lies about 400 miles southeast. The populations of both islands have been relatively isolated from Western influences. Their native diet and culture remain much as it has for centuries. Pukapuka and Tokelau are among the more isolated Polynesian islands and have had relatively little interaction with non-Polynesians.

The coral sands of these atolls are porous, lack humus, and will not support the food plants that flourish on other tropical islands. Coconut palms and a few starchy tropical fruits and root vegetables supply the vast majority of their diets. Fish from the ocean, pigs, and

chickens make up what little meat they eat. Some flour, rice, sugar, and canned meat are obtained from small cargo ships that occasionally visit the islands.

The standard diets on both islands are high is saturated fat derived from coconuts, but low in cholesterol. The diet is high in fiber, but low in sugar. The major food source is coconuts. Every meal contains coconut in some form: the green nut provides the main beverage; the mature nut, grated or as coconut cream, is cooked with taro root, breadfruit or rice; and small pieces of coconut meat make an important snack food. Plants and fruitfish are cooked with coconut oil. In Tokelau, coconut sap or toddy is used as a sweetener and as leavening for bread.

The studies were begun in the early 1960s and included the entire populations of both islands. This was a long-term multidisciplinary study set up to examine the physical, social, and health consequences of migration from the atolls to New Zealand which has jurisdiction over the islands. The

Table 8-1.   BODY FAT COMPARISONS

Fatty acid composition of the adipose tissue lipids of Tokelauans, Pukapukans, and New Zealand Europeans

Fatty acids	Tokelauans	Pukapukans	NZ Europeans
10:0	0.1	0.3	0.1
12:0	10.4	11.5	0.3
13:0	Trace	0.3	0
14:0	17.3	16.4	4.2
15:0	0.3	0.5	0.5
16:0	20.0	20.4	23.3
17:0	0.3	0.5	0.6
18:0	2.8	2.5	5.0
20:0	0.4	0.2	0.5
Total saturated	**51.6**	**52.6**	**34.5**
12:1	1.2	1.1	0
14:1	3.3	3.0	0
15:1	0.1	0.1	0
16:1	10.0	9.6	9.0
17:1	0.6	0.6	0
18:1	27.8	29.0	49.4
18:2	3.8	3.2	3.0
18:3	0.4	0.1	0.8
19:1	Trace	0.1	0.3
20:1	0	0	0
20:4	1.2	0.6	1.0
Total unsaturated	**48.4**	**47.4**	**63.5**

Source: Shorland FB, Czochanska Z, Prior IAM. Studies on fatty acid composition of adipose tissue and blood lipids of Polynesians. Am J Clin Nutr 1969; 22:594.

total population of the two islands consisted of about 2,500 people.

The overall health of both groups was good. There were no signs of kidney disease nor hypothyroidism that might influence fat levels. No hypercholesterolemia (high blood cholesterol). All inhabitants were lean and healthy despite a very high saturated-fat diet. In fact, the populations as a whole had ideal weight-to-height ratios as compared to the Body Mass Index figures used by nutritionists. Digestive problems are rare. Constipation uncommon. They average two or more bowel movements a day. Atherosclerosis, heart disease, colitis, colon cancer, hemorrhoids, ulcers, diverticulosis, and appendicitis are conditions with which they are generally unfamiliar.

Table 8-1 compares the body fat of the islanders with that of New Zealanders of European decent. In column one the first number designates number of carbons the second number identifies number of carbon bonds. So 12:0, which is lauric acid, is a saturated fat with no double bonds; 18:1 is an unsaturated fat with one double—a monounsaturated fat; 18:2 is an unsaturated fat with two double bonds and 18:3 is an unsaturated fat with three double bonds—both polyunsaturated fats.

Note that the islanders have a significantly greater saturated fat content in their body tissues than the New Zealanders of European decent. New Zealanders have 15-16 percent more unsaturated body fat. This is important because unsaturated fat is more prone to oxidation and free-radical damage and, consequently, cancer and numerous other degenerative conditions. A higher saturated-fat diet helps to protect them from the aging processes caused by free-radical degeneration. Medium-chain fatty acids, such as those found in coconut oil, protect against high blood-fat levels and cardiovascular disease.

Even the chickens and pigs raised on these islands eat large amounts of coconut. This is reflected in the unusually high concentration of medium-chain fatty acids in their fat which, in turn, contributes to the saturated fat intake of the islanders who eat them. See table 8-2 for a comparison.

Since these animals have a relatively high lauric acid and total saturated fat content, they are healthier foods than the unsaturated animals we eat feed on a diet high in unsaturated fat. In comparison, the fat profile of pigs raised on farms in other parts of world average 41% saturated fat and 59% unsaturated; for chickens it's 31% saturated and 69% unsaturated.

Saturated Fat Consumption

The American Heart Association recommends that we get no more than 30 percent of our total calories from fat and that saturated fat should be limited to no more than 10 percent. The Tokelauans apparently aren't aware of these guidelines, because 57 percent of their energy is derived from fat and most all of that is saturated fat largely derived from coconuts. The fat in the Pukapukan diet is also primarily from saturated fatty acids from coconut with total energy from fat being 34 percent.[40] Most Americans and others who eat typical Western diets get 34-40 percent of their calories from fat, most of which is in the form of *unsaturated* vegetable oils. And they suffer from numerous degenerative conditions and weight problems. The islanders in this study consumed as much or more total fat and a far greater amount of saturated fat. Yet, they are relatively free from degenerative disease and are generally lean and healthy.

Considering the amount of saturated fat in their diet, Dr. Ian A. Prior and colleagues calculated their cholesterol

Table 8-2
FAT COMPOSITION IN PIGS AND CHICKENS

Fatty acid composition of lipids of pig and chicken fat from Tokelau, percentage fatty acid.

Fatty acids	Pork fat	Chicken fat
10:0	0.3	1.7
12:0	9.6	39.1
13:0	0.2	0.2
14:0	20.0	18.8
15:0	0.2	0.2
16:0	25.3	13.3
17:0	0.1	0.3
18:0	6.4	4.0
20:0	0.1	0.1
Total saturated	62.2	77.7
12:1	0.1	0.2
14:1	1.1	0.7
15:1	0	0
16:1	7.1	2.0
17:1	0.1	0
18:1	26.3	16.2
18:2	2.0	2.5
18:3	0.6	0.7
19:1	Trace	0.1
20:unsaturated	0.3	0
22:unsaturated	0.2	0
Total unsaturated	37.8	22.3

Source: Shorland FB, Czochanska Z, Prior IAM. Studies on fatty acid composition of adipose tissue and blood lipids of Polynesians. Am J Clin Nutr 1969; 22:594.

Table 8-3
PREDICTION OF CHOLESTEROL LEVELS FROM DIET DATA

Measured in milligrams.

	Pukapuka		Tokelau	
	Observed	Predicted	Observed	Predicted
Males	170	238	208	290
Females	176	251	216	296

Source: Prior, I.A., Davidson, F., Salmond, C.E., Czochanska, Z., Cholesterol, coconuts, and diet on Polynesian atolls: a natural experiment: the Pukapuka and Tokelau island studies. American Journal of Clinical Nutrition 34 (8): 1552-61, 1981 Aug.

levels. The calculations they used were based on rates observed in Western countries. The islanders had much lower cholesterol levels than predicted (see Table 8-3).

Actual blood cholesterol levels were 70 to 80 mg lower than predicted. Cholesterol levels were higher in Tokelau because they derived 57 percent of total calories from fat. Their total food consumption, including imported flour, rice, sugar, and meat was also higher. Dietary cholesterol and polyunsaturated fatty acids of both groups were low. These were primarily the long-chain highly unsaturated fatty acids from fish. Blood cholesterol level was believed a result of the myristic acid (14 carbon long-chain fatty acid) content of coconut fat and of the pork and chicken fat eaten on both atolls.

Pukapukans ages 25-54 consumed about 63 grams of saturated fat per day and only 7 grams of unsaturated fat. Tokelauans consumed about 130 grams of saturated fat per day and only 6 grams of unsaturated fat.

Dietary Changes Affect Health Status

The migration of Tokelau Islanders from their island atolls to the very different environment of New Zealand is associated with changes in fat intake that indicate increased risk of atherosclerosis. This is associated with an actual *decrease* in saturated fat intake from 57 percent to around 41 percent of energy, an increase in dietary cholesterol intake to 340 mg and an increase in carbohydrate and sugar. Fat changes include increased total cholesterol, higher LDL (bad cholesterol) and triglycerides, and lower HDL (good cholesterol) levels.[41]

Blood cholesterol becomes higher when they migrate to New Zealand despite the fact that the *total* fat content of

their diet drops, declining from 63% in Tokelau, with 80% of that from coconut oil, to around 43% in New Zealand.[42] They eat more white bread, rice, meat, and other Western foods and less of their high-fiber, coconut-rich foods.

Ian Prior, who headed some of the studies on these two island populations, stated: "Vascular disease is uncommon in both populations and there is no evidence of the high saturated-fat intake having a harmful effect in these populations."[43]

The conclusion we can make from these island studies is that a high saturated-fat diet, particularly one consisting of coconut oil, is not detrimental to health and does not contribute to arteriosclerosis. It appears that something else, rather than saturated fat, which is in the Western diet, but missing in traditional diets, is the primary problem. What are the foods we eat, or don't eat, that are the real problem? The biggest changes the islanders made was to reduce total fat, saturated fat, fiber, and complex carbohydrates and to increase polyunsaturated fat and simple carbohydrate (sugar and white flour) consumption. This pattern of dietary change followed by increased incidence of degenerative disease has been documented throughout the world and is discussed more fully in the next chapter.

THE TROPICAL OIL WARS

In the late 1980s, the media was in a swarm warning the public about a newly discovered health threat—popcorn. Yes, popcorn emerged as the new menace on the block. Why? Because up until that time most popcorn was popped in coconut oil. It wasn't so much the popcorn, but the coconut oil that was attacked. Coconut oil, they proclaimed, was a saturated fat and would cause heart attacks. Everywhere you turned, any product that contained coconut or palm oils was criticized as being "unhealthful." In response to the seemly overwhelming public response, movie theaters began cooking their popcorn in soybean oil. Food makers began switching from the tropical oils they had used for years to soybean oil. Restaurants stopped using tropical oils in favor of soybean and other vegetable oils. By the early 1990s, the tropical oil market had dwindled to a fraction of what it once was. The promoters of this media frenzy declared a victory in their fight against tropical oils.

This war of oils, unfortunately, made every man, woman, and child in America its victim. The only winner was the soybean industry. Why are we the victims? Because the oil that replaced coconut and palm oils was *hydrogenated* vegetable oil (principally from soybeans)—one of the most health-damaging dietary oils in existence. It's ironic that these hydrogenated replacements contain as much saturated fat as the tropical oils.[44] But they are not made from easily digested medium-chain fatty acids, but of the toxic trans fatty acids. The result has been to replace healthy tropical oils with some very nasty, chemically altered vegetable oils. We are all victims because when we eat foods containing these oils our health suffers.

Why is hydrogenated oil being used rather than ordinary vegetable oil? Saturated fat has long been the preferred ingredient in baked and prepared goods to enhance flavor and texture and prevent rancidity. Over time, tropical oils gradually replaced animals fats in many food products. Polyunsaturated vegetable oils are too liquid and spoil too quickly and, therefore, make less desirable replacements for saturated fat. Hydrogenated vegetable oils are resistant to spoilage, impart a similar taste and texture as saturate fat, and they're much cheaper to use.

Since the 1950s, research has shown the health benefits of coconut oil. So how did coconut oil become a despised artery-clogging villain? Credit the American Soybean Association (ASA) and its friends. The entire campaign was actually a carefully orchestrated plan by the ASA to eliminate competition from imported tropical oils. In 1986 the ASA sent a "Fat Fighter Kit" to soybean farmers encouraging them to write government officials, food companies, etc., protesting the encroachment of "highly saturated tropical fats like palm and coconut oils." The wives and families of some 400,000 soybean growers were encouraged to fan out across the country in a lobbying effort touting the health benefits of soybean oil. Well meaning, but misguided health groups joined in the fray, issuing news releases referring to palm, coconut, and palm kernel oils as "rich in artery-clogging fat."

Researchers familiar with tropical oils were called on to testify on the health implications of these products. "Coconut oil has a neutral effect on blood cholesterol, even in situations where coconut oil is the sole source of fat," reported Dr. George Blackburn, a Harvard Medical School researcher who testified at a congressional hearing about tropical oils held on June 21, 1988. "These (tropical) oils have been consumed as a substantial part of the diet of many groups for thousands of years with absolutely no evidence of any harmful effects to the populations consuming them," said Mary G. Enig, Ph.D., an expert on fats and oils and former research associate at the University of Maryland.[45]

Dr. C. Everett Koop, former Surgeon General of the United States, called the tropical-oil scare "foolishness." Commercial interests either trying to divert blame to others or ignorantly following the saturated-fat hysteria were "...terrorizing the public about nothing." Many misguided public interest groups have also condemned coconut oil because they believed all saturated fats were bad.

In October 1988, Nebraska millionaire Phil Sokolof, a recovered heart attack patient and founder of the National Heart Savers Association, began running full-page newspaper advertisements accusing food companies of "poisoning America" by using tropical oils with high levels of saturated fat. He staged a blistering national ad campaign attacking tropical oils as a health danger. One ad showed a coconut "bomb" with a lighted wick and cautioned consumers that their health was threatened by coconut and palm oils.

Meanwhile, tropical oil exporters from Malaysia prepared a public relations campaign against what it called "vicious scare tactics" being used against its product. The tropical oil war was in full swing. At stake was the $3 billion-a-year vegetable oil market in the United States, where the dominant domestic soy oil producers were squaring off against foreign competitors.

Major newspapers and networks picked up the anti-saturated-fat ads and developed alarming news stories. After a few weeks, McDonald's, Burger King, and Wendy's restaurants announced they would replace the saturated fat they used with more "healthful" vegetable oils. The switch to the new vegetable oils actually *increased* the fat content of the fried foods—hardly a healthful move. Tests by the Food and Drug Administration (FDA) and others found that French fries cooked in beef tallow absorbed less fat than those cooked in vegetable oil, which led to estimates that the switch to vegetable oil would more than double the fat content of fries and increase fat consumption by half,[46] plus the fat was hydrogenated.

The ASA succeeded in producing a health crisis where none had existed. The general ignorance about nutrition by most people swayed them into siding with the soybean industry, which proves money and politics can override truth. In reality, there was no public outcry; the change was mainly brought about by an aggressive negative campaign. As a result, most major food companies, sensitive to consumer fear, reformulated hundreds of products, replacing tropical oils with hydrogenated oils. Since 1990, the fast food industry has been cooking French fries in hydrogenated vegetable oil instead of beef tallow and tropical oils. They made the change because of the prevailing opinion that vegetable oils were healthier than the other oils.

Even now the cinders of this war still burn. Many ill-informed writers and speakers continue to condemn coconut oil as containing "artery-clogging" saturated fat.

The only studies on coconut oil that indicate any possible negative effect on cholesterol levels have been shown to be flawed. These studies often used hydrogenated or chemically altered coconut oil. Later studies confirmed that natural coconut oil as a part of a normal diet has a neutral effect on blood cholesterol. Natural coconut oil has absolutely no adverse health effects. This has been proven in the lab and in nature. Epidemiological studies show conclusively that populations that consume large amounts of coconut oil experience almost no heart disease as compared to other populations in which coconut oil is only a small part of the diet. If coconut oil did have any adverse health effects associated with it, we would see it reflected in the morbidity and mortality of countries which are high consumers of coconut oil. Yet they are among the healthiest peoples in the world.

Jane Heimlich, the wife of Dr. Heimlich the inventor of the Heimlich maneuver, and author of the best-selling book *What Your Doctor Won't Tell You,* stated: "The next time you go to the movies or a ball park and want to snack on popcorn, ask the vendor what kind of oil the kernels are popped in. If it isn't coconut, it's probably partially hydrogenated vegetable oil, and that isn't good for you."

Chapter 9

NUTRITION AND PHYSICAL DEGENERATION

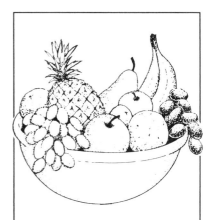

MALNUTRITION: A MODERN EPIDEMIC
Food for Thought

A few generations ago, before the industrial revolution came into full swing and before people began moving to the cities to work in factories, most lived on farms. They subsisted on diets of fresh natural foods they made, killed, gathered, or grew. As long as they could get enough to eat, they enjoyed relatively good nutritional health.

Although nutritional deficiencies occurred from time to time, the most prevalent diseases were those caused by infectious microorganisms. Pneumonia and tuberculosis were the dreaded diseases of the day. Degenerative disease was comparatively rare. Most of the degenerative diseases that are common today were so rare that they were not even identified at that time.

Louis Pasteur ushered in a new era in science and preventative medicine with the discovery of germs—microscopic organisms that can cause disease. The cause of infectious illnesses that had plagued mankind from the beginning of time was at last discovered. The attention to sanitation and hygiene put a stop to many diseases that had plagued the world. In hospitals, the simple act of washing hands saved the lives of thousands of patients each year. Before that time, it was common for doctors when treating new patients to simply wipe their hands off on a towel after administering to a sick patient or even after dissecting a cadaver. As you might expect, people would come into a hospital for one condition and often die of another.

At the same time, a revolution in food technology began to take place. Food processing enhanced taste and prolonged shelf life. Rice was polished to remove the brown, fibrous outer layer. Wheat milling methods were developed that allowed a more thorough separation of fiber for a purer, whiter flour. Sugar production became more cost-efficient and production rates soared.

The dietary habits of the population began to change from one based on the natural foods of our ancestors to one based on the highly processed foods of today.

Cold breakfast cereals, some of our first convenience foods, made their appearance in the 1890s, along with soda pop, ice cream, and other junk foods. By the 1950s and 1960s, the traditional breakfast cereals like Grapenuts and Shredded Wheat took a back seat to Sugar Frosted Flakes, Sugar Crisps, and other highly sweetened cereals.

Refined vegetable oils started to become widely available in the early 1900s. Margarine made its debut in the mid-1930s. Vegetable oil production steadily increased after World War II. By 1958 world oil production exceeded 60 billion pounds yearly.

"Hypertension is a disease of civilized life. Growing up in New Guinea or the northern forests of Brazil is a fine way to avoid the disease."
—Harvard Medical School Health Letter

"Your body isn't programmed to develop disease."
—Dr. M. Ted Morter, Jr. Your Health, Your Choice

"When I graduated from medical school in 1911, I had never heard of coronary thrombosis which is one of the chief threats to life in the United States and Canada today—an outstanding development in one's own lifetime."
—Dr. Paul Dudley White, Whitehouse Physician

"The ultimate cause of human disease is the consequence of our transgression of the universal laws of life."
—Paracelsus (1493-1541)

Foods were processed and packaged to look appetizing, to tantalize the taste buds, and to have as long a shelf life as possible. In the process, nutrients were destroyed and natural and synthetic chemicals were added. You go to the store now and it's near impossible to find a packaged food that doesn't have preservatives, dyes, emulsifiers, anticaking agents, flavor enhancers, sweeteners or other things added to it.

We learned as early as the late 1800s, after the practice of polishing of rice became common, that food processing can cause deficiency disease. This didn't stop the practice, we just added back some of vitamins that were removed. This was a quick fix, but not a good solution. Some 22 nutrients are removed in the processing of wheat into white flour. Only four or five are added back. Scientists have now identified some 90 nutrients that are important to health. Modern food processing methods remove most of them.

In his book, *Nutrigenetics*, Dr. R.O. Brennan lists how much of each nutrient is lost when whole wheat is converted into white flour, for example: magnesium (85 percent), vitamin A (90 percent), vitamin B-1 (77 percent), vitamin B-2 (80 percent), vitamin B-3 (81 percent), vitamin B-6 (72 percent), folic acid (67 percent), calcium (60 percent), vitamin E (86 percent), zinc (78 percent), and selenium (16 percent).[1] If you are like most people, you eat bread of one type or another at every meal. This could be pancakes, tortillas, breakfast cereal, donuts, bagels, noodles, etc. You might be surprised at how many flour products you eat every day. Wheat comprises the bulk of most of our foods. These products are almost always made from white flour.

Processed vegetable oils, sugar, and white-flour products make up 73 percent of the average American diet and supply almost no vitamins or minerals. When animals are placed on diets of refined and processed foods, they develop a long list of degenerative conditions which increase in number and severity in successive generations. The relationships are so strong that specific nutrient deficiencies frequently can be shown to cause defects in specific parts of the body.[2]

The infectious diseases that plagued mankind in ages past have been controlled for the most part and in some cases almost eliminated. But a whole new breed of illness has taken their place. Degenerative diseases are now on the rampage. Diseases that were rarely seen before throughout all of history have now become commonplace.

Modern Civilization and Degenerative Disease

The transformation of the major cause of death from infectious disease to degenerative disease began to take place in the early 1900s. At the beginning of the 20th century, heart disease was still rare, accounting for approximately 8 percent of all deaths in the United States. Today coronary heart disease accounts for about 45 percent of all deaths. Incidence of heart disease rose dramatically between 1920 and 1960 and is the number one cause of death today.

The cancer rate at the beginning of the century was about 1 in 30; it's now risen to 1 in 4. The incidence of cancer continues to increase year after year.

The United States is number one in the world in colon cancer rates and diverticulitis. This is due to too much fat and sugar (24% of calories). Dr. Dennis Burkitt in his research on tribal Africans could find only four cases of diverticulosis out of 4,000 cases studied and yet this disease is epidemic in the west.

Rural areas in less developed countries have literally no dental cavities in their children, yet almost every child in the United States has some cavities even though we have the finest dental care and put fluoride in the water, which is supposed to harden teeth and make them more resistant to decay.

Fat consumption, especially vegetable oils, continues to increase.

FAT CONSUMPTION
Pounds per person per year

Source: Liebman, B. *Nutrition Action Healthletter* 26 (3):8

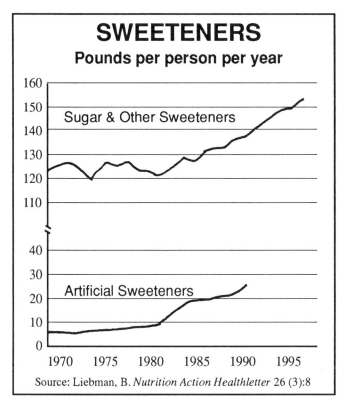

SWEETENERS
Pounds per person per year

Sugar consumption continues to rise.

Source: Liebman, B. *Nutrition Action Healthletter* 26 (3):8

Prostate problems have risen from an obscure malady to a world crisis. Seventy percent of men past the age of sixty require prostate surgery.

While breast cancer in women is very rare in less developed areas of the world, in the United States one out of every eight women will develop breast cancer at some time in her life. This rate is similar in other Western countries.

If you go to areas of the world where the people eat the foods they produce themselves, separated from industrial pollution and hectic lifestyles, you will find that people have a dramatically lower incidence of all types of degenerative disease. Because sanitation and hygiene often isn't up to our standards, they do suffer more with infectious illness. Many of these people, however, like the Hunza of Pakistan; Vilcabamba and Titicaca Indians of South America; the Russian Georgians, Abhazians, Azerbaijanis and Armanians; and the people of the Lhasa Valley in Tibet; to name a few, are known for their long life spans and relative freedom from modern degenerative disease. They don't know what heart disease, cancer, or diabetes are because they have never seen them. At least not until recently. Now, however, as modern processed foods are being introduced into these societies, degenerative disease has followed. This pattern has been repeated time and time again throughout the world. As soon as a culture abandons its traditional lifestyle and diet and begins eating processed foods, degenerative disease creeps in.

Dr. Hugh C. Trowell, a British physician, was one of the first to identify this tread. Dr. Trowell worked among the primitive peoples of East Africa from 1930 to 1960. He was part of an extensive research project sponsored by the British government to study the prevalent diseases of the area. When he started his research back in 1930, the people lived as they had for thousands of years. They ate only what they foraged or killed. Except in the larger cities, Western culture had little impact on the people.

In their research, Dr. Trowell and fellow workers noted that there was absolutely no evidence of diabetes, high blood pressure, stroke, or coronary artery disease. In those early years, autopsies showed no evidence of atherosclerosis or heart disease. Over the next thirty years all this changed. Degenerative disease slowly started to appear and became more and more prevalent over time. The natives still lived in a relative wilderness, away from industrialization, but they became increasingly dependent on processed foods shipped in from Western countries.[3]

Another researcher who studied tribal Africans in the 1930s and 1940s was Weston Price. Price, a retired dentist, went to Africa to study why people developed tooth decay. He went to remote areas to find people who didn't have dental problems in an attempt to discover their secret.

Price found that the more isolated a native population was, the less tooth decay and other degenerative disease he found. In areas that were almost totally isolated, the natives had almost no tooth decay and the people were healthy and strong. Degenerative disease was virtually unknown to them. In areas that were easily accessible and Western influence greater, tooth decay and disease was much more prevalent.

Price soon began to see a pattern developing. Tooth decay became particularly common among children in areas where modern processed foods were available. Price found that wherever white flour, white rice, and sugary foods were sold, tooth decay and degenerative disease were prevalent. He got to the point where he could tell how many years the local store had been in operation by the age of the children with the most tooth decay. He would go into a new area and, after examining the teeth of the children and comparing their ages, he could tell the year in which their store had opened.

One of the frightening things about Price's discovery is that it didn't take much of a change in the people's diets in order to cause notable changes in health. While their diet remained primarily the same as it had always been, the addition of even a small quantity of processed food made dramatic differences in their health.[4]

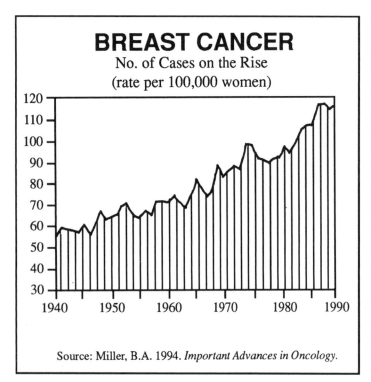

BREAST CANCER

No. of Cases on the Rise
(rate per 100,000 women)

Source: Miller, B.A. 1994. *Important Advances in Oncology.*

The effect of modern processed food is nowhere more dramatic than it has been on the Eskimos of North America. Prior to 1955, the Eskimos lived a nomadic life, living off the land. Their food consisted predominantely of fish, caribou, fowl, musk ox, rabbit, and fox. Occasionally they would supplement their diet with some vegetable foods such as roots, seaweed, and leafy greens according to the season. Starting in the mid-1950s, Eskimos were recruited to work on military and civilian airports across the Alaskan and Canadian Arctic.

By the late 1960s, almost all of the Eskimos had given up their nomadic lifestyles and were living in permanent communities. They also gave up their traditional foods and began eating the same things most North Americans eat—processed flour, sugar, and vegetable oils. The Eskimos rarely ever saw sugar and never used vegetable oil before that time. They ate ox fat and whale blubber by the pound, but had never even tasted margarine or corn oil. These new oils took the place of the animal fats they had been eating. They started eating less meat and fat and replaced it with more processed vegetable foods.

Before living in permanent communities, the Eskimos' health was like most other isolated peoples. Degenerate diseases like diabetes and heart disease were extremely rare. Within one decade, the Eskimos began experiencing degenerative disease at an alarming rate. Dia-

betes tripled. Dr. Schaefer, who worked among the Eskimos, noted that in one group of Eskimos living in the Canadian Western Arctic, there were more new cases of diabetes than had occurred in all the Eskimos of Canada a few years earlier.

Diabetes wasn't the only problem; diseases of the arteries among men over 40 increased five-fold. Gallbladder disease skyrocketed. Even acne, which was previously unknown to the Canadian Eskimos before the mid-1950s, began afflicting the youth.

With a civilized diet came also civilized disease. The Eskimos had few health problems with their high saturated-fat and cholesterol diet. But as soon as they began eating processed foods, diseases of all types, including heart disease, began to plague them. What saturated fat and cholesterol couldn't do over generations of time, sugar, white flour, and vegetable oil did in just a few years.[5]

What has happened to the Eskimos can be seen in many different parts of the world. When a Western diet is adapted, degenerative diseases common in the Western countries eventually follows. Ian Prior, M.D., a cardiologist and director of the epidemiology unit at the Wellington Hospital in New Zealand, says this pattern has been very clearly demonstrated with Pacific Islanders, "The more an Islander takes on the ways of the West, the more prone he is to succumb to our degenerative diseases." He states, "Our evidence now shows that the fur-

Cancer, diabetes, and other degenerative diseases have been increasing among those populations who eat modern processed foods.

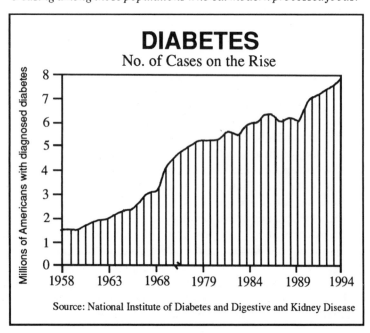

DIABETES

No. of Cases on the Rise

Millions of Americans with diagnosed diabetes

Source: National Institute of Diabetes and Digestive and Kidney Disease

ther the Pacific natives move from the quiet, carefree life of their ancestors, the closer they come to gout, diabetes, atherosclerosis, obesity, and hypertension."[6]

Dr. Prior has studied the differences in health of the Islanders in and around New Zealand. He documented that Islanders who live with the least western influence have the least incidence of degenerative disease. As island populations become more Westernized and import more processed foods, their health begins to deteriorate. Islanders who have migrated to New Zealand and who have taken on the Western lifestyle, have disease rates similar to the population of European origin.

Before the American Indians began to eat white man's food, they ate foods consisting of beans, squash, corn, cactus, seed, acorns, and game. After World War II, the U.S. government began giving the Indians U.S. surplus commodities, consisting of white flour, vegetable oils, sugar, and other foods typical of the modern Western diet. The Indians replaced their high-fiber, complex carbohydrate diet for one dominated by simple carbohydrates and vegetable oils and other processed foods. As a consequence, the incidence of obesity and diabetes became epidemic.

There are now over 250,000 Indian diabetics in Arizona. The Pima tribe residing in south central Arizona has the highest incidence of diabetes in the world. More than 50 percent of all adults over 35 year of age are diabetic. Diabetes in this population has increased over 40 percent in the last 20 years. Along with the increase in diabetes is an increase in atherosclerosis, heart disease, stroke, and other degenerative conditions. The Indians in the American Southwest are sixteen times more likely to have kidney disease and need dialysis machines than their non-Indian neighbors.

SUBCLINICAL MALNUTRITION

According to the World Health Organization, 70 to 80 percent of people in developed nations die from lifestyle- or diet-caused diseases.[7] The majority of cancers is caused by what we put into our bodies. Heart disease, stroke, and atherosclerosis, the biggest killers in industrialized nations, are dietary diseases. Diet is a significant factor in most all degenerative disease. Plainly put, a poor diet leads to ill health.

A major cause of disease in the world is malnutrition. Advanced stages of malnutrition can exhibit themselves in a number of characteristic diseases such as scurvy (vitamin C deficiency), beriberi (thiamin deficiency), pellagra (niacin deficiency), and others. Such conditions leave the body vulnerable to infections, depress immunity, and stifle healing, normal growth, and body functions. A malnourished body is subject to premature degeneration and disease.

If you read a newspaper headline that announced, "Most Americans Malnourished" you would probably be shocked. A similar headline could also be broadcast in Canada, Britain, and most every other industrialized country. When we think of malnutrition, we usually think of drought victims in Africa or starving people in India, but not the Western world where food is in abundance.

Yes, we have plenty of food, but food and nutrition are two different matters. While we may have plenty to eat, the food we eat is seriously lacking in important nutrients. As a consequence, many of us suffer from what is called *subclinical malnutrition*. Subclinical malnutrition is a condition in which nutrient intake is at a bare minimum; we get enough nutrients to keep from developing severe symptoms of malnutrition, but not the amount our bodies want or need for optimal health.

In Third World countries, malnutrition is primarily due to famine, poverty, and politics. In more affluent countries, the problem is masked by the abundance of foods and medicines. In order for symptoms of malnutrition to manifest themselves, a diet must be lacking in essential nutrients for an extended period of time. The body maintains reserves of essential nutrients to protect itself during periods when foods are less readily available. It can take months for signs of malnutrition to become evident. Methods of diagnosing deficiency diseases require malnutrition to be in an advanced stage before it can be detected.

Subclinical malnutrition is a condition where a person consumes just enough essential nutrients to prevent full-blown symptoms of severe malnutrition, but the body is still nutrient deficient and prone to slow, premature degenera-

"Think back over the years of cancer research, of the millions spent, the time consumed, the pains extended...and where are we today? Is it not time to take stock of our basic conception of cancer to see if there is not something radically wrong with this, to account for the years of utter and complete failure to date? Cancer had been consistently on the increase. Is it possible that the cause of cancer lies in our departure from natural foods? It would surely look so to any man from Mars, but we have lived so long on processed foods deficient in vitamins and tissue salts that we are in a state of unbalanced nutrition almost from birth. We have come to regard our [refined] foods as the hallmark of civilization, when it is a fact that these very foods set the stage for every sort of ill, including cancer."

—W. Howard Hay, M.D.

tion. This condition can go on unnoticed indefinitely. In Western countries the problem of subclinical malnutrition is epidemic. Our foods are sadly depleted of nutrients. We eat, and even overeat, but we can still be malnourished because our foods do not contain all the essential nutrients our bodies need to function optimally. As a result, the body cannot fight off infections well, the immune system is chronically depressed, toxins build up, free-radical chain reactions run wild, and disease slowly consumes the body.

Many people eat three so-called "balanced" meals a day and falsely believe they should be healthy. Eating processed convenience foods stripped of vital nutrients and loaded with artificial food additives and incidental contaminants contributes to toxic buildup and degenerative stress in our bodies. Many of the foods we eat actually drain nutrients from our body. Sugar, for example, has no nutrients, but it does use up nutrients when it is metabolized. Eating sugary foods can drain the body of chromium, a mineral vital to making insulin. Without insulin, diabetic symptoms can result which can lead to disease and death. The more processed the food we eat, the more nutrients we need to metabolize it. Polyunsaturated oil eats up vitamin E reserves, certain food additives burns up vitamin C, etc. A diet loaded with white-flour products, sugar, and vegetable oil quickly depletes nutrient reserves creating a condition of subclinical malnutrition.

Food cravings often are initiated as a result of the body's need for certain vitamins and minerals, but when processed foods are eaten loaded with meat, dairy, and sugar, the few vitamins that are consumed are used up to process the foods just eaten, so a deficiency remains. Cravings continue and more food is eaten and more calories consumed, setting up a vicious cycle that leads to obesity. People are eating more but becoming less nourished.

> All that Nature requires of [mankind] is that he keep his body fed and resupplied with all of these chemical elements in thier natural organic state. If he will do this he is obeying the law under which Nature built the primitive man and if he does not do this he is disobeying the law. The reward for obeying this law is health, strength, vitality and the preservation of youth. The penalty for disobeying this law is sickness, pain, misery, suffering, and permature death. These, my friends, are propositions so obvious that they do not admit of argument. They simply must be accepted if we give them thought.
>
> —Dr. Eugene Christian

The U.S. Department of Agriculture states that most all of us don't get enough (100% RDA) of at least 10 essential nutrients. Only 12 percent of the population obtains 100 percent of seven essential nutrients. Less than 10 percent of us gets the recommended daily servings of fruit and vegetables. Forty percent of us eat no fruit and 20 percent no vegetables. And most of the vegetables we do get are fried potatoes (cooked in heat-damaged vegetable oil).

In November of 1993, the *Journal of the American Dietetic Association* reported a study of 1,800 second- and fifth-graders in New York State which found that on the day they were surveyed, 40% of the children did not eat any vegetables, except potatoes or tomato sauce; 20% ate no fruit, and 36% ate at least four different types of snack food. With dietary habits like this, it is no wonder we suffer from subclinical malnutrition.

It's bad enough that foods are stripped of their nutrients and fiber, but when these foods are eaten, they displace or replace nutrient-rich foods like fresh vegetables and whole grain products. The higher the sugar and white flour content of the diet, the less you eat of vitamin-rich foods.

Besides lacking nutrients, processed foods also contain toxins—food additives and contaminants that increase free-radical generation. For example, vitamin E is used up to fight free radicals generated by polyunsaturated oils. Eating a lot of vegetable oil will deplete vitamin E reserves and can contribute to vitamin E deficiency. This can happen to any of the antioxidant vitamins. A person can get the RDA of antioxidants C, A, E, but if they also eat foods that cause free radicals—typically proceed foods containing vegetable oils, food additives, and contaminants or exposed to cigarette smoke and other environmental toxins—they can use up these antioxidants and become vitamin deficient even if they are getting the RDA. A person who isn't exposed to free-radical substances doesn't need as much antioxidant nutrients. A person who doesn't eat as much animal protein doesn't need as many B vitamins, and so forth. This is why people who lived a hundred and fifty years ago and people who are now living in areas of the world where they depend entirely on the foods they produce themselves do not experience the degenerative disease like those in modern industrialized countries. They don't eat vegetable oils. If they eat any pure oil at all it is of animal origin, rich in saturated fat and cholesterol.

DIETARY FIBER

Fiber is that portion of plant foods that cannot be digested by enzymes in the human digestive tract. Because fiber is not digested, it does not provide any nutrients. For this reason, it was at one time thought to be unimportant to health. We now know that fiber plays a significant role in the digestive process and can dramatically affect our state of health.

Fiber is important because it regulates bowel activity. It absorbs water, providing a medium that is moist and mobile which can effectively sweep the inside of the bowel clean. A diet lacking in fiber will result in a toxic, constipated colon. The colon is the sewage pipe of the body, and when debris gets bogged down, toxins can be absorbed into the bloodstream, causing all types of mischief.

The richest source of fiber in our diet is found in whole grains. Both brown rice and whole wheat bread are excellent sources of fiber; however, in the refining of these grains most of the fiber is removed. White bread and white rice are, consequently, high in empty calories, but low in fiber.

The importance of fiber in our diet was first noted by physicians working in Africa. They observed that as long as the people remained on their traditional diets they enjoyed extraordinarily good health. But when they begin eating refined grains and sugar, their health deteriorated. Where fiber intake is high, like in rural Africa, degenerative disease is low. Where fiber consumption is low, due to the use of refined grains, disease rates are much higher. This observation led to what is known as the "fiber hypothesis" which states that the consumption of unrefined, high-fiber foods protects against many diseases common in Western countries such as colon cancer and arteriosclerosis.

People in rural communities in Africa, India, and other parts of the world, who have healthy gastrointestinal tracts, consume approximately 60 grams of dietary fiber a day. Nutritionists recommend that we should eat at least 20 to 35 grams daily. This is about twice as much as we currently get. Most of the foods we eat consist of products made with refined white flour (e.g., bread, pasta, crackers, cake, etc.) which has had most of the fiber removed, and sugar, meat, eggs, and dairy products which contain absolutely no fiber.

Eating whole foods rich in fiber are thought to be beneficial with respect to the following:

- Weight control
- Constipation and diarrhea relief
- Hemorrhoid prevention
- Appendicitis prevention
- Diverticulosis prevention
- Colon cancer prevention
- Cardiovascular disease prevention
- Blood glucose and insulin modulation
- Diabetes control

HEART DISEASE AND MODERN FOODS

Despite decades of research and a significant decrease in animal fat consumption, heart disease is still our number one killer. Continuous attempts by an army of researchers over this time have failed to show a definitive link between blood cholesterol and heart disease. Much to the chagrin of researchers and their sponsors, studies have shown only a very mild and even questionable relationship between cholesterol and heart disease.

If saturated fats and cholesterol don't cause heart disease, what does? There are a number of factors that have been found that tie into heart disease far better than these fats.

In the 1940s and 1950s, researchers Yudkin and Lopez discovered a link between consumption of refined sugar and heart disease. Sugar consumption depresses the immune system, lowering the body's resistance to bacteria and viruses that may cause inflammation in the heart and arteries.

With the use of packaged, processed foods, our vitamin C intake has declined over the years. Vitamin C is necessary to maintain integrity of connective tissue including those in the arteries. One of the signs of vitamin C deficiency is atherosclerosis. The B vitamins, which have also declined in our food supply, are necessary in order to keep arteries strong and healthy. Research has shown that vitamin B deficiency is a major cause of atherosclerosis and heart disease (see graph on page 160). Heart disease has also been correlated with mineral deficiencies. Coronary heart disease rates are lower in regions where drinking water is naturally rich in trace minerals, particularly magnesium, which acts as a natural anticoagulant and aids in potassium absorption, thereby preventing heart-rate irregularities. Vitamin D is important in protecting the heart. It is essential for absorption of many minerals, particularly calcium and magnesium. Our bodies can manufacture vitamin D from cholesterol by the action of sunlight on the skin, but we have reduced our cholesterol consumption and our exposure to the sun in fear of developing skin cancer.

Excess sugar consumption also drains B vitamins needed to maintain healthy arteries. Research at the U.S. Department of Agriculture indicates that fructose may be even more dangerous than sucrose (table sugar). Fructose, mainly in the form of high-fructose corn syrup, has become the sweetener of choice for soft drinks, snacks, and many so-called health foods. Fructose is often touted as a "natural" sugar derived from fruit. This is a lie to make people believe it is harmless. Fructose is made from sugar cane, sugar beets, and corn, the same sources as sucrose. In fact, manufacturers take sucrose and refine it even further to get fructose. It can in no way be considered a "natural" sugar.

In the 1950s, Dr. Annand discovered that heat caused a change in milk protein that encouraged the formation of blood clots. Raw milk did not have this effect. He noted that since the laws requiring milk pasteurization began in the 1920s, heart disease rate has risen dramatically.

In recent years studies have confirmed that excessive protein, not fat, consumption is a major factor in the development of atherosclerosis and heart disease. The combination of subclinical vitamin deficiency with excess protein, particularly animal protein, has emerged as the primary factor in the cause and development of heart disease.

Another major factor is the excessive consumption of vegetable oils. This causes an imbalance in the production of prostaglandins that control many factors associated with our circulatory system. Vegetable oils encourage blood clotting, constriction of arteries which narrow passageways, and inflammation, all of which contribute to heart disease. Vegetable oils contain free radicals that damage the arteries, thereby initiating plaque deposits.

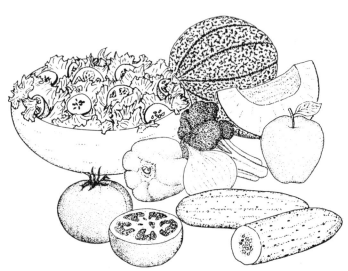

The key to good health is found in eating fresh whole foods that have undergone as little processing as possible. Manufactured foods are dead foods and do not supply the nutrients necessary to maintain health and vitality.

THE PRITIKIN DIET

Nathan Pritikin began a revolution in the way many people think about food in relation to their health. When he failed a treadmill test in 1958, he asked his doctor what he could do for his heart condition. Surgical procedures such as angiograms and heart bypass surgery were not yet available, so the doctor had nothing to offer and simply told him to come back when he had more trouble.

Pritikin didn't go home and wait for a heart attack. He knew that there must be something he could do and began researching the medical literature. While there wasn't much he could do medically he did find that heart disease was rare among primitive people. What was it that protected them he asked? The most obvious answer was their diet. Most primitive people based their diets around fruits, vegetables, seeds, and grains. They didn't use vegetable oils at all. The only oil they ate was animal fat and milk, and even those were usually eaten in moderation.

Between 35-45 percent of the calories in the typical Western diet comes from fat. The American Heart Association recommends reducing that amount to 30 percent. Pritikin noted that most primitive peoples eat even less than that. Influenced by the cholesterol theory, he reasoned that the less fat he ate, the better, and developed a diet that eliminated almost all fat. In order to accomplish this all meat, dairy, and eggs would have to be eliminated as well as vegetable oils. His diet was based on fresh fruits, vegetables, and whole grains. He claimed that the only fat we need we can get from our foods. Eating this simple diet brought about remarkable changes and his condition dramatically improved.

Inspired by his own success he began teaching others how to reverse the destructive effects of heart disease. In the mid 1970s the Pritikin Longevity Center was opened in Santa Barbara, California. Under medical supervision, patients entered a four-week program. This involved an extremely low-fat diet, the elimination of processed foods, and walking up to six miles a day at a leisurely pace.

Pritikin advocated eliminating sugar, white flour, and all processed foods from the diet, and recommended the use of fresh raw foods, whole grains, and a strenuous exercise program; but it was the low-fat aspects of his regimen that received the most attention in the media.

The success of the Pritikin diet was due to a number of factors having little to do with reduction in dietary fat. Pritikin soon found that the fat-free diet presented many problems, not the least of which was the fact that the people just could not stay on it. Those who possessed enough will power to stay fat-free for any length of time developed a variety of health problems, including low energy, difficulty in concentration, depression, weight gain, and signs of mineral deficiencies.[8]

After problems with the no-fat regimen became apparent, Pritikin introduced a small amount of fat into his diet to about 10 percent of total caloric intake.

Adherents to this new regimen found that they lost weight and that their blood cholesterol levels and blood pressures declined. Angina pains went away. People who were too ill to walk when they arrived, regained their ability to move around as they pleased. EKGs and treadmill tests improved. People who followed the program began to enjoy living again. Under the direction of Nathan Pritikin the program flourished.

Pritikin died in 1985 at the age of 69, much longer than he would have if he followed his doctor's advice to simply come back when symptoms got worse. He lived with a malignant lymphoma during his last 27 years. When his body was examined after death, his arteries were described as resembling a newborn baby's—a remarkable achievement for a man who had a history of coronary artery disease.

DEAN ORNISH HEART DISEASE REVERSAL DIET

While Nathan Pritikin demonstrated that people eating a primitive diet could reverse heart disease, it was not yet scientifically proven. Dr. Dean Ornish's studies in the 1980s and 1990s provided the scientific proof that verified the positive effects of eating fresh wholesome foods.

The results of Ornish's first major study, known as the Lifestyle Heart Trial, were reported in the medical journal *Lancet* in 1990 and in his book *Reversing Heart Disease*. Patients with significant coronary artery disease problems were randomly divided into two groups. The lifestyle-change group followed a vegetarian diet that contained only 10 percent fat. People in that group also stopped smoking, meditated one hour per day, exercised, and underwent lengthy group-therapy sessions. The control group followed the standard American Heart Association diet (fat intake under 30 percent of diet and cholesterol less than 300 mg per day) and received routine medical care from their own physicians. All patients received a quantitative angiogram at the beginning of the program and after one year.

Patients on Ornish's program did far better in relieving symptoms and in opening obstructions in their arteries than control patients. Most study patients were free of angina within one month of starting the program. Those patients who followed the program the closest showed more improvement than those patients who were not so strict.

Ornish's program was compared with other more standard medical approaches to see which were most effective. In one study in which a cholesterol-lowering drug was used, 16 percent of the patients showed some improvement. In the second study a cholesterol-lowering drug and niacin (vitamin B-3) was used, resulting in a 39 percent improvement. In Ornish's study 85 percent of patients showed improve-

ment. Ornish's dietary approach was clearly far superior.

Ornish's Reversal Diet has no animal products at all except egg whites and nonfat dairy products. Like Pritikin's diet, total fat calories are limited to 10 percent. Most of the fat we get in our diet is from cooking oil and oil used in processing foods. Most of us eat way too much, nearly 40 percent calories from fat. To cut total fat intake to only 10 percent, you must eliminate all meat, fish, dairy, eggs, cooking oil, and all processed, packaged foods, which are loaded with added oil. Basically you must eat a natural, vegetarian diet of fresh fruits, vegetables, and grains. You get nearly 10 percent fat just from the foods you eat. Such a diet eliminates not only saturated fat and cholesterol but most all processed vegetable oils. This is a key element to the success of the Pritikin and Ornish programs.

Pritikin and Ornish both designed their diets with the cholesterol theory in mind. They reasoned that the less fat eaten the better, particularly saturated fat and cholesterol. The positive results they experienced were, for a large part, attributed to the low-fat diet. Many people assume low-fat diet means simply low saturated fat and cholesterol and it's the elimination of these two fats that bring about the dramatic improvement in health. This is a false impression. People can't go on a 10 percent fat diet without making drastic changes in the type of foods they eat. Such a diet must also be extremely low in vegetable oil as well. Processed, nutrient-poor foods are replaced by high fiber, vitamin-rich fresh vegetables, fruits, and whole grains. These latter changes make all the difference in the world, as you will see in the next few chapters. People often forget that primitive diets *never* include vegetable oils (with the exception of coconut and olive oils) but often do include animal fat, raw milk, and eggs. As you have seen in Chapter 8, the Tokelauans and Pukapukans consume a diet consisting of as much as 63 percent fat, yet do not experience heart disease or other degenerative conditions. Their saturated fat-rich primitive diet has kept them healthy for generations.

The key to good health is not reducing total fat, but eliminating vegetable oils and processed foods from the diet and replacing them with fresh vitamin- and fiber-rich natural foods. A natural foods diet or primitive diet can have 20 or 30 percent fat as long as it does not include refined polyunsaturated vegetable oil.

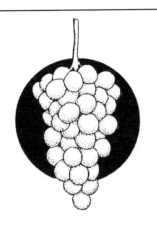

Chapter 10

THE ANTIOXIDANT CONNECTION

THE GRAPE CURE

Juicing or juice fasting has become a popular method for improving health. The theory behind juicing is that fresh fruit and vegetable juices contain a high concentration of essential minerals, vitamins, and disease-fighting phytochemicals. A person can consume much more nutrient-rich juice than he can solid food, so juice fasting provides a way to get lots of nutrients without the calories and bulk that accompany foods. It's like a concentrated source of liquid vitamins.

The idea that fresh juices contained great healing powers was first discovered by Johanna Brandt in the 1920s. By this time white flour and sugar had became the dominant foods in many people's diets. At this time, Brandt was diagnosed with stomach cancer. X-rays clearly showed the cancerous growth overtaking her body. Nothing could be done to help her, and she resigned to the fact that death would soon follow. She was introduced to fasting by a little book called *The Fasting Cure* by the novelist Upton Sinclair. This book gave her new hope for relief from her suffering. She began fasting. Her battle lasted for several years. She would fast up to three weeks at a time, drinking only water. Repeated fasting brought about a slight improvement, but not relief. The cancerous tumor persisted. She suffered violent attacks of vomiting and purging with excruciating pain which brought up half-digested blood. Doctors eventually recommended an immediate operation as the only means of prolonging her life. She refused and decided to go on another fast. It was then that she accidentally discovered a food that destroyed the growth and eliminated the poisons from her body.

She lived in an area in South Africa surrounded by vineyards. Grapes were readily available. She was so sick at this time that she knew she couldn't fast on water alone, so she allowed herself to eat only grapes and drink grape juice to provide some nourishment to her weakened body.

After eating grapes exclusively for six weeks, her symptoms as well as her cancer miraculously disappeared. X-rays which had clearly shown the cancer before, now showed no trace of the growth. Fasting on water alone had not been able to dissolve the cancerous mass. Grapes, she reasoned, contained elements that were able to penetrate the cancer, break up the tissue, and purify the blood. She witnessed that, "abnormal growths, cancers, tumors, abscesses, and fibrous masses seem to be dissolved by the powerful chemical agent in the grape. Diseased tissues and fatty degenerations and every form of morbid matter are apparently broken up into minute particles and thrown into the bloodstream to be carried to the organs of excretion."[1]

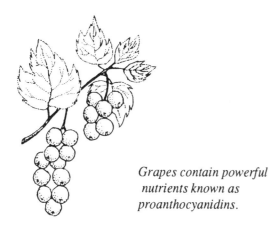

Grapes contain powerful nutrients known as proanthocyanidins.

As a result of her miraculous healing, she began advocating the grape fast as a cure for cancer and other degenerative conditions and traveled around the world with her message. She supervised many grape fasts which typically lasted one to two months, and many people testified to the effectiveness of her methods.

Johanna Brandt helped many people with incurable degenerative disease recover their health by teaching them about the grape cure. She used grapes in the diet and as poultices topically when the disease was manifest in the flesh. She recorded her experiences in the book *The Grape Cure*. This book recounts the effects grape juice had in healing numerous people, even those who seemed on the verge of death. Patients who were given up as hopeless by their doctors reclaimed their health through Brandt's grape cure. She found that it helped not only against cancer but most every other form of degenerative disease that had become common in modern industrialized societies. Even dental problems could be successfully treated. She stated, "The organic acids of the grapes are strongly antiseptic and their effect on the gums is perhaps more valuable than any other result of the diet. For it means preservation of the teeth, on which mankind is dependent, not alone for health but for beauty. Would that I had the tongue of a saint to warn against the evil of having sound teeth extracted because of poison at the roots! It is not always necessary. Every tooth may be loose in its socket and pus may be pouring from the gums, but after a few weeks on the exclusive grape diet it will in time be found that the teeth are firmly set in the jaws and that every trace of pyorrhea poisoning had disappeared."

Because Brandt had no medical training and her methods were unconventional, she was frequently criticized and her grape cure ridiculed as unproven. She insisted that her methods do work and had helped hundreds of people regain their health. She issued a challenge to anyone who doubted, "Do not take my word for this. Try it. Prove it. Demonstrate the diet." If the grape cure was valid, all that was necessary was to simply try it. The medical community ignored her challenge.[2]

Because the refined, processed foods we eat are nutritionally deficient, we suffer from varying degrees of subclinical malnutrition. Some of the most vital nutrients to our health and well-being are collectively known as antioxidants. The best known are vitamins A, C, and E. Antioxidants are used to fight free radicals. Without their protection, free-radical chain reactions would run wild, tearing our cells apart and greatly accelerate aging and disease.

Johanna Brandt was the first person to recognize that grapes contained a group of vitamins that had substantial healing properties. The grape seed and skin, it was later discovered, contains bioflavonoids, including proanthocyanidins, a group of powerful antioxidants that are many times more powerful than Vitamins A or C in neutralizing harmful free radicals. As a result of Johanna Brandt's discovery, fasting clinics began experimenting with grape and other juices. The results have proved quite favorable. Today juicing is a common method used by nutritionists and natural health practitioners to restore health, and numerous books have been written on the subject. The secret behind the success of juicing is that it provides a concentrated dose of antioxidants and other healing nutrients. People who are ill because they are nutritionally "challenged" find juicing to work miracles for them if the juice is fresh and uncontaminated by additives and sweeteners.

FREE RADICALS AND NUTRITION

When an apple is cut open, it will normally turn brown as it becomes oxidized by the air. Coating the apple with lemon juice, which is rich in antioxidants, can prevent oxidation from happening and keep the apple from turning color. Antioxidants work the same way in our bodies. They prevent oxidation by stopping free-radical reactions. Tissue aging and injury is thus slowed down or prevented.

We are exposed to free radicals from the food we eat, the air we breathe, chemicals in which we come in contact, and metabolic processes within our bodies. Because free-radical generation is a part of our everyday life, our bodies are equipped with a defensive force to intercept them and to prevent destructive chain reactions from running out of control. This defensive force is composed of a variety of antioxidant compounds scattered throughout the body. In fact, every cell contains antioxidants for their protection.

Some of our antioxidant defenders are manufactured in our bodies, others come from the foods we eat. Even the ones synthesized in our bodies need certain nutrients from our diets in order for them to be made.

Free-radical damage is a common factor in a host of degenerative diseases. Those who have low antioxidant reserves experience premature aging and suffer more from degenerative disease.

Collagen, a tough, fibrous protein, is the single most common protein in our bodies. It forms the connective tissues that hold cells, tissues, and organs together. Free radicals destroy collagen, weakening tissues throughout the body.

As we age, our skin loses its elasticity and begins to wrinkle and sag. This is a result of free-radical destruction of the collagen in our skin. The less elastic your skin is, the more free-radical damage has occurred. You can test the amount of free-radical damage that has occurred to the collagen throughout your body by taking the Skin Elasticity Test in Chapter 2. This test gives you a rough idea of the functional age of your skin and, consequently, the rest of the tissues in your body. Compare the functional age from this test to your actual age. How well are you holding up?

Collagen is what holds arteries and capillaries together and gives them strength. Free radicals can weaken the collagen causing deterioration of the circulatory system that leads to the development of microscopic lesions and the deposition of plaque in these lesions. Antioxidants protect collagen and allow the body to repair collagen that has been damaged by injury or free-radical action. They protect the collagen in our arteries and keep them strong and flexible. They also help prevent and heal bruising, varicose veins, and edema (swelling caused by leakage of fluids from blood vessels into surrounding tissues). They can prevent abnormal platelet adhesion which encourages blood-clot formation. They can help improve mental function, reduce some of the side effects of diabetes, speed healing, reduce the risk of stroke, improve vision, and protect against cancer. Antioxidants provide protection against inflammatory diseases (including allergies), rheumatoid arthritis, osteoarthritis, hepatitis, Crohn's disease, lupus, and ulcerative colitis which all involve free radicals. Joint tissue is composed of collagen, so antioxidants can improve joint flexibility and health.

It should become clear to you by now that the most common degenerative diseases we face today are in some way connected with low antioxidant reserves and free-radical destruction. Degenerative disease is, for the most part, a result of chronic subclinical malnutrition. Surgery and drugs can bring an immediate change, but this is usually done by removing the symptoms without addressing the underlying cause. Often simply getting the missing nutrients and avoiding things that create free radicals are all that is needed to bring about healing and to prevent premature degeneration.

There are two major factors that deplete antioxidant reserves and leave us vulnerable to free-radical deterioration. One is exposure to substances that encourage free-radical formation and the other is eating a diet deficient in antioxidants.

Free radicals can occur from many sources: pesticides, radiation, cigarette smoke, air pollution, industrial chemicals, and even some forms of atmospheric oxygen. For many of us, some of our greatest exposure to free radicals comes from the foods we eat. The number one source of free radicals in our food is from polyunsaturated oils. By simply eliminating them from your diet, you prevent a great deal of free-radical activity.

We are exposed to free radicals every day and must continually replenish our supply, of antioxidants if we are to maintain some reasonable level of protection. Refined, overly processed foods are deficient in antioxidants as well as other important nutrients. A diet of packaged convenience foods leads to antioxidant deficiency because it is both low in nutrients and high in free-radical causing substances (e.g., vegetable oils and other food additives).

Simply adding more antioxidants by eating more fresh whole foods or taking dietary supplements can greatly improve health. Many people can attest to the effectiveness of this approach. For some it has been the means in which they have overcome crippling disease and regained their health.

CASE HISTORIES

"My experience in the field of nutrition dates back to 1952," says Dr. Lamar Rosquist. "I've been practicing nutrition ever since that time with tremendous success." Antioxidant therapy brought a new dimension to his practice. "It has produced a myriad of results that I have never seen with any other nutritional approache that I used in the past."[3]

Some years ago Dr. Rosquist was given a sample of Pycnogenol (a special blend of antioxidant bioflavonoids) and literature describing its therapeutic effects and uses. At this time, Pycnogenol was relatively new in the United States, although it had been studied and used therapeutically for a couple of decades in Europe, especially France where his sample was manufactured.

In reading the literature, he learned that Pycnogenol, especially when combined with other antioxidants such as vitamins C and E, beta-carotene, and selenium, was extremely effective in reversing many degenerative conditions so prevalent in our society. He was particularly interested in the studies that showed antioxidants as useful in treating all types of inflammatory conditions. Like most men in their 60s, he had been experiencing symptoms of prostitis—inflammation and swelling of the prostate gland. Prostate enlargement affects one out of every four men and is characterized by the frequent urge to urinate and the inability to completely void the bladder. This caused him to get up several times in the night to relieve himself.

Since his prostitis involves inflammation, Dr. Rosquist decided to try out the antioxidant treatment and see what it would do for him, and started taking the recommended dose. He took it faithfully for six months without experiencing any noticeable difference. A great disappointment. He was still getting up at night as he had been doing for the past several years. It was beginning to look like antioxidant therapy was just another passing fad.

He then learned that many who have regained their health through antioxidant therapy did so using a saturation or therapeutic dose. He had been taking only two tablets a day. So he increased his dose to a total of 11 tablets, dividing them through the day, so he took some with each meal.

Within one week after starting the therapeutic dose, he noticed that he didn't have to get up at night to void his bladder. This was the first time in years he could sleep through the night undisturbed. He hasn't had any prostate problems since.

But this wasn't all. For the several years he had been experiencing increasing pain in his arms, shoulders, and knees. The pain intensified during the cold winter months. Over the previous three years, he had been in almost constant pain. After taking the antioxidant supplements, the pain vanished.

Dr. Rosquist said he felt so good that "I decided I was going to stay on this continuously for the rest of my life."

After his own success, he began recommending antioxidant supplements to his patients, and achieved what he described as "phenomenal results."

One of the first patients he had try antioxidant therapy was a man with terminal lung cancer, with tumors in both lungs. The cancer had enveloped so much of his lungs and surrounding tissues that the doctors wouldn't even attempt an operation. They thought he was too far gone for chemotherapy and radiation. They sent him home to die. He came to Dr. Rosquist, to see if there was an alternative therapy that might be of some help. "Here was a man in a very bad condition," says Dr. Rosquist. "His nose was purple, his hands were purple, his face was purple, his lips were purple. He was breathing in short pants, really struggling for oxygen."

After looking at him, Dr. Rosquist said, "I didn't know what I could do." He had been having some success with antioxidant therapy, so gave the patient some supplements, told him to take a therapeutic dosage, and sent him home.

The patient called back in 60 days and said he had good news and bad news. The bad news was that they discovered that in addition to cancer he also had a heart problem. So his doctor sent him to the Mayo Clinic in Rochester, Minnesota, because his case was too complicated for them to handle. After seven days of extensive examinations,

they told him that the tumors in his left lung had totally disappeared. That's the good news. Knowing what his condition was before coming to them, the doctors at the Mayo Clinic asked him what he had been doing. He told them his doctor had him taking a special compound. They told him to continue to take it and come back in 30 days. Because one lung was now better, they might be able to do surgery, and if his heart was okay, an angiogram.

In 30 days he went back and they ran him through their testing procedures again. After the examinations, they took him aside and asked, "Tell us again, what have you been doing?"

"Well, I told you, I've been taking these vitamins from this doctor and this compound from France. Why do you ask?"

"Your tumors are gone in your right lung as well. Because your tumors are gone in the right and left lungs and your breathing is so much better, we don't have to do the angiogram."

"Well what do I do now?"

"Go home and continue to do what you are doing and don't stop," they told him. "Come back and see us in three months."

He was feeling so good that he thought he was cured and didn't need the vitamins anymore, and stopped taking the antioxidants. The cancer came back.

The man was a smoker and during this whole time he continued to smoke. Even though he kept smoking, when he took the antioxidants his cancer went into remission. But when he stopped taking the supplements, the cancer returned. Many people don't realize that it is their lifestyle and habits that bring on much of the disease they face, and if they don't change their habits, they will never rid themselves completely from degeneration.

This man wouldn't give up smoking even when cancer ravaged his body. But, he said he would continue to take antioxidants for the rest of his life.

Some people who take antioxidants take enough to neutralize most of the new free radicals they are exposed to every day, but not enough to reverse degenerative conditions already raging inside them. They need to take enough to handle both the daily influx of free radicals and support the body's healing and recuperative processes.

Glen A. Halvorson, M.D., considers antioxidants to be the key in reversing the aging process naturally.[4] Dr. Halvorson, a diabetic, was introduced to antioxidant therapy while fighting an illness that involved his respiratory and gastrointestinal tract. The illness sapped his energy, affected his memory, and interfered with insulin production and control of his blood sugar. As part of a nutritional treatment plan, his personal physician prescribed Pycnogenol.

The antioxidant supplement worked miracles. Not only did it help him regain his health, but many chronic problems also showed remarkable improvement. He suffered for several years with chronic aching knee pain that resulted from six knee surgeries due to sports-related injuries. After taking the supplement for a few months he said, "That knee pain has almost completely resolved. Recurrent swelling in my left knee during exercise, including golf, has completely disappeared."

He continues, "I was on allergy shots and antihistamines for nearly two years with no improvement prior to taking Pycnogenols, which have relieved my allergic symptoms so that I no longer take medications...I've also experienced a similar decrease in blood-sugar levels anecdotally reported by many diabetics. I'm taking less in the evening to control morning blood-sugar levels that increased whenever I stopped taking Pycnogenols."

Impressed by the results he experienced, he began to investigate the medical literature to find out as much as he could about the healing powers of antioxidants. "My research and personal experience substantiate claims that Pycnogenol is a potent antioxidant that boosts immune defense, improves health, and even rejuvenates aging skin. As a physician, I was trained to diagnose and treat disease, not prevent it." He now advocates preventative medicine, and to all who will listen he tells them, "I encourage you to examine the evidence yourself and take responsibility for your current and future health." It's a lot easier to prevent a disease from happening than it is to remove it after it has become established in the body. Antioxidants can do that.

Dave Shook, president of the Chronic Fatigue Syndrome Foundation in Greensborough, North Carolina, says that antioxidant therapy "has made a dramatic difference in my life. I've suffered from chronic fatigue syndrome for the past seven years...Since I've been taking Pycnogenols I've noticed I have much less fatigue and a lot more energy."

Even more important to him was what it did for the rest of his body. He suffered continually with arthritic pain in his left shoulder. Four orthopedic surgeons told him surgery was his only hope for improvement. "Well, after about two weeks on Pycnogenols I found that the pain was reduced to the level that I was able to function again. I can use my arm or raise my shoulder without any problem whatsoever." Needless surgery was avoided by simply taking antioxidants.

In 1989 Bill Gleason was diagnosed with non-Hodgkin's lymphoma cancer stage four. This disease is almost always malignant and characteristically causes enlargement of the lymph nodes in the neck and other regions. It often spreads causing cancer to develop anywhere in the body. He underwent chemotherapy for 18 months and the doctors said it was in partial remission. Treatment was stopped for a year and a half. In that time the cancer came back, spreading to his kidney and stomach. He didn't want to endure chemotherapy again and opted to try antioxidant therapy. After taking supplements for about seven months he went in for a CAT scan. The scan showed no signs of cancer. "Until this day I'm living normal," Bill says, "no cancer to be found."

Twelve-year old Angie had asthma since she was five years old. Antioxidants helped her break free from the binding chains of this illness and allow her to run and play like other children. "I don't have to take any more of my inhalers," she happily explains, or "any more of my medicine, and I'm more free to do what I want to do."

Benefits from antioxidants can be obtained even without taking supplements. After looking at the MRI, the doctors told Donna her results were one of the worst ever seen at that clinic. Donna suffered from multiple sclerosis (MS). She was told to expect to be wheelchair bound within five years, blind within eight, and probably dead in ten to twelve. This wasn't a positive prognosis. Multiple sclerosis is an autoimmune disease in which nerve cells slowly deteriorate and harden, leading to the loss of muscle control and function. There is no cure.

She learned that many people with MS have gained a great deal of improvement without drugs using a dietary approach. The approach is basically a low-fat diet with almost no meat or dairy products and a heavy emphasis on lots of fresh fruits and vegetables rich in antioxidants and other nutrients. The diet worked miracles. "Nutrition has had a profound impact on my battle with MS." Says Donna with conviction, "Five years ago they said by now I'd be in a wheelchair. I'd like to go back to the doctor and say, 'Look!'" She continues to remain physically active and free from crippling pain.

Michelle first noticed something was wrong when she began experiencing shooting pain in her fingers and knees while hanging drapes. She brushed it off as just strain from her job as an interior decorator. The pain persisted off and on for some time. One morning she woke up, and two of her fingers had become swollen for no apparent reason. She began to suspect that something other than just strain might be involved. When she went to the doctor, he told her she had lupus—an autoimmune disease.

Lupus is a chronic inflammatory disease in which the immune system attacks connective tissue as if it were foreign or diseased. Because connective tissue is an integral part of most every organ in the body, lupus can cause prob-

Antioxidants protect us against the health-destroying effects of free radicals.

lems anywhere and is usually accompanied by chronic pain. A characteristic sign of lupus is a red rash that often develops on the cheeks and nose.

Like most other degenerative diseases in our society, there is no cure. The doctor recommended drug therapy to help her cope with the symptoms. Michelle didn't want to rely on drugs for the rest of her life and sought the counsel of a nutritionist. Under the nutritionist's guidance, Michelle altered her eating habits. Meat and dairy were almost completely eliminated. Packaged foods were avoided. Whole-grain products and fresh fruits and vegetables were stressed. She began a detox program which involved drinking lots of fresh vegetable juice rich in antioxidants and other vital nutrients. She consumed seven to nine glasses of freshly made juice every day. She also took vitamin supplements.

For over a year now Michelle has been free of pain. The disease that once engulfed her body and threatened her health has now vanished from sight. This would not have happened if she had decided to treat her disease with drugs. "I want people to know," she says "that there is an alternative and that the alternative does work. Degenerative disease, no matter its name, is the result of a body that's just not working properly. Drugs don't help a body work better. They don't fix anything. They just mask the problem."

THE ANTIOXIDANTS

The major dietary antioxidants are vitamins A (beta-carotene), C, and E, the trace mineral selenium, and bioflavonoids (vitamin-like compounds found in plants). Our bodies make many of its own antioxidants but in order to do so it must get the proper amount of nutrients from foods. In this section, the key antioxidants necessary for optimal health are described.

Vitamin A and Beta-Carotene

Beta-carotene belongs to a group of plant pigments known as carotenoids. These pigments give carrots their orange color and are found abundantly in apricots, cantaloupe, squash, sweet potatoes, and pumpkin. They are also found in broccoli, spinach, and other dark, leafy greens. Beta-carotene is often added to foods as a coloring agent.

Carotenoids are found only in plants and are converted into vitamin A by the liver. Beta-carotene is the most biologically active of the carotenoids. Our bodies split the beta-carotene molecule in half to form two molecules of vitamin A. Vitamin A, itself, is found only in animal products like meat, eggs, and milk. There is no vitamin A in plants. When people speak of the vitamin A content in plant foods they are really referring to its precursor, beta-carotene.

Vitamin A is an essential nutrient involved in maintaining and regulating eye function, bone and tooth growth, reproduction, hormone synthesis, digestion, and immunity. It is also one of our primary antioxidants. As an antioxidant its use has proven beneficial for the improvement of many health conditions associated with the destructive action of free radicals.

Vitamin A is important to our immune system. It is required for the growth of tissues such as the lymph glands where antibodies are produced. It protects the linings and membranes in our body and cells against invasion from bacteria, viruses, and carcinogens such as free radicals. Children with even mild vitamin A deficiencies develop respiratory diseases and diarrhea at two and three times the rate of children with normal vitamin A status.[5]

Mega doses of vitamin A are not recommended. Vitamin A is a fat-soluble compound and, therefore, is easily stored in the fatty tissues of the body and particularly in the liver. If taken in excess, it can cause severe liver damage and numerous other health problems. Beta-carotene, on the other hand, is converted into vitamin A only in the amount needed by the body. Because it is nontoxic even in large amounts, it is preferred in supplemental form. Although not fully understood yet, beta-carotene also has health benefits aside from its association with vitamin A. This is another reason why beta-carotene is preferred over vitamin A.

Cancer is one of the diseases that is associated with free-radical reactions, and a number of studies have suggested that beta-carotene might reduce cancer risk. Since 1925, researchers have noted a relationship between vitamin A deficiency and cancer. Experiments up through the 1950s confirmed this relationship. Since then, scientists have learned that cancer-causing free radicals can react strongly with DNA in vitamin A-deficient cells. It has been seen that animals with adequate amounts of vitamin A do not get cancer easily when injected with cancerous cells.[6] Dr. Frank Chytill of Vanderbilt University stated: "Recent dramatic findings about vitamin A and its effects on cancer have opened up a whole new approach to cancer therapy. With vitamin A therapy, doctors may some day have a way to restore body cells to normal—rather than destroy them with surgery, chemotherapy, or radiation. We now have laboratory evidence that, under certain laboratory conditions, cancers such as breast, lung, and skin tumors can be cured by treatment with vitamin A."[7]

Harvard Medical School initiated a large study to determine the effects of beta-carotene on the occurrence of cancer. A total of 22,000 physicians were recruited as volunteers. Half took supplements of beta-carotene and half took a placebo. The study lasted ten years.

Researchers were disappointed to find little difference in the rate of cancer between the beta-carotene and placebo groups. However, something unexpected happened. Physicians in the study who had a history of coronary artery disease and took beta-carotene experienced a 50 percent reduction in all major cardiovascular events, such as heart attacks and strokes."[8]

While this study did establish beta-carotene as an important nutrient in the fight against heart disease, it raised some questions about its ability to protect against cancer. Numerous studies performed earlier had already shown beta-carotene to be of benefit against cancer. So why the discrepancy? Some believe it's due to the type of beta-carotene used. Naturally derived beta-carotene is always associated with a mix of other carotenoids. Synthetic beta-carotene is pure. Pure beta-carotene appears to be potent against the conditions that lead to heart disease, but to fight cancer a mixture of carotenoids may be necessary. The cancer fighting effects attributed to beta-carotene may actually be the result of a synergistic mixture of beta-carotene with other naturally occurring carotenoids.

Research on other carotenoids which include alpha-carotene, lutein, lycopene, zeaxanthin, and cryptoxanthin has shown a strong anti-cancer effect. Only beta-carotene is converted into vitamin A, but some of the other carotenoids have stronger antioxidant effects. Studies of alpha-carotene drastically reduced the number of tumors in an animal study of liver, lung, and skin cancer. The cancer-fighting ability of alpha-carotene exceeded that of beta-carotene. Lycopene, a pigment which gives tomatoes their red color, reduced the risk of prostate cancer by nearly 45 percent in men who consumed at least 10 serving a week of tomato-based foods. In contrast, those who ate four to seven servings a week had only a 20-percent reduction in their risk of prostate cancer. Lycopene has shown to protect against cancer of mouth, pharynx, esophagus, stomach, colon and rectum. Lycopene was much more potent than beta-carotene in quenching singlet-oxygen, a type of free radical. However, the antioxidant-quenching ability of these nutrients depended on the dietary intake of both carotenoids.[9]

The greatest protection comes from a complete mix of carotenoids. Blood levels of total carotenoids were measured in 1,899 men and their cardiovascular health was followed for 13 years. The men with the highest blood levels of carotenoids had 36 percent fewer heart attacks and deaths than those with the lowest levels of carotenoids.

The dietary intake of several carotenoids in 332 lung cancer patients was compared to that of 865 cancer-free controls. After adjusting for smoking and other risk factors, researchers reported that the lowest risk of lung cancer occurred in those with the highest intake of mixed carotenoids.[10]

The conclusion that can be drawn from all this is that a mixture of all carotenoids provides the greatest range of protection against free-radical-induced disease, and the more that is consumed the greater the benefit.

There is no dietary minimum set for beta-carotene or other carotenoids. The Recommended Dietary Allowance for vitamin A is set a 800 mcg RE for women and 1000 mcg RE for men. This is equivalent to about 8,000-10,000 IU of beta-carotene. Comparing vitamin A with beta-carotene is confusing because vitamin A is measured in RE or retinol equivalents while beta-carotene is measured in IU (international units).

Vitamin C

Before the 19th century people on long ocean voyages feared the mysterious disease known as scurvy more than they did marauding pirates or devastating hurricanes. In those days scurvy killed more sailors than wars or natural disasters. As many as two-thirds of a ship's crew might die of scurvy on a long voyage. Although not known at the time, the cure that could have saved them was to simply eat fresh fruits and vegetables. The rations of fresh fruits and vegetables, which unknowingly provided protection from the disease, were used up early, requiring them to subsist on grains and meat for the remainder of the voyage.

Scurvy is characterized by bleeding gums, loosened teeth, bone fragility, muscle degeneration and weakness (including the heart muscle), rough skin, spontaneous bruising, failure of wounds to heal, anemia, and pain. For centuries the disease was a complete mystery. Food was suspected by some. James Lind, an 18th century British physician, put this theory to the test. He took 12 sailors with scurvy and divided them into six pairs. Each pair received a different supplement to their normal sea rations: cider, vinegar, sulfuric acid, seawater, oranges and lemons, or a laxative mixed with spices. Why Lind chose these particular items is not clear, but the sailors who received daily portions of vinegar, sulfuric acid, and laxatives must have had a very rough time of it. They were already suffering from the effects of scurvy, and to consume these unpleasant items must have greatly added to their misery. The sailors who received the oranges and lemons, on the other hand, quickly recovered. Despite Lind's discovery, it took the British Navy another half century to implement a program to ward off scurvy. At that time all British ships were required to carry a daily ration of oranges and lemons—formerly called "limes" for every sailor. The nickname "limey" was given to British sailors because of this practice. The antiscurvy substance in citrus fruits, which we now call vitamin C, was not actually discovered until 1928.

Vitamin C is necessary for the production of certain hormones. It is used in the synthesis of several amino acids that end up being converted to hormones, most notably norepinephrine and thyroxin. Thyroxin is of particular interest because it is the hormone produced by the thyroid gland which regulates the metabolic rate of the entire body. Lack of either vitamin C or vitamin A can adversely affect the thyroid and thyroxin production. Low thyroxin production lowers metabolism which, in turn, slows down healing and encourages body fat deposition.

Vitamin C plays an important role in the health of the cardiovascular system. A deficiency causes blood vessels to deteriorate and lose integrity. Capillaries under the skin spontaneously break, producing pinpoint hemorrhages. Bleeding occurs easily—especially in the gums, which is one of the classic signs of scurvy. Arteries are damaged, leading to clotting and the rapid growth of atherosclerotic plaques. Muscles, including the heart muscle, degenerate, increasing susceptibility to heart attack.

It is interesting to note that one of the symptoms of vitamin C deficiency is atherosclerosis. Without this antioxidant, free-radical reactions run wild and cause damage to the circulatory system. One study of vitamin C deficiency in humans almost came to a tragic end. Human volunteers who consumed a vitamin C deficient diet for several months ran into serious complications that caused a termination of the study. Some suddenly developed cardiac emergencies before any signs of scurvy became obvious.[11]

It's easy to get enough vitamin C in your diet to prevent scurvy. Vitamin C is found abundantly in most fresh fruits and vegetables. Meat contains very little vitamin C, and grains like wheat and rice contain none. Vitamin C is sensitive to heat and is destroyed in cooking, so processed foods are sadly deficient in this important nutrient. The only way we can get sufficient quantities of vitamin C in our diet is from eating raw fruits and vegetables. Frozen fruits and vegetables are also deficient because they are usually blanched (a heating process) before freezing to inactivate all the enzymes.

Although scurvy is relatively rare in Western countries where vitamin C-rich foods are plentiful, people who do not eat enough raw produce can develop subclinical deficiency conditions. They get just barely enough of the vitamin to prevent full-blown symptoms of scurvy, but the body is suffering and slowly degenerating with life-threatening atherosclerotic plaques forming. Moderate vitamin C deficiency can lead to a slow death by way of any number of cardiovascular conditions.

Modern food processing destroys vitamin C as does the heat involved in ordinary cooking. A person who does not eat any raw fruits or vegetables can easily become vitamin C deficient. In a society that subsists primarily on restaurant foods and packaged prepared meals, which are lacking in vitamin C, it's no wonder why diseases of the heart

WHAT DO DOCTORS DO TO PREVENT A HEART ATTACK?

What do cardiologists—medical doctors who specialize in treating heart and related illnesses—do for themselves to prevent heart disease? Most of them take antioxidant vitamins.

A survey among members of the American Academy of Cardiology revealed that 54% routinely take antioxidants. The most common dosages: 400 IU of vitamin E, 500 mg of vitamin C and 20,000 IU of beta-carotene. Why are so many cardiologists taking antioxidant vitamins? Studies are showing promising results. For example, among the more recent studies:

• A population-based study conducted in Canada with 2,313 men demonstrated vitamin supplement use was associated with a 69% reduced risk of death due to coronary artery disease and a 47% reduced risk for a non-fatal heart attack. (*Canadian Journal of Cardiology* 1996, 12:930)

• In the Cambridge Antioxidant Heart Study, 2,002 patients with coronary artery disease were given either vitamin E or a placebo for 510 days. Vitamin E supplementation reduced the number of patients experiencing a heart attack by an impressive 77%. (*Lancet* 1996, 347:781)

More cardiologists take vitamins than low-dose aspirin—the standard preventive treatment for heart disease. Aspirin, like omega-3 fatty acids, works by thinning the blood. Most cardiologists, however, believe that preventing oxidative damage to the arteries to be a better solution to the problem—they must or they wouldn't take the vitamins themselves.

Another interesting statistic revealed by this survey is that while most cardiologists recommend aspirin to their patients to prevent heart attack, They themselves take antioxidants instead of aspirin for the same purpose. An interesting discrepancy. Vitamins have no adverse side effects, unlike drugs—including aspirin—so why do they recommend a substance that can be harmful and one they prefer not to use themselves? ♥

Source: Mehta, J. 1997. Intake of antioxidants among American cardiologists. *Am. J. Cardiol.* 79:1558.

and circulatory system are a major health problem.

Like the carotenoids, vitamin C has gained a reputation for its cancer-fighting ability. Dr. Linus Pauling, a two-time Nobel prize winner, advocated the use of vitamin C as a means to prevent and treat cancer. He conducted clinical studies with cancer patients showing that high doses of vitamin C significantly prolonged the life of cancer patients. Similar results were noted in subsequent studies with a variety of different cancers. This led Dr. Pauling to claim that vitamin C could cut the death rate from cancer by 75 percent. In the U.S. that would amount to 420,000 lives saved each year. Other researchers have verified the benefits of vitamin C against cancer.[12]

A few years following Pauling's findings, the Mayo Clinic attempted to repeat one of his studies using large doses of vitamin C on terminally ill cancer patients. Their results showed no difference between those who took vitamin C and those who didn't. Pauling's theory was brought into question. Pauling, however, explained that the difference was due to the fact that the patients at the Mayo Clinic had also undergone chemotherapy, which his did not and, consequently, their immune systems were destroyed. Vitamin C works against cancer by increasing the effectiveness of the immune system. If the immune system has been destroyed by drugs and radiation, vitamin C will be much less effective.

Vitamin C is an important nutrient in maintaining the health of our immune system. Vitamin C aids in the production of white blood cells when microscopic invaders attack our bodies. Studies have shown that vitamin C can strengthen the body's immune defenses, thus shortening the duration of viral infections. Taking vitamin C at the first signs of a cold is now a common practice.

Vitamin C is a powerful antioxidant and acts like a bodyguard against oxidization from free radicals. Its antioxidant properties aid in its fight against the effects of menacing microorganisms and renegade cancer cells.

The amount needed to prevent scurvy is just 10 mg a day. Recommended daily levels vary among countries. In the United States and Canada, the RDA is 60 mg. In Great Britain it is 30 mg and in Germany it's 75 mg. Although these amounts vary widely, they are all generously above the requirement to prevent scurvy. Keep in mind that these minimums are established to maintain health in healthy individuals, not to restore health in sick people. Circumstances may increase nutrient needs.

When we are sick, our bodies use up vitamin C quickly and so more than the recommended amount may be necessary to maintain optimal health. When we have a cold or other illness, taking extra vitamin C helps give the immune system a boost. Smokers are advised to take 100 mg per day.

Likewise, stress, toxins, injury, and pollution all increase our need for vitamin C.

Since vitamin C is water-soluble, it is needed every day. What the body does not immediately use is washed away in the urine. For this reason, some people take large quantities just to be sure they are getting enough. Dr. Linus Pauling recommended mega dosages up to 2,000 to 4,000 mg a day. Such large quantities, however, may cause unpleasant side effects such as nausea, abdominal cramping, and diarrhea. Most authorities feel that the safe maximum dose under normal circumstances is between 100 and 500 mg a day.

Vitamin E

Thelma Van Arsdel had taken vitamin E from the time she was in her early 50s until her death at age 93. The only time Van Arsdel stopped taking it was in her late 60s, and she said that during this time she began feeling the typical aches and pains of her age. But as soon as she began using vitamin E again, she regained her flexibility and was unusually alert and active the rest of her life. Like Van Arsdel, many people swear that vitamin E makes a dramatic difference in the quality of their lives.

Probably no other single nutrient has gained such widespread acclaim as vitamin E. In recent years, vitamin E has gained a reputation as a super nutrient and by some it has been hailed as a miracle vitamin. It is one of our most important aids in combatting the effects of eating modern processed foods saturated with health-damaging vegetable oils. Because vitamin E is a fat-soluble antioxidant, it battles free radicals within the fatty tissues of the body and is an effective warrior against one of our biggest health threats—polyunsaturated oils.

A multitude of studies have suggested that vitamin E provides some degree of protection from the effects of aging and degenerative disease. It has shown to be beneficial in protecting against cancer and heart disease as well as relieving symptoms associated with menopause; it enhances healing, prevents scarring on wounds, boosts efficiency of the immune system, improves sexual potency, and increases athletic performance, among other things. Benefits associated with vitamin E are continually being reported in the medical literature.

Vitamin E is an essential nutrient. A deficiency can lead to degeneration of red blood cells and anemia, muscle degeneration and weakness, and fibrocystic breast disease. Our white blood cells, the workforce of our immune system, require vitamin E to function in our defense against cancer and disease-causing microorganisms. Without adequate vitamin E reserves, the entire body quickly deteriorates, accelerating the aging process.

A major factor in the efficiency of vitamin E in protecting us from the ravages of disease is its ability to act as an antioxidant. Vitamin E is found in every cell where it functions as a bodyguard against renegade free radicals. Within the cell membrane (the outer covering or "skin" around our cells) it provides a first line of defense against free-radical attack. The cell membrane is composed predominately of fatty acids, the *unsaturated* portion being easy prey to free radicals. When the body has enough vitamin E, this antioxidant is found liberally within the membranes of the cells. Vitamin E also patrols the inside of the cells protecting delicate organelles (cell organs) and DNA, both of which are highly vulnerable to oxidative destruction from free radicals.

A deficiency of vitamin E can leave cells without sufficient bodyguards to protect them, and the cells succumb to free-radical attack and quickly break down. It's no wonder why vitamin E has been labeled an anti-aging nutrient. Without enough of it, every cell in your body deteriorates as a result of a constant bombardment from free-radical invaders.

A deficiency can be caused by not eating enough foods with the vitamin, or excessive exposure to substances that generate free radicals. Vitamin E reserves are quickly used up in fighting free radicals and, if they are not replenished, our cells are left defenseless.

One of the most vulnerable places in the body to free-radical attack is the lungs. Air pollutants and some forms of oxygen, such as ozone, are strong oxidizing agents. Oxidation occurs when carcinogens react with polyunsaturated fats in our bodies, forming free radicals. Polyunsaturated fatty acids within the cell membranes of our lungs are readily exposed to oxidative elements in the air we breathe.

Free radicals play a key role in the development of all types of cancer. Lung cancer is the most deadly of all. More people die from it than any other form of cancer. One of the primary reasons why tobacco smoke is toxic is that it creates free radicals. Not everyone that smokes gets cancer, and cancer is not limited to just smokers. Nonsmokers also get lung cancer. Diet also plays a big part. Those smokers who do not get adequate amounts of vitamin E in their diet and consume lots of vegetable oil are the ones most vulnerable to lung cancer. Some smokers, knowing that vitamin E and other antioxidants afford some degree of protection against lung cancer, take heavy doses of antioxidant supplements; although it helps, a better option would be to quit smoking.

Vitamin E is a valuable aid in the fight against heart disease. Recent epidemiological surveys have suggested that diets or supplements containing abundant vitamin E are of benefit in reducing the risk of coronary heart disease.[13]

Since vitamin E is fat-soluble, its effects are most pronounced within fatty tissues of the body where you would expect to find cholesterol and polyunsaturated fats. Vitamin E protects these fats from becoming oxidized. As you recall from Chapter 7, only *oxidized* fats are incorporated into arterial plaque. Normal fats are never associated with atherosclerotic arteries. If you have adequate vitamin E reserves, you are protected to some degree from the deposition of these fats in the arteries. Vitamin E helps protect arteries from free-radical injury that may initiate the atherosclerotic process and the development of plaque. Vitamin E also reduces platelet adhesion, thus reducing blood pressure and the tendency of blood to clot and clog arteries.[14, 15]

The World Health Organization conducted a study that compared death rates from coronary artery disease with several well accepted risk factors. The association between elevated blood cholesterol, or blood pressure, and coronary artery disease death rates was minimal. The best predictor of heart attack risk turned out to be low blood levels of vitamin E, and the lower the level the greater the risk. The authors concluded: "The differences in coronary artery disease mortality are primarily attributable to plasma status of vitamin E, which might have a protective function."[16]

Vitamin E has been reported to reduce the incidence of heart disease in long-term users. In studies conducted by Richard Passwater, Ph.D., this vitamin's protective qualities were impressively demonstrated. The studies involved two groups. One group took 400 IU or more of vitamin E daily for at least ten years. The study involved 2,508 people from 50 to 98 years in age. Out of this number of people, statistics indicate that 836 of them would develop heart disease. The actual number in this group developing the disease was only four! Less than one percent of the expected number. The second group consisted of 1,038 people taking 1,200 IU or more of vitamin E daily for at least four years. In this group 323 would be expected to get heart disease. Only seven did.[17]

Numerous studies have shown that dietary intake of vitamin E either in fresh vegetables and whole grains or in supplements decreases risk of coronary disease by as much as 50 percent.[18, 19]

Vitamin E has shown to have beneficial effects on certain diseases that are known to be associated with the overconsumption of vegetable oils. The autoimmune diseases lupus and rheumatoid arthritis are two examples. Studies also show promising results in slowing neurological problems in older people, preventing them in children, and in treating Parkinson's and Alzheimer's patients.[20] A study published in *The New England Journal of Medicine* put 341 Alzheimer's patients on daily regimen of vitamin E or a placebo. For up to two years researchers charted the pace of the patients' deterioration. The result: those taking vitamin E showed a 25 percent less decline in mental ability. Research at the University of South Florida has shown that Alzheimer's disease is associated with free radicals. When these scientists added beta-amyloid, an abnormal protein that's one of the characteristics (and maybe a contributing factor) of Alzheimer's, to a lab slide containing blood vessels, it sparked the production of free radicals; these, in turn, constricted the vessels. In the brain, the same reaction would starve brain cells of oxygen and essential nutrients, killing brain tissue. When researchers treated the blood vessels with antioxidants like vitamin E, the vessels stayed wide open.[21]

Free-radical damage can affect brain function by limiting oxygen delivery to the brain by contributing to atherosclerosis or by damaging individual brain cells. In a series of experiments conducted by D. Harman, mice were give different types of fat in their diet and their mental function was measured. When young mice were given vegetable oil containing vitamin E, they showed significant improvement in mental capacity over those fed oils lacking the vitamin. This demonstrated that free-radical damage, even at young ages, can affect mental capacity and that vitamin E can provide some protection against mental deterioration from free-radical damage.[22] It also demonstrated that unsaturated oils cause free-radical reactions that affect brain function. Adding vitamin E prevented free-radical formation.

Like vitamin C, vitamin E can give our immune system a boost to fight off foreign invaders and clean out dying and diseased cells. Jeffrey Blumberg, a human-nutrition researcher at Tufts University in Boston, tested the effects of vitamin E on the immune system of healthy older people. In a four-month study, different amounts of vitamin E were added to volunteers' diets. Each of 88 volunteers, 65 and older, was assigned to one of four groups: members of the first group got 60 IUs (international units) of vitamin E per day; a second group got 200 IUs; a third got 800 IUs, and the fourth got placebos.

Although they theorized that vitamin E would produce positive results, what they discovered was startling. Normally, immune cells become less efficient as we age and don't protect our bodies as well against disease. But the cells of the vitamin E groups didn't act their age. "The responses of 65- and 70-year-olds looked more like those of 40-year-olds," Blumberg says.

Subjects taking 200 IUs got a bigger immune-system boost than the ones who got only 60 IUs. But the 200-IU group also fared better than those on 800 IUs. Why? The researchers suspect 200 IUs may be the optimal dose for immune system benefit.

With results like those described here it's no wonder why people such as Thelma Van Arsdel, who took vitamin E regularly, lived to be 93. Like others, she found that the vitamin helped to prevent the typical aches and pains so often associated with aging.

Vitamin E consists of several different types of compounds collectively known as tocopherols. The most active of these is alpha-tocopherol. Most vitamin E supplements are made using only synthetically derived alpha-tocopherol. The other tocopherols also have health benefits and studies suggest that when used together, as they are found in nature, their effects are enhanced. The best vitamin E supplements to use are those that combine alpha-tocopherol with mixed tocopherols.

Vitamin E is found most abundantly in green and leafy vegetables, wheat germ, whole grains, liver, egg yolks, nuts, and seeds. Vitamin E is destroyed by heat and food processing. Eleanor Noss Whitney, Ph.D., R.D., former associate professor at Florida State University and president of Nutrition and Health Associates, states, "Vitamin E is readily destroyed by heat processing and oxidation, so fresh or lightly processed foods are preferable as sources of this vitamin. Processed and convenience foods do not contribute enough vitamin E to ensure an adequate intake." Dr. Whitney also states, "A person's need for vitamin E is higher if the amount of polyunsaturated vegetable oils consumed is higher."[23] So those who eat vitamin E-deficient processed foods, which are usually full of free-radical-producing polyunsaturated oils, are likely to be vitamin E-deficient to some level.

The RDA for vitamin E is 30 IU, or 10 mg for men and 8 mg for women. If you eat a lot of vegetable oils or foods cooked in or with vegetable oil, your need is greater.

Studies indicate that between 200 and 400 IUs of vitamin E is the optimal range for enhancing the immune system and lowering risk for certain diseases. Like any supplement, vitamin E may be less safe at extremely high doses, and may throw off the balance of other nutrients in your body. Vitamin E supplements are considered safe for most people up to about 1,000 IUs, but some people should check with their doctors before taking vitamin E or any other supplements. If you take aspirin to protect against heart disease, or if you take any other prescription drug, check with your doctor. Vitamin E, like aspirin, is a blood thinner, so your physician may want to adjust how much you take.

Selenium

The mineral selenium was first discovered in 1817 in the refuse of a sulfuric acid factory. Since its discovery and until the 1950s, selenium was considered a toxin dangerous to health. In large doses, it can cause digestive disorders, loss of hair and nails, skin lesions, tooth damage, and nervous system disorders.

Selenium's bad reputation changed abruptly in 1957 when it was found to be an essential trace element in lab animals. Deficiency symptoms include abnormalities in the vascular system, cataracts, hair loss, and degeneration of the pancreas. The news of this discovery was quickly followed by numerous reports of farm animals from around the world that appeared to have selenium deficiency.

There is a significant relationship between soil levels of selenium and deficiency. Animals that live in areas where the selenium content of the soil is poor often became sick. A correlation was later discovered in the human population as well. Animals and humans get selenium from plants which absorb the mineral from the soil. If the soil has little of this mineral, the plants will also. Animals and humans subsisting on foods grown in selenium-deficient soils will, likewise, be deficient.

Selenium's importance as a dietary nutrient was significantly demonstrated in the Chinese province of Keshan. It was here that a troubling heart and circulatory condition called Keshan disease became a serious problem. It is most evident in children. The people in Keshan ate only the foods grown in the selenium-poor soils of the region. It wasn't until the 1970s that the cause of the disease was linked to a selenium deficiency.

There are large regions in the world that are selenium deficient, and some areas where it is relatively abundant. Deficiency disease is not as pronounced in other selenium-poor areas as it was in Keshan because most people eat foods brought in from other regions where selenium levels are greater. While their deficiency may not be as great as those seen in Keshan, many do develop a variety of illnesses that could be prevented if adequate amounts of selenium were available to them.

The importance of selenium to cardiovascular health was demonstrated in the provinces of China where the mineral was deficient. This correlation can be seen throughout the world. Ray Shamberger, M.D., and Charles Willis, M.D., of the Cleveland Clinic in Ohio, reported in 1976 that people who live in low-selenium areas have three times more heart disease than those living in areas where the soil and water are rich in the mineral.[24]

One of the most striking correlations with selenium and human health is in relation to the incidence of cancer. Dr. Shamberger and colleagues have documented an inverse relationship between the incidence of cancer and the amount of selenium in patients' blood samples. Also, the lower the level of selenium in locally grown crops, the higher the incidence of cancer. For these reasons, some scientists believe selenium helps to protect against cancer.

An analysis of cancer incidences in 34 American cities found that cancer is greater in areas where selenium content in the soil is poor. Rapid City, South Dakota, has the lowest cancer rate of any city in the United States. The people of Rapid City also have the highest measured blood selenium levels in the nation. But in Lima, Ohio, which has twice the cancer rate of Rapid City, the people have only 60 percent of the blood selenium levels of those in Rapid City.[25]

Researchers from around the world have found that selenium protects against various forms of heart disease and stroke; strengthens the immune system; reduces the risk of cancer; detoxifies environmental pollutants; and helps to defend against arthritis, Crohn's disease, respiratory infections, asthma, infertility, and a variety of skin diseases among other things.

Selenium's ability to protect against a variety of health problems is to a large extent due to its function as an antioxidant. Free radicals are associated with most all of the above conditions. Controlling the damage these troublemakers cause can limit the destructive effects of free radicals and allow the immune system to function more efficiently.

Technically, selenium itself is not an antioxidant. It is a trace element that functions as part of the antioxidant enzyme glutathione peroxidase. We don't get glutathione peroxidase from our food; it is synthesized inside our bodies. Selenium is a necessary component of glutathione peroxidase and, without it, the body could not manufacture this enzyme. So in that respect it can be considered as contributing to the antioxidant capacity of the body.

Glutathione peroxidase is a powerful antioxidant and, like vitamin E, is important in protecting the polyunsaturated fatty acids in our cells from oxidation. Its effects as an antioxidant are enhanced when combined with vitamin E and, likewise, vitamin E becomes more effective when adequate amounts of selenium are available.

Polyunsaturated fats from vegetable oils are known to cause cancer in lab animals. The cancer being caused, in whole or in part, by free radicals. Giving the animals antioxidants can block free-radical production and thus prevent the disease from developing.

Selenium and glutathione peroxidase seem to provide humans antioxidant protection against cancer. Asian women have a rate of breast cancer significantly lower than women from Western countries. Dr. Christine S. Wilson from University of California, San Francisco, compared the nutrient content of foods typically eaten in the United States and certain regions in Asia. She found that the Western diet contains about a fourth of the selenium of the Asian diet. She also noted that the Asian diet contained significantly less "easily oxidizable" polyunsaturated oils, 7.5 to 8.7 grams a day compared to 10 to 30 grams in Western diets. Because selenium is a vital element in the antioxidant glutathione peroxidase which protects against the oxidation of fatty acids, Dr. Wilson concluded that the combination of high selenium and low polyunsaturated fatty acids protects the Asian women against breast cancer.[26]

Exposure to certain environmental chemicals and heavy metals may increase our need for selenium. For example, oil refinery workers were found to have low selenium levels, in spite of taking 217 mcg per day; this was over three times the RDA of 55-70 mcg established by the Food and Nutrition Board.[27] Exposure to any toxic chemical that produces free radicals uses up selenium quickly. The greater the exposure to toxins, including polyunsaturated oils, the greater the drain on our antioxidant system and the greater the need.

Selenium content in food varies greatly. The best sources are from seafood, meat, and butter if the animals ate a diet high in selenium. Whole grains are the best plant sources, but again this depends on the selenium content of the soils in which they were grown. Fruits and vegetables generally supply very little selenium, regardless of the soil content. When whole grains are refined or polished, much of the selenium is removed. White flour is a poor source for selenium even if the wheat from which it came was grown in selenium-rich soil.

The RDA for selenium is 70 mcg for men and 55 mcg for women. If you are exposed to air pollutants, including outgassing of formaldehyde and other toxic chemicals from carpets, particle board, draperies, bed sheets, etc. and you eat vegetable oils or other chemical food additives, your need for selenium will be greater.

Like many other trace minerals, selenium can be toxic in large quantities. Selenium intakes in people up to nearly 750 mcg per day have been shown to have no toxic side effects.[28] This amount is far more then the RDA and more than even a therapeutic dose which is usually between 200-400 mcg.

Bioflavonoids

Bioflavonoids are a group of phytochemicals (plant chemicals) with antioxidant properties. Major sources include citrus fruits, grapes, plums, apricots, buckwheat, cherries, blackberries and rose hips. They are found abundantly in the white lining inside the rinds of citrus fruits.

Bioflavonoids are usually found in plants along with vitamin C and have much of the same properties. They are important complements to vitamin C because they enhance each other's effects. This can be illustrated from a study involving the herpes virus—the virus which produces cold sores. Cold sores tend to get better by themselves on average after nine and a half days. When vitamin C was supplemented at 1,000 mg per day, there was a slight reduction in the duration of the cold sores to about seven days. When

vitamin C and bioflavonoids were administered together at levels of 1,000 mg each, the length of time dropped from nine and a half to about three and a half days. The bioflavonoids and vitamin C mixture was significantly more effective than the vitamin C by itself.[29]

Bioflavonoids were originally classified as vitamins and given the name vitamin P. They were given the designation "P" in reference to their observed ability to strengthen and tighten connective tissue and prevent excessive capillary permeability.

By definition, vitamins are substances that prevent a diagnosable deficiency disease in the body. Bioflavonoids are like vitamins, but since the lack of them in the diet does not lead to any overt deficiency symptoms, the designation of vitamin P was dropped in 1950. Since that time, these substances have been termed bioflavonoids. Because there is no recognizable deficiency disease associated with bioflavonoids, there is no set recommended daily minimum requirement.

There are over 20,000 different bioflavonoids that have been identified so far, but only relatively few have been studied to any extent. It is estimated that the actual number of bioflavonoids is in the millions. Some are very powerful antioxidants, even stronger than either vitamins E or C in their ability to neutralize free radicals. The most well-known are rutin, hesperidin, quercetin, and epicatechin.

One of the major health benefits associated with citrus bioflavonoids is their ability to improve capillary-wall integrity. The capillaries, or small blood vessels, normally maintain a barrier between the blood and surrounding tissues. Pore spaces in the capillaries are very tiny and allow only certain substances to pass from the blood into surrounding tissues and vice versa. In this way, substances that don't belong in the blood are kept out and those that are supposed to stay in the blood remain. When the capillaries lose their integrity, due primarily from free-radical injury, they become weakened and substances from surrounding tissues can migrate into the bloodstream. This would allow materials inside the intestinal tract or respiratory tract to penetrate the capillary barrier and enter the blood. This is how many allergies are created. Undigested food particles in the intestines or pollen in the lungs can penetrate the capillary wall and enter the blood. These particles are recognized as foreign bodies by the immune system and an allergic reaction kicks in as the body attempts to rid itself of these invaders. This is why bioflavonoids have been suggested as useful in the management of asthma, hay fever, and some food allergies.[30]

Isoflavones are a group of bioflavonoids that are found exclusively in soybeans and soy products. Epidemiological studies have consistently found that Japanese people, who eat up to 110 times more isoflavones than Americans, are less likely to develop breast or prostate cancer. More than 1,000 studies conducted over the past few years illustrate the cancer-protective effects of soy isoflavones. Research also suggest that the earlier a person starts consuming soy foods, the greater will be his or her lifelong resistance to cancer.

One particular class of bioflavonoids known as proanthocyanidins or PCOs has been shown to be particularly powerful antioxidants. A patented blend of proanthocyanidins derived from the bark of the European coastal pine is known as Pycnogenol. Pycnogenol has become a very popular antioxidant supplement which users and researchers have attributed many health benefits beyond that of other antioxidants.

The benefits of proanthocyanidins demonstrated in studies and clinical experience include:[31]

• improves skin smoothness and elasticity
• strengthens capillaries, arteries and veins
• improves circulation and enhances cell vitality
• reduces capillary fragility and improves resistance to bruising and strokes
• reduces risk of phlebitis (inflammation of veins)
• reduces varicose veins
• reduces swelling of the legs
• helps restless-leg syndrome
• reduces diabetic retinopathy
• improves visual acuity
• helps improve sluggish memory
• reduces the effects of stress
• improves joint flexibility
• fights inflammation in arthritis and sports injuries

Pycnogenol derived from the European coastal pine is not the only source for these powerful proanthocyanidins. This mix of bioflavonoids can also be extracted from grapes, cranberries, beans, cola nuts, and other fruits and vegetables. The most common source for proanthocyanidins in North America is grape skins and grape seeds. You will often see supplements containing grape skin or grape seed extract. These extracts can be just as effective as Pycnogenol and in some cases even better.

Fresh grapes and grape juice are rich sources of proanthocyanidins. This was, undoubtedly, the secret ingredient in grapes that made Johanna Brandt's grape cure so effective against cancer and other degenerative diseases. It also explains why populations that drink a lot of wine, which

also is a good source of grape bioflavonoids, have a low death rate from heart disease.[32] As early as 1957 it had been shown that wine protected animals that were fed high-fat diets.[33] Researchers say that red wine may reduce the risk of Alzheimer's disease. A March 1997 study by France's National Institute of Health and Scientific Research showed that moderate drinkers who consumed two to four glasses of wine a day were 80 percent less likely than tea drinkers to develop senile dementia, and 75 percent less likely to develop Alzheimer's.[34]

Supplement advertisers love to announce the fact that the antioxidant effects of proanthocyanidins, either as Pycnogenol or grape seed extract, are 20 times more powerful than vitamin C and 50 times more powerful than vitamin E. For this reason, Pycnogenol is known as a super antioxidant. Pycnogenol is the most concentrated antioxidant known. The benefit of a highly concentrated antioxidant is that it enables the body to obtain protection against free radicals in tissues that have limited blood flow, such as the linings of inflamed joints, the elastin under the skin, the brain, and the spinal cord. Proanthocyanidins are one of the few dietary antioxidants that can readily cross the blood-brain barrier. Brain cells are very sensitive and can be injured easily by a number of substances in our foods and in our blood. The blood-brain barrier protects the brain from these substances, many of which normally circulate in the blood and may be necessary elsewhere in the body.

Brain tissue is composed predominantely of fatty tissues, most of which is cholesterol. Saturated and polyunsaturated fats are also present in abundance. Oxidation of the polyunsaturated fatty acids in the brain are a concern. Antioxidant body guards are vitally important in keeping our mental abilities youthful. As we age, mental ability declines. A great deal of this deterioration is due to free-radical damage that accumulates over the years.

Because proanthocyanidins can penetrate the blood-brain barrier, they provide antioxidant protection to our central nervous system and may be an important nutrient that can be useful against Alzheimer's and Parkinson's disease and other neurological disorders. People have reported that this antioxidant complex has been effective in reducing senility and improving memory.

No recommended daily amounts of any bioflavonoids have been established. How much is recommended as being safe, yet still beneficial? Pycnogenol appears to be very safe. It has been used for decades with no signs of toxicity even at mega dosages.[35] The consensus among several researchers is that people start with about 100 to 150 milligrams of Pycnogenol or equivalent daily for a few months and then switch to a maintenance level of 50 milligrams per day.

Other Antioxidants

Besides the major antioxidants listed above, there are numerous others both known and unknown. A few of the most recognized include zinc, CoQ10, superoxide dismutase (SOD), glutathione, catalase, glutathione peroxidase, BHA, and BHT.

Out of all of these, zinc is of the greatest dietary importance. Zinc is an active participant in nearly every organ of the body and is necessary for the activation of more than 70 enzymes, some of which have antioxidant capability. Like Selenium, zinc itself is not an antioxidant, but forms a critical part of other compounds that function as antioxidants. Zinc as well as copper forms a part of the antioxidant superoxide dismutase (SOD). Zinc is also involved in the making of proteins, immune system function, processing of vitamin A (a deficiency of zinc can cause a vitamin A deficiency), wound healing, the making of sperm, and the normal development of the fetus. A deficiency of zinc can lead to numerous symptoms ranging from growth retardation and night blindness, to thyroid dysfunction and anorexia. Significant sources of zinc in our foods come from fish, meat, and whole grains. In processed grains, much of the zinc is stripped away.

Our bodies manufacture many different types of antioxidant compounds which include CoQ10, superoxide dismutase (SOD), glutathione, catalase, glutathione peroxidase, and others. A few of these antioxidants are sold as dietary supplements. In the case of CoQ10, some studies show supplementation may be of benefit, but the rest are questionable. SOD, for example, is often billed as the ultimate antioxidant. However, there is no way that SOD supplements could be helpful; the enzyme is completely broken down by stomach acids during digestion.[36] If you eat the foods that have all the right vitamins and minerals, the body will have all the building blocks it needs to synthesize these antioxidants, and supplementation is unnecessary.

You may recognize the antioxidants BHA and BHT from the ingredient label of packaged foods. They are some of the most common food additives and are put in packaged foods as preservatives. Being antioxidants, they protect packaged foods from oxidizing and thus retard spoilage. BHA and BHT are sometimes sold as dietary supplements in health foods stores. While they do act as antioxidants, they are not found in nature. They are man-made chemicals and, because of this, their function in the body is not fully known. Man-made chemicals, including those added to foods, often have adverse side effects. It is best to stay away from them.

BHA and BHT are potent synthetic antioxidants with possible toxic side effects. They are totally unsuitable as dietary supplements. Polyunsaturated fats are in one form or another in most all packaged food. They are also the major cause of food deterioration. That is why when you go to the grocery store, a huge percentage of the products contain one or more of these synthetic antioxidants.

Many types of foods and herbs are also spoken of as antioxidants. While these substances aren't really antioxidants, they do contain antioxidant phytochemicals both known and unknown. Extracts of these are often used in antioxidant supplements.

Plants contain a variety of antioxidant compounds. Many herbs and spices are known as antioxidants because they contain a high percentage of these compounds. Some of the most popular are ginkgo biloba, green tea, milk thistle, bilberry, turmeric, rosemary, cloves, oregano, nutmeg, and vanilla. Some of these are used in foods, not only for the flavor they provide, but also to act as antioxidants to extend shelf life. Oats, the common grain used in many foods, also has antioxidant properties; however, its activity is rather low so it's not used commercially for this purpose. Vanilla is used extensively as a flavoring agent in sweetened foods and cereals. It was only recently that its antioxidant potential was discovered. Rosemary has been long recognized for its antioxidant properties and has received a lot of attention. The first scientific reports on rosemary as an antioxidant go back to 1952, and research on it has been reported at regular intervals over the years. These herbal antioxidants are being used to some extent by the food industry to preserve packaged foods, but as yet have not been utilized to their full potential. Ginkgo, green tea, milk thistle, bilberry, and rosemary are often used in combination with other antioxidants in the formulation of dietary supplements.

Research has shown that a diverse selection of dietary antioxidants function synergically to offer better protection against free radicals than do large amounts of single antioxidants. The effects of beta-carotene are enhanced when combined with other carotenoids. Alpha-tocopherol (vitamin E) works better in the presence of other tocopherols and is reenergized by vitamin C. Vitamin C effects are stronger when combined with bioflavonoids, and vice versa. Vitamin C enhances the absorption of selenium which is used to make glutathione peroxidase. Glutathione peroxidase along with vitamin E helps to protect the polyunsaturated fats in our cells from free radicals. They both complement each other, yet can not replace one another. To get the best antioxidant protection, you need a full spectrum of these vital nutrients. Consuming just one or two, even in large quantities, won't do much for you.

ANTIOXIDANT HEALTH

Antioxidants of all types are available as dietary supplements. They can be purchased individually or as mixtures. The best source for a complete spectrum of antioxidants is directly from our foods. That's the way people have gotten their antioxidants throughout history. The foods with the highest concentration of antioxidant nutrients are fresh fruits, vegetables, and whole grains.

Over the past century, however, our foods have been stripped of these vital nutrients in the course of refining and processing. To make matters worse, free radical-producing toxins have been added to our foods in the form of food additives. Polyunsaturated fatty acids from vegetable oil is a major contaminante. Air pollution, chlorinated water, pesticide residue on foods, and an assortment of other man-made chemicals in our environment have all placed a heavy demand on our antioxidant reserves. We have become an antioxidant-depleted society. The result is tissue degeneration and premature aging as a consequence of unrestrained free-radical attack. It is no wonder why degenerative disease of all types has become our most dreaded health concern. The gradual increase in degenerative disease has paralleled the increased use of processed foods. This phenomenon has been repeated time and time again throughout the world as manufactured foods have replaced traditional diets.

Study after study have shown that eating plenty of fruits and vegetables lowers the risk of heart disease, stroke, cancer, and other common degenerative conditions. For example, in a study reported in the *Journal of the American Medical Association*, researchers surveyed 832 male participants in the ongoing Framingham Heart Study. The men had no cardiovascular disease and were 45 through 65 years old when enrolled in a dietary assessment study from 1966 to 1969. During that time, the interviewers documented the men's food intake. The information was kept on file, and the participants were monitored for the next 18 to 22 years for, among other things, any episodes of strokes. The results: there were 97 stroke-related incidents, and researchers found a substantial decrease in stroke risk among those who had consumed higher quantities of fruits and vegetables. For each increment of three half-cup servings a day, there was a 22-percent decrease in stroke risk. The average number of servings among participants was 5.1. These results, the researchers conclude, provided support to programs aimed at widespread increases in the consumption of fruits and vegetables. When we eat more fruits and vegetables we eat less nutrient-deficient white bread, sugar, coffee, and other health-destroying foods. Likewise, the more we eat of processed foods, the less we eat of fresh produce and whole grain products. Researchers have determined the more fresh fruits, vegetables, and whole grains we add to our diet, the lower our risk of developing degenerative disease.

Look at all the diseases that are in some way connected with free radicals: cancers of all types, atherosclerosis, heart disease, stroke, varicose veins, arthritis, cataracts, allergies, asthma, lupus, colitis, Alzheimer's, senility, psoriasis, and many, many others. The number of people afflicted with these conditions has increased over the past several decades. And they are not affecting just older people but the young as well. Most teenagers and young adults now show signs of atherosclerosis. Cancer among young people is rising. These diseases aren't conditions that are limited to the elderly. It's true that the longer a person lives, the greater the degree of free-radical damage, but age isn't an excuse for disease. Autopsies on older people who had lived on primitive diets show no signs of atherosclerosis or other degenerative disease.

Researchers have shown that adding antioxidants, principally vitamins C, E, beta-carotene, and selenium, can provide protection against and reduce symptoms of these conditions. In one study, for example, eighty men received either an antioxidant compound or a placebo for five months. people in the study group consumed 600 mg of vitamin C, 300 mg of vitamin E, 27 mg of beta-carotene, and 75 mcg of selenium daily. Free radicals in the blood went down by 20 percent and the tendency of platelets to stick together went down by 24 percent.[37] Studies are coming out all the time showing the protective effects of one antioxidant or another. Why are these antioxidants so useful? The reason is because we aren't getting them in our diets. Degenerative disease doesn't wander the earth like a troublesome virus waiting to pounce on any unsuspecting person it encounters. It is, for the most part, a result of subclinical malnutrition and free-radical damage. The solution is simple: remove the cause and the body will heal. In other words, replace the overly processed foods you're eating now with wholesome natural foods. Returning to a more basic or primitive diet will provide the body with all the vitamins and minerals and other nutrients it needs just as it has done for millions of others throughout history.

One problem we face in our modern world that our ancestors did not encounter to any great extent is pollution. In the 19th and early 20th centuries coal miners often suffered from an affliction called black lung disease. This condition was a result of breathing in coal dust day after day. They may have eaten a relatively good diet, yet still become afflicted with this disease. Others may have worked in factories surrounded by smoke or chemical fumes which led to numerous degenerative health problems. Cigarette smoke has long been associated with cancer and heart disease. Pollutants in the smoke burn up antioxidant reserves in our body at an accelerated pace. In our world today, we encounter free-radical generating pollutants to a much greater degree than in times past. Stress also increases free-radical production and we live in a world full of stress.

The greater your exposure to pollutants, the more your

antioxidant reserves are used up, and the greater your need. This is why people living today need to supplement their diets with antioxidants, while those living in centuries past got all they usually needed from their foods. We must have two or three times the amount our ancestors had and much more than the RDA.

It is a well-known fact that vegetarians as a whole are healthier and experience less disease than nonvegeratians. Most vegetarians are very conscience of the types of foods they eat. They have better health, not because they don't eat animal products which are high in saturated fat and cholesterol, but because they are more likely to eat lots of fruits, vegetables, and whole grains which supply the body with ample antioxidants to counter free-radical formation.

Dr. Hermann Esterbauer at the University of Graz has reported that low antioxidant reserves lead to the oxidation of polyunsaturated fatty acids, which in turn oxidizes cholesterol.[38] Oxidized polyunsaturated fatty acids and cholesterol are the only fats found in arterial plaque. As long as antioxidant defenders are in ample supply, oxidation, which causes the formation of free radicals, is kept under control.

"Most of us should be paying more attention to our intake of antioxidant nutrients," states Richard Passwater, Ph.D. "My point is that even in cholesterol-sensitive people, antioxidant protection is more important than cholesterol level. Don't concentrate on the minor problem and ignore the major factor."[39]

Free-radical damage can be rampaging in the body because the antioxidant defenders are in short numbers. The only way you're going to get complete antioxidant protection is from eating wholesome foods and taking dietary supplements.

Chapter 11

IRON AND YOUR HEALTH

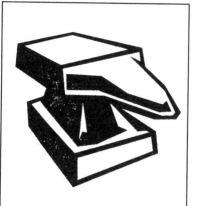

One of the classic examples in nature of free-radical deterioration is that of rust. Iron exposed to the elements in the air readily oxidizes. In this process, the corroded iron expands, becomes brittle, and falls apart. The process is one of dis-integration or decay. This reaction is often used as an analogy with the processes that occur inside our arteries with oxidative stress and the development of athero-sclerosis. The rust that builds up inside a weathered iron pipe is similar to the plaque that forms inside the arteries. Both processes involve free radicals.

Many other metals are also affected by oxidation—copper turns green, silver tarnishes, aluminum becomes darkened. Some metals are more susceptible to oxidation than others. In human tissues, some metals actively promote oxidation and act as catalysts, accelerating the process.

Exposure to iron, copper, nickel, cobalt, cadmium, chromium, mercury, and lead can cause antioxidant depletion and free-radical generation.[1, 2] Many of these metals are dangerous pollutants in our environment. Some are nutrients necessary in tiny amounts for optimal health. But too much of any of them can turn deadly.

Cadmium, mercury, and lead are recognized toxins at even minute levels. One of the destructive aspects of these toxins is their ability to generate free radicals. Lead compounds, for example, increase fat oxidation. This was clearly observed in a study in Taiwan. Blood analysis of factory workers who were exposed to lead were compared to workers who were not exposed. Those exposed to lead had a much greater degree of fat oxidation.[3] These workers were at a much greater risk of developing heart disease and other conditions associated with free-radical de-generation.

Iron is of special concern because it is one of the most abundant minerals in the environment and one of the most reactive. Iron is not only highly susceptible to oxidation, but in human tissues actively promotes it.[4] Iron and copper acceler-ates the oxidation of polyunsaturated oils and cholesterol. This process creates the highly reactive hydroxyl radical—the most powerful and destructive free radical known.

Excess levels of iron and copper in the body can lead to an increased produc-tion of free radicals, which can lead to an increase in oxidative damage. Most of the iron and copper in our bodies is bound to special proteins in our blood and causes no harm. But excess iron and copper that roam around our system freely can create a free-radical nightmare, contributing to heart disease, liver damage, dia-betes, joint inflammation, cancer, and other problems.[5, 6] Men who donate blood on a regular basis, thus reducing their iron reserves, have been found to have fewer heart attacks.[7]

"Moreover ye shall eat no manner of blood, whether it be of fowl or of beast."
—Leviticus 8:26

Iron is found in most all fresh fruit, vegetables, and whole grains. It's most abundant in meats and especially liver and blood products. We also consume it in dietary supplements and in fortified foods. Ironically, many people purposely consume it in various forms in hopes of improving health and in the process actually degrade it.

THE IRONY OF IRON

Iron is an example of a good mineral gone bad. It's not that the iron itself is bad really, but modern food processing and dietary habits have turned it into a monster.

Iron is a necessary nutrient. Every living cell contains iron. Without iron, cells could not generate energy to fuel metabolic processes. New cells could not be made, neither could hormones and enzymes. In fact, without iron every cell in the body would quickly die because iron is required for the delivery of oxygen throughout the body.

Too much iron, however, can spell trouble, and lots of it. Just like most other essential nutrients taken in excess, it can be hazardous. But how can we get too much? Isn't iron deficiency one of our major health concerns?

In terms of nutrition, when you think of iron, what comes to mind? Most of us envision iron as a necessary nutrient that gives us energy and strength. It fights "iron-poor blood" and prevents anemia that causes fatigue. We are advised to eat spinach and liver because they are good sources of iron. The cartoon character, Popeye, would instantly transform himself from a scrawny weakling into a mighty superhero just by eating iron-rich spinach. If we are fatigued, all we need to do is take Geritol, a vitamin formula packed with extra iron, to get more energy.

Iron has become linked in our minds with strength and endurance. Most of these ideas stem from aggressive advertising by supplement manufacturers. One company, the makers of Geritol, capitalized on this prevailing myth and through aggressive advertising persuaded millions of people to take excess supplements of this potentially dangerous mineral. Geritol advertisements loudly proclaimed "has twice the iron as a pound of calf's liver" and will make you "feel strong fast."

Recent scientific findings have shown that, contrary to popular belief, most of us get way too much iron already, so much so that it has now been recognized as a major health concern. Nobel prize winner Baruch S. Blumberg, M.D., Ph.D., states: "Over the years, numerous experimental studies showed that, in animals and in humans, greater amounts of available iron increase the possibility of infection and the development of cancer and other forms of illness."[8]

The Fox Chase Cancer Center in Philadelphia began investigating the possible connection between iron and disease after discovering links with the mineral to hepatitis and liver cancer. Dr. Richard Stevens embarked on a series of epidemiological studies comparing the level of iron in blood samples to death rates. The first study used data collected from people living in the Solomon Islands who had been the subjects of an intensive health survey conducted in the 1960s and early 1970s. These studies included the collection of blood samples. A repeat visit to the island established who was still alive. This study showed that increased body stores of iron were associated with *decreased* survival rate.[9]

Because of dangers of excessive iron consumption, The Food and Drug Administration (FDA) in 1998 started requiring a warning on all supplements containing 30 mg or more of iron which reads:

> "Warning: Accidental overdose of iron-containing products is a leading cause of fatal poisoning in children under 6. Keep this product out of reach of children. In case of accidental overdose, call a doctor or poison control center immediately."

Iron is the only nutritional supplement that I am aware of that carries such a warning. According to an FDA report, in the past 11 years, 110,000 children have been poisoned and 35 have died after eating adult iron supplements. Nearly half the estimated 21,150 iron products on the market contain more than 30 mg. of iron per dose (the amount the FDA links to serious poisonings).

THE BANTU

The link between iron and increased incidence of disease and death has been documented for decades. Evidence linking dietary consumption of iron and disease was strikingly noted with certain Bantu-speaking people of South Africa.

The Bantu-speaking people comprise a large and culturally and ethically diverse population that includes the Zulu and Swazi in South Africa, the Kuba in Angola, and the Ganda of Uganda. Much of the southern half of Africa is populated by Bantu-speaking tribes.

In 1924, A.S. Strachan of Glasgow, Scotland, began studying the health of the native peoples in South Africa. He found that a large number of people in the hospitals had highly elevated iron levels. He later reported that roughly half of 745 autopsies performed showed excess iron in the liver, spleen, and other organs. Ten percent had liver cirrho-

---

Blood is our richest natural source of dietary iron.
Diets containing blood products can quickly lead to
iron overload.

sis and 3 percent had liver cancer. For some unknown reason iron seemed to be associated with an increased rate of death.

Studies of Bantu-speaking people in other areas of Africa showed them to have normal iron levels and to be completely free of degenerative disease. Why were the people in South Africa which Dr. Strachan studied so different? What led to the iron overload?

Diet was the most obvious suspect. But their diet was typical with those of other cultures in Africa, which consisted largely of grains. Measurements of the iron content in these foods was no higher than anywhere else.

The iron problem remained a mystery until 1950. The key factor was not in the types of foods they ate, but in the way they prepared it. The Bantus in this area used iron pots for almost all their cooking. Large quantities of iron leached out of the pots into the food. Their diet ordinarily would supply them with roughly 10-30 mg of iron per day, which falls within guidelines set by nutritionists. After cooking, however, the daily iron intake shot up to 100-200 mg. This is like taking a large iron supplement every day for life.

Nowadays steel pots have replaced the crude iron pots and the incidence of iron overload among the South Africa Bantus has decreased by 50 percent over the last 25-30 years.[10]

IRON OVERLOAD

Iron plays an essential role in the distribution of oxygen throughout the body. Our red blood cells are specifically designed to pick up oxygen in the lungs and release it in the tissues. Each red blood cell carries about 300 million molecules of hemoglobin, the iron-containing substance that grabs the oxygen. Hemoglobin allows our blood to carry seventy times more oxygen than could be dissolved in water alone, making for more efficient oxygen delivery.

We have over 25 trillion red blood cells in our bodies. They are so numerous that if they were placed end to end, the red blood cells from a single person could encircle the world six times—almost enough to reach the moon. Red blood cells dash through our veins and arteries for about 120 days. After being squashed and shoved and pushed through tight capillaries, they become tarnished so to speak, like a car after many years of heavy use. Worn out red blood cells are gathered up by the liver, spleen, and bone marrow and recycled.

Our bodies are the ultimate recycling machine. Proteins, fats, minerals, and other substances are broken down and recycled to make new compounds. Iron is extracted from old red blood cells and stored in special compounds called ferritin. Ferritin is a huge spherical protein molecule. Inside there is room for up to 4,500 iron atoms. We have

millions of ferritin molecules roaming around in our blood and organs. This iron is used to make new red blood cells, enzymes, and other compounds.

Iron is so vital to life that it is stockpiled as a safety precaution. This protects us if the diet periodically becomes low in iron. Such a situation may have been common to our ancestors during winter or famine when food was scarce.

The body goes to great lengths to recycle iron once it is absorbed into the bloodstream and doesn't want to give it up. In fact, the body has no mechanism for getting rid of iron. Almost all the iron we consume is stored away in the body.[11]

Because of the efficiently of the recycling of iron, our daily requirement for iron from food is really very small. We do lose iron, about 1 mg per day, in the form of sweat and urine, as well as in cells that naturally slough off from the intestinal wall, hair, skin, and nails. The biggest loss of iron occurs with the loss of blood. Iron-filled red blood cells and ferritin molecules are lost and the body pulls out iron from its storage sites to replenish what was lost.

Premenopausal women lose iron on a regular basis, which is why women are considered more at risk of low iron levels than men. The Recommended Dietary Allowance (RDA) of iron for premenopausal women is 15 mg and for postmenopausal women and men is 10 mg. The body absorbs approximately 10 percent of the iron in our foods so consumption of 10-15 mg of dietary iron would supply 1 to 1.5 mg to body stores. This gain equals about the same that is lost every day. Consuming more than 10-15 mg of iron means that all of the excess will go into storage.

If the diet becomes iron deficient, a signal is sent to the digestive tract and more iron is absorbed from the food in the intestines. It's an efficient system to make sure the body gets all the iron it needs when dietary intake decreases. Most menstruating women are not iron deficient because this absorption mechanism performs effectively. In addition, if more iron is needed, the body can pull more out of its ferritin reserves.[12]

The average diet supplies more than enough iron for all our needs. Most of us eat far more than the RDA which is roughly equal to the amount we lose. All excess iron is packed neatly away in our tissues. Because we normally take in more iron than we lose, iron reserves increase with age, even in most premenopausal women.

The fact that humans accumulate excess iron over time was clearly demonstrated in a study published in 1976.[13] James Cook, Clement Finch, and Nathan Smith of the University of Washington and the University of Kansas collected and analyzed blood samples in over 1,500 people. The study found that blood ferritin levels and thus, iron stores, increase as we age. The graph on the following page summarizes their results.

The graph shows the average amount of stored iron for men and women. Iron levels for both men and women start out the same. The lines split at the time of puberty when menstruation commences. Rapidly growing bodies need more iron, so reserves remain moderate for both sexes until about the age of 18. At this age full growth is reached and iron stores in men increase dramatically. Iron levels in women remain modest until about the age of 45-50 or the time of menopause. Since women no longer lose iron from menstruation, iron stores rapidly increase, approaching the value of men.

The results of this study has been confirmed by other researchers.[14, 15]

Iron stores of between 100-300 mg or so seems to be enough to satisfy our needs. Most premenopausal women have this amount without suffering from anemia or other deficiency problems. The extra 600-800 mg or so just sits there inside the body because it has no useful function. Iron accumulates, waiting to be used if needed.

At this moment almost all of us could live for a significant period of time without any iron in our diet whatsoever. Premenopausal women can do fine without iron for roughly three to seven months before depleting their iron stores of 200-300 mg. Most men and postmenopausal women, with stores of only 600 mg, could go without iron for two years or more before they become deficient.[16]

We've all heard the advertisements warning us to make sure to get enough iron to avoid "iron poor blood." We all know that without iron we suffer with anemia. The real problem we face, however, is not from an iron deficiency, but from an iron overload. It is this excess iron that can wreak havoc on our bodies. In the United States it has been estimated that the incidence of real iron-deficiency anemia is *lower* than that of undiagnosed iron-overload disease.[17] The same is probably true in other Western countries.

THE PROBLEM WITH IRON

So what's so terrible about having a little extra iron stored away in our body? It might come in handy if we ever need it. And if iron is such an important nutrient that the body makes special efforts to stockpile it, how can it bad?

Some of the iron stored in ferritin molecules leaks out and roams around the body as free iron. The larger our iron reservoirs, the more free iron we have wandering about inside our body.

The trouble with free iron is that it is a powerful oxidizer. It acts as a catalyst, which means it speeds up an otherwise slow chemical reaction. The reaction in this case unleashes a horde of destructive free radicals. Polyunsaturated fatty acids, cholesterol, and other compounds quickly fall prey to these molecular renegades. This damage caused by an iron-catalyzed reaction is extensive and can affect all cells and tissues. A growing number of scientists now believe that tissue damage initiated in this fashion is at the core of a wide range of human disease, including heart disease and cancer as well as being a significant player in the aging process.[18]

Randall Lauffer, Ph.D., professor biochemistry at Harvard Medical School, describes iron this way: "Free iron can unleash a destructive chain reaction that makes use of iron's special property of combining with different forms of oxygen. When bound to hemoglobin, iron is a little chemical angel, carefully escorting oxygen in the blood and benevolently delivering it to the neediest tissues. But free— alone and bare—iron is a little devil, a neighborhood brat playing with a dangerous chemistry set and a tank of oxygen. The interaction between iron and oxygen then becomes destructive, and our tissues are the victims."[19]

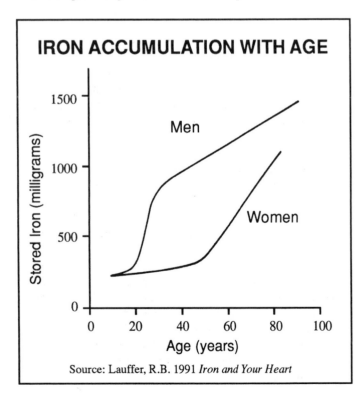

IRON ACCUMULATION WITH AGE

Men

Women

Stored Iron (milligrams)

1500

1000

500

0

0   20   40   60   80   100

Age (years)

Source: Lauffer, R.B. 1991 *Iron and Your Heart*

Iron accumulates in our bodies as we age. Iron stores for males and females are the same until puberty. The iron stores in men build up rapidly and appear to continue to rise throughout their lifetime. This process is delayed about 20 or 30 years in women because of the regular iron loss due to menstruation. After menopause is reached around the age of 45-55, women begin to accumulate iron rapidly.

Iron is recognized as a carcinogen. Some researchers suspect increased iron reserves may be involved in the development of cancer, arthritis, diabetes, Parkinson's disease, Alzheimer's disease, stroke, and heart disease.[20] This is because iron can cause the formation of potent free radicals that promote fat oxidation.[21]

Another mechanism whereby iron can cause oxidative damage is when we encounter injury. Mechanical or chemical injury to tissues can cause cells to rupture and release their contents into the surrounding area. These contents will include metal ions such as iron which accelerate free-radical reactions in extracellular fluids. These radicals can accelerate fat peroxidation since fats are the most vulnerable segments of our tissues.

It has been proposed that injury to the brain by mechanical means (trauma) or by oxygen deprivation (stroke) can result in release of iron ions into the surrounding area. Iron ions could facilitate further damage to these surrounding areas by accelerating free-radical reactions.

Because disease causes tissue injury and the release of iron, almost any disease is likely to be accompanied by increased formation of free radicals. It is not, therefore, surprising that the list of diseases in which their formation has been implicated is long and is growing.[22]

Since the iron content of human tissues increase as we age, injuries to older tissues result in the release of a greater amount of iron. Free-radical damage, therefore, increases as we age.[23]

THE LINK TO HEART DISEASE

Life expectancy for men is about 72 years and for women its 79—a seven-year difference. Why do women live longer than men? No one has yet to figure it out. Many theories have been proposed but none of them have withstood the test of time.

Heart disease is the major contributor to the gender gap in life expectancy. Women experience a far lower rate of heart disease than men, until they reach menopause, at which time their heart disease rate begins to approach that of men.[24]

The current belief is that estrogen, a female hormone, endows women with some degree of protection against heart disease. During childbearing years, women's ovaries actively secrete estrogen. When they reach menopause, the rate of secretion slows down to a mere trickle by comparison. Since the protection women enjoy is during the time when estrogen production is at its highest, it is logical to assume that perhaps it is the key.

There are some major problems with this theory. For one, if it were estrogen that gave protection then men of *all* ages would have a high rate of heart disease. But this isn't the case.

In the early 1970s, an effort was made to test the estrogen theory. When estrogen was administered to men, the results were alarming: it *increased* the heart attack rate rather than lowering it.[25]

The theory took another blow with data from the Framingham Heart Study. In agreement with many other studies, the investigators found an increased risk of heart disease in women within two years after menopause. Heart attack rates for women that had hysterectomies (removal of the uterus and sometimes the ovaries) were recorded. Most all of the estrogen in the body is produced in the ovaries. Those who had hysterectomies without the removal of the ovaries were compared with those that did have their ovaries removed.

On the basis of the estrogen protection theory, you would expect the women who had their ovaries removed to have higher heart attack rates. However, both groups had a similar increase in risk compared to premenopausal women. Somehow the removal of the uterus, not the ovaries, strips women of their natural protection.[26]

A better explanation for the reason why women don't suffer as many heart attacks as men during childbearing age is due to their lower iron reserves. Menstruation keeps their iron levels low, while iron continues to pile up in men. As a consequence, men suffer a much greater degree of cellular damage by the oxidative reactions of iron. Polyunsaturated fat and cholesterol being highly susceptible to free-radical damage would be readily oxidized.

Dr. Jerome Sullivan, a professor of pathology at the Medical University of South Carolina, showed that iron could explain the Framingham results in a way that fit the data. He was the first to propose that the protection exhibited by premenopausal women might be due to their lower level of iron, which results from regular blood loss. He noted that the different patterns of iron accumulation in men and women seemed to mirror trends in heart disease mortality rates.[27]

Dr. Sullivan's data is summarized on the following page. Cholesterol levels for men and women are essentially the same at all ages. This shows that cholesterol has little, if any effect on risk for heart disease. But iron concentration corresponds remarkably well with heart disease rate.

It has long been known that vegetarians exhibit fewer heart disease deaths than the general population. A variety of vitamins and phytochemicals (plant chemicals) have been credited with this protective quality. Another explanation may involve iron. Meat is the primary source of iron in our diet. While many vegetables contain respectable amounts of iron, it isn't absorbed as well as the iron in meat.

This theory is substantiated by studies with Seventh-Day Adventists. Seventh-Day Adventists were chosen because they avoid eating meat, fish, and poultry, but do eat

IRON AND HEAD DISEASE

**IRON AND
HEAD DISEASE**

*The graph on the upper left shows the difference in iron levels
between men and women as they age. A ratio of 1:1 is indicated as 1
on the graph, a ratio of 2:1 is indicated as 2, and so on. Between the
ages of 25-35, for example, men have nearly four times the iron that
women have. The graph on the lower left shows the difference in
heart disease death rate between men and women. At age 30 men
die four times more frequently from heart disease than women. After
age 40 the ratio begins to even out until age 75 when death rates are
about the same. Notice that these two graphs have a similar pattern,
strongly suggesting a correlation between iron level and heart
disease.*

*The graph below shows the difference in cholesterol levels
between men and women. If cholesterol was important in the
development of heart disease it should show that women have less
cholesterol than men until they reach 75. However, there is very
little variation in cholesterol levels between men and women at any
age. This indicates that when compared to iron levels, cholesterol
has very little influence on heart disease.*

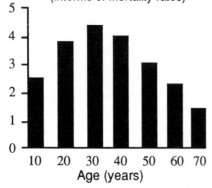

Male/Female Iron Level Ratios
(in terms of serum ferritin levels)

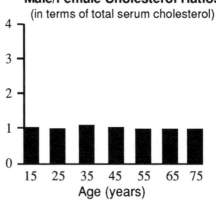

Male/Female Heart Disease Ratios
(interms of mortality rates)

Male/Female Cholesterol Ratios
(in terms of total serum cholesterol)

Source: Lauffer, R.B. 1991 *Iron and Your Heart*

some high-cholesterol foods such as dairy products and
eggs. Adventist men exhibit 40-50 percent fewer heart disease related deaths than non-Adventist men. The reason is
usually ascribed to reductions in cholesterol and saturated
fat. However, the Adventist men, even though they abstain
from eating meat, still get a lot of saturated fat and cholesterol from dairy products and eggs. Studies have shown that
their blood cholesterol levels are only slightly lower than
those of other men, roughly 6 percent, far too small a difference to account for the dramatically lower heart disease
rates.[28]

A more likely explanation for the lower disease rate
in Adventist men is their avoidance of meat, which leads to
lower body iron stores.[29]

So why haven't we heard more about the dangers of
iron overload and why is iron still added to enriched foods?

Randall Lauffer, Ph.D. author of *Iron and Your Heart* responds, "Often an accumulation of a large body of evidence
is required before the public is motivated to change health
practices. For example, even though significant evidence that
cigarette smoking was detrimental began to accumulate in
the 1950s, it wasn't until recently that there were changes
in public health practice. And increased awareness of the
possible hazards of increased iron intake may now be developing, and this could stimulate additional research and
ultimately public action."[30]

WHERE DO WE GET IRON?

Except for sugar and oil, most all of our foods contain iron. Iron is found naturally in all produce, grains, nuts,
and seeds. Meat contains about the same amount as most

fruits and vegetables, but the iron in meat is much more readily absorbed by our intestines. While we absorb only about 10 percent of the iron in plants, dairy, and eggs, we absorb 23 percent of the iron in meat. Shellfish and organ meats, like liver and heart, are the richest natural sources of iron. Blood probably contains the highest concentration of iron. Therefore, meat should be completely drained and rinsed of blood before cooking. Foods containing a lot of blood such as blood sausage are extremely rich in iron and should be completely avoided.

When meat is cut or ground, it not only increases its exposure to oxygen, but iron is also released from the cells. This iron attacks the fat within the meat, greatly accelerating oxidation. Ground meat would be affected most because more tissues are broken and exposed. The older the meat, the more time is allowed for lipid peroxidation to occur. Freshly ground meat would have essentially no oxidation, while meat that has been sitting around for several days may have a significant amount. The degree of oxidation will also vary with fat content. The more polyunsaturated fat in the meat, the more peroxidation will occur. Saturated fat is resistant to oxidation, so meat with a higher saturated fat content will be safer to eat. Unfortunately, most animals nowadays are given feed high in polyunsaturated fats and so their tissues also contain more of this fat. So the meat we eat has undergone more lipid peroxidation than that eaten by our grandparents.

One of the problems with living in an industrialized and prosperous country, as most western nations are, is that we eat too much meat. Meat is often eaten two or three times a day. This high meat consumption drives up our iron stores fast. This, many believe, is one reason why eating meat has also been associated with increased risk of heart disease as well as other degenerative conditions. Eating meat is worse for your health than eating either saturated fat or cholesterol.

Another food source that contributes even more iron than meat is white flour. When whole wheat flour is processed, iron and several other nutrients are removed. In a society where wheat constitutes the main source of food, taking out vital nutrients has had a drastic effect on health. For many people bread is the staff of life. When the processing of white flour and bread became common, the lack of nutrients resulted in people developing deficiency diseases. The government mandated that white flour be "enriched" with certain nutrients to prevent these diseases. One of these nutrients was iron. Although some 20 nutrients are removed in the process, only four or five are added back. To make the bread even "healthier" more iron is added than was present in the original whole wheat. A few slices of bread can supply all the iron you need for an entire day.

Most all white flour has been enriched with iron. So any product made with white flour is also enriched with iron.

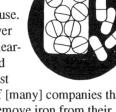

Iron should not be included in any multi-nutrient formula intended for daily, long-term use. Supplemental iron should never be taken, except in cases of clear-cut iron deficiency as assessed by laboratory testing. The most likely reason for the failure of [many] companies that sell vitamin supplements to remove iron from their multi-nutrient formulas is that they simply have not been reading the scientific literature about the dangers of iron.

—Life Extension Foundation

Think about it. How many items do we eat every day that are made from refined wheat flour? We usually just think of bread and rolls, but must include cookies, crackers, pretzels, pancake mix, breakfast cereal, flour tortillas, burritos, pizza, macaroni, spaghetti, frozen dinners, pot pies, the list can go on and on. These are the types of foods most of us live on!

Most all of the hot and cold breakfast cereals are "fortified" with additional iron. Many of the cold cereals are predominantely sugar and sugar has no nutritional value other than providing calories. Some breakfast cereals are as much as 60 percent sugar. So in effect, when you eat these products, you're eating fortified sugar. The worst cereals, in terms of iron content, are those that appear to be the best, such as Total and Product 19. These cereals have 100 percent of the RDA with each serving. One serving will supply all the iron you need for an entire day, but everything else you eat during the day will supply additional iron, all of which will be stockpiled in your body.

With all the iron we get it's no wonder why iron-induced free-radical destruction has been identified as a major source of concern.

If this weren't enough iron, many of us intentionally add more to our body's stores by taking iron tablets, multiple vitamin supplements, and enriched drinks. Most multiple vitamins contain iron. However, now that people are becoming aware of the iron problem, some manufacturers are making multiple vitamins with reduced amounts of iron or with no iron at all.

There is one more source of iron that affects a few people, and that is from cookware. The Bantu of South Africa became overloaded with iron leached from metal pots, cast iron cookware may be doing the same thing to you. Using iron or copper pots to cook foods not only increases the amounts of these metals in our bodies, but also destroys vitamin C and other antioxidants in the food.[31] It's safer to use stainless steel or glass.

GET THE IRON OUT

Now that you are aware of the iron problem, how do you protect yourself from overload? If you're an adolescent or a premenopausal woman you have little to worry about. The young have not had time to build up iron stores to any great amount and women of child-bearing age continually lose iron with their periods. Some women may lose so much iron that they may even develop an iron deficiency. Those who should be most concerned about excess iron are adult men and postmenopausal women.

For those who are at risk, the best way to avoid iron overload is to watch what you eat. Avoid all enriched foods—primarily breakfast cereals and white flour products. Meat, including fish and chicken, should be eaten sparingly.

The American Cancer Society recommends a diet with less meat and more fruits, vegetables, and whole grains because study after study have shown these foods to have protective properties.[32] This diet also happens to be low in iron.

Another reason why whole natural foods are beneficial is because they contain fiber and phytic acid. Fiber helps to move food through the digestive tract and quickly rids the body of carcinogenic substances. Phytic acid binds to heavy metals, including iron, and pulls it out of the digestive tract with the fiber. So the amount of iron absorbed is reduced. Whole grains and beans contain the most fiber and phytic acid. Vegetables and fruits contain much lower amounts of both and were not found to be as important in preventing colon cancer.[33]

Regular aerobic exercise also helps to reduce iron stores. A small amount of iron is excreted in sweat. So a vigorous workout can help unload extra iron. A single bowl of cereal for breakfast can replenish the iron lost in two hours of strenuous exercise. So you can't depend on exercise alone to reduce iron reserves.

Alcohol increases iron absorption. A number of studies have shown that drinkers have higher iron levels than nondrinkers.[34, 35] Alcohol damages the intestinal lining, disrupting the body's ability to regulate nutrient absorption, including iron. When this self-regulating mechanism goes awry, iron absorption can be increased.

Oral contraceptives partially rob younger women of the protection they get through menstruation. Oral contraceptives decrease menstrual blood flow in most women to a third or half the normal rate. This reduces the amount of iron that would normally be lost. So those who use oral contraceptives are more likely to build up their iron stores earlier in life. This has been confirmed in studies, which show that the amount of stored iron in women who use oral contraceptives for two years or more is roughly double that of non-users.

Any loss of blood will reduce iron loads. Donating blood has been suggested as a means to lower iron reserves. Donating blood a couple of times a year is sufficient for most people to keep iron reserves within bounds as long as iron intake is kept moderate.

LIVER SPOTS

Have you ever noticed that as people age they often develop brown, freckle-like spots on their skin? This pigment is called lipofuscin. It is also known as aging spots or liver spots. The appearance of lipofuscin is one of the classic signs associated with aging along with wrinkles and sagging skin. It is also a sign of free-radical deterioration.

Iron-induced oxidation of fats and protein in the skin are recognized as a cause of liver spots.[36, 37] Increasing the iron levels of both animals and people increases the amount of lipofuscin deposition. Experimentally, lipofuscin has been shown to accumulate within the cells of animals deprived of dietary vitamin E which retards free-radical reactions. So iron is associated directly with processes involved in aging.[38, 39]

Lipofuscin is produced by the reaction of free radicals on the fats and proteins within cell membranes. Because cells cannot dispose of the lipofuscin pigment, it gradually accumulates within many cells of the body during aging.

On the surface of the skin, lipofuscin forms the so-called liver spots. While these spots are clearly seen on the skin, they also form in other tissues throughout the body—intestines, lungs, kidney, brain, etc. They represent areas that are damaged by free-radical reactions. The more you have on your skin, the more you have inside of you and the more damage or "aging" your body has undergone. You can judge to some degree your antioxidant status by the size and number of liver spots on your skin. The more you have and the bigger they are, the more free-radical damage has been done in your body and the greater your need for antioxidant nutrients.

Lipofuscin or liver spots don't ordinarily hurt or show any signs of discomfort. If we couldn't see them we wouldn't even know they were there. But they do affect our health. All the tissues affected are damaged, aged, and to some degree dysfunctional. If this occurs in your intestine, it can affect the organ's ability to digest and absorb nutrients. In the brain it will affect mental ability.

Once lipofuscin pigment develops, it tends to stick around for life. Little can be done to remove the spots even after dramatic dietary and lifestyle changes. That doesn't mean that all the tissues in the body are beyond hope. You can prevent further oxidation by making wise dietary and lifestyle choices.

Chapter 12

THE HOMOCYSTEINE REVOLUTION

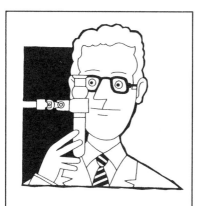

PROTEIN AND ATHEROSCLEROSIS

A highly significant factor in the development of atherosclerosis and heart disease was uncovered by M.A. Ignatovsky's rabbit-feeding experiments in 1908. By feeding rabbits a diet composed of high amounts of animal protein, he caused them to develop atherosclerosis.

In 1913 Nikolai Anitschkov attempted to show that cholesterol, rather than protein, was the cause of atherosclerosis. Anitschkov's studies looked convincing, but it took another 60 years before researchers discovered the errors in his experiments.

While the cholesterol hypothesis proposed by Anitschkov gradually gained favor, not all researchers accepted it. In 1922 Harry Newburgh, a professor at the University of Michigan School of Medicine, became intrigued by the fact that atherosclerosis could be induced in rabbits by manipulating their diet. He wanted to determine if it was protein or fat that was the primary factor in causing the disease. He reasoned that if protein was at fault then feeding rabbits a high protein diet devoid of all fat would produce atherosclerosis. He prepared lean beef muscle that was dried, powdered, and extracted with solvents to remove all traces of fat and cholesterol. He fed increasing doses of the powdered meat protein to rabbits. Within just a few months the rabbits all developed atherosclerosis. Newburgh also found that the higher the protein content of the diet, the sooner and more severe atherosclerotic changes in the rabbits' arteries occurred.[1]

Since atherosclerosis was induced in rabbits by feeding them animal protein devoid of all fat and cholesterol, protein was obviously suspect. Protein is composed of amino acids. Scientists today have identified 20 amino acids that are found in foods and that are important to human health. Newburgh took on the challenge of finding out which one or more of these amino acids was the culprit.

Newburgh reasoned that if he intravenously injected one amino acid at a time into test animals, he would eventually identify those involved in the development of atherosclerosis. He did this, but to his disappointment, none of the amino acids he used caused atherosclerotic plaque to develop.

Unexpectedly, however, he did find that the amino acids cystine, lysine, histidine, tyrosine, and tryptophan all caused kidney damage.[2]

Newburgh's failure to find an amino acid that caused the development of atherosclerotic plaque only provided more support for the lipid hypothesis. The results seemed to contradict his earlier studies which showed that protein, containing all the amino acids, was a causative factor in the development of atherosclerosis. At the time of Newburgh's studies, however, not all of the amino acids were known. The amino acid methionine was just discovered in 1922, a couple of years earlier, and was not considered to be an essential component of proteins. Homocysteine, another amino acid closely related to methionine, was not discovered until 1932. So neither of these were among those tested by Newburgh. Years later it would be found that these two amino acids have a very pronounced effect on cardiovascular health and are the key elements in protein that lead to atherosclerosis. Proof of this did not come until after the cholesterol theory became firmly entrenched, and shaking established ideas has always met with fierce resistance even in the face of indisputable facts. This is the case with the cholesterol theory.

VITAMINS AND ATHEROSCLEROSIS

The riddle of atherosclerosis and heart disease is more complex than simply eating a certain type of food. If eating excessive amounts of cholesterol or animal protein were the sole cause, Eskimos and other heavy meat and fat-eating cultures would show signs of severe cardiovascular disease associated with atherosclerosis, but they haven't. There are other factors involved.

The possibility of a vitamin deficiency being linked to atherosclerosis came from the studies of James Rinehart in the early 1950s. Rinehart had been trying to produce cirrhosis of the liver in monkeys by feeding them a diet deficient in various vitamins. His experiments initially failed to produce cirrhosis, but he discovered that a deficiency of vitamin B-6 led to the development of atherosclerosis after 6 to 18 months.[3]

In his initial studies Rinehart found no evidence of cholesterol deposits in the atherosclerotic arteries. Only with prolonged intermittent or partial deficiency of vitamin B-6 were deposits of fats eventually found in some of the plaques. When the diet contained adequate amounts of vitamin B-6, the monkey's arteries remained healthy. Deficiencies of other vitamins did not cause atherosclerotic plaques. Rinehart's studies were reproduced and confirmed by other researchers.[4] Cholesterol researchers tried to induce atherosclerosis in various animals by feeding them diets composed of large quantities of fat. They found that fatty deposits* did accumulate in vegetarian animals, but dogs and other carnivores were unaffected. Dogs given a diet deficient in vitamin B-6 and with normal amounts of fat, however, did produce atherosclerotic plaques.[5] These studies led researchers to conclude that a widespread deficiency of vitamin B-6 in the human population might be a factor in causing atherosclerosis.

*These fat deposits are not like those found in humans, see page 96.

During the 1960s and 1970s the cholesterol theory was gaining in popularity, and there was no theory that could relate a vitamin B-6 deficiency with atherosclerosis, so the studies by Rinehart and others were simply ignored. Also, the dogs and monkeys that developed atherosclerosis from eating vitamin B-6-deficient diets had normal blood cholesterol levels and only a small amount of fat and cholesterol were found in the plaque of the arteries, which went contrary to the cholesterol theory.

In the late 1960s, George Mann a believer in the cholesterol theory at the time, attempted to repeat Rinehart's experiments.[6] The diet he and his associates fed their monkeys was so deficient in vitamin B-6 that the animals quickly lost weight, became severely anemic, and died within a few months. On autopsy of the monkeys' bodies, no fatty plaque deposits were found. Mann and his associates at Harvard concluded that vitamin B-6 deficiency does not produce atherosclerosis and that cholesterol and fat must be necessary for development of the disease. As a result of this study, interest in vitamin B-6 research in connection with atherosclerosis died.

A major discrepancy with the atherosclerosis found in Rinehart's test animals was the absence of fat and cholesterol deposits. Fat is usually present in human plaques. Only when the monkeys were subjected to intermittent periods of complete vitamin B-6 deficiency and prolonged periods of partial vitamin B-6 deficiency, allowing the animals to survive for periods as long as 23 months, did fatty deposits develop. Prolonged intermittent or partial deficiency of 6 to 12 months allowed enough time for changes to occur in the arteries and hardening to develop, and the longer the animals survived, the greater the likelihood of developing fatty deposits. In the studies performed by Mann, vitamin B-6 deficiency was so severe the animals died within 4 to 9 months. Although arteries were losing elasticity, they had not had time to develop fatty deposits. The logical conclusion is that perhaps prolonged partial vitamin B-6 deficiency in humans also is the reason why fatty deposits frequently develop and why atherosclerosis becomes more severe with age. But the question now was how does a vitamin B deficiency relate to protein consumption?

HOMOCYSTINURIA

The big breakthrough in understanding the connection between protein, B vitamin deficiency, and atherosclerosis came from the discovery of a rare genetic disease called homocystinuria.

In 1968, Dr. Kilmer McCully, a newly-appointed Harvard pathologist, listened to a presentation that sparked an interest in an area of medical research that is now revolutionizing the way medicine looks at atherosclerosis and heart disease.

The presentation was on a rare genetic disease that had only been discovered a few years earlier called homocystinuria. One of the first suspected cases was an eight-year-old boy who had died 35 years previously in the very hospital where the meeting was taking place. The boy exhibited all signs of advanced atherosclerotic disease and died from a stroke—a curious death for an 8-year-old. Atherosclerosis and stroke are considered diseases of aging because they are normally found only in the elderly. This case was so unusual that it was published in the *New England Journal of Medicine* in 1933.[7]

Intrigued, McCully looked up the musty files of the boy's original autopsy report, and pulled out pieces of the boy's tissues embedded in paraffin blocks. Although the wax had melted together, technicians were able to salvage enough tissue to reexamine under a microscope. The boy's arteries had undergone the same destructive process McCully had seen hundreds of times before, only this time it was in an 8-year-old boy rather than an 80-year-old man. The only difference in the boy's arteries and those of others he had examined was that the boy's arteries did not contain fat deposits.

In homocystinuria, the patient's urine contains elevated levels of homocysteine, an amino acid derived from the normal breakdown of proteins in the body. Homocysteine is *not* one of the 20 amino acids that comprise the human body, but is derived from the metabolic breakdown of methionine, one of our essential amino acids. In a healthy body, the liver converts homocysteine back into methionine or into other substances, so the concentration is normally very low. In homocystinuria, a genetic defect in the liver prevents the formation of enzymes which are necessary for homocysteine metabolization, and homocysteine concentrations build up in the body. The problem with homocysteine is that it is toxic. People with homocystinuria typically have mild mental retardation, are tall in stature*, and develop atherosclerosis which can lead to heart attack, stroke, and kidney disease.

A NEW THEORY FOR ATHEROSCLEROSIS

People with homocystinuria are deficient in certain enzymes that metabolize homocysteine. These enzymes are dependent on vitamins B-6, B-12, and folic acid. When those suffering from this genetic disease were given high doses of vitamin B-6 and folic acid, a significant percentage showed remarkable improvement even to the point of reversing the effects of atherosclerosis.

McCully theorized that in the general population, a deficiency of these vitamins would raise homocysteine levels, leading to the development of atherosclerosis. If the deficiency was intermittent and prolonged, fatty deposits would also develop as was the case with Rinehart's monkeys.

McCully further reasoned that excess consumption of animal protein would also raise homocysteine levels. The amino acid methionine, which is much more abundant in animal protein than it is in plant protein, is converted into homocysteine. When animal protein is eaten, homocysteine levels increase. The more protein that is eaten the higher the homocysteine level.

The homocysteine theory predicts that a dietary imbalance between too much methionine from protein and a deficiency of vitamins B-6, B-12, and folic acid is the underlying cause of death and disability from vascular disease. Elevated levels of homocysteine set in motion many processes that lead to loss of elasticity, hardening and calcification, and narrowing of the artery and the formation of blood clots. The homocysteine theory considers atherosclerosis a disease of protein intoxication. The cholesterol theory considers the disease to be caused by intoxication from fats.

If the underlying cause of atherosclerosis was the result of eating too much fat and cholesterol, prevention would be easily achieved simply by decreasing the consumption of the foods that are rich in these substances. However, if the underlying cause was from intoxication by homocysteine, then prevention could be achieved by consuming foods that provide a limited quantity of methionine and an abundant supply of vitamins B-6, B-12, and folic acid.

McCully began a series of experiments to test his new theory. He injected homocysteine into rabbits while feeding them a normal diet. His initial experiments were designed to study the effects of moderate doses of homocysteine comparable with the dose that a human adult might receive when eating a diet consisting predominantely of animal protein. Within only three to five weeks of daily injections, the rabbits developed atherosclerotic plaques in their arteries.[9]

He then tested the effects of vitamin B-6 deficiency. He found that if the animals were given a diet that was deficient in vitamin B-6 and also injected with homocysteine, the plaques become more prominent and more widespread. If the animals were fed cholesterol and also injected with homocysteine, the atherosclerotic plaques were found to

---

*Many of the children with homocystinuria grow rapidly in childhood, achieving taller stature than their unaffected relatives. Homocysteine is involved in stimulating the growth of normal cells and tissue. Cancer cells accumulate excess homocysteine which reacts with and alters the structure and function of proteins and the nuclear material containing DNA.[8]

contain fat deposits. For the first time in medical science, atherosclerosis had been induced by injection of an amino acid, reproducing the same features of atherosclerotic plaques found in humans. The results were clear. McCully found the amino acid that eluded Newburgh 40 years earlier.

The homocysteine view of cardiovascular disease is that atherosclerosis is caused by a diet low in B vitamins and high in protein. A balance between the two are necessary to reduce risk of heart disease. If fats are a part of the diet, as they are for most people, they will also be incorporated into the plaque, but fat isn't necessary for atherosclerosis to develop.

Dr. McCully has referred to atherosclerosis as "protein intoxication" because homocysteine is derived from the amino acid methionine which is most plentiful in meat. Grains, legumes, and vegetable protein contains less methionine than meat and dairy foods and does not pose as great a threat. This is another reason why vegetarians tend to be protected against atherosclerosis.

A diet lacking adequate amounts of B vitamins combined with excessive meat consumption leads to cardiovascular disease. This is exactly the situation with our modern diet. Modern food processing has destroyed or removed so many nutrients that many of us suffer from chronic subclinical malnutrition. We eat too much meat and dairy and not enough fruits and vegetables. It's no wonder cardiovascular disease kills more people in Western countries than all other diseases combined.

Rejection

Despite the clear evidence gathered by McCully, his new theory was difficult for most of those in the medical community to accept. They had become so enamored with the cholesterol theory that any other explanation for atherosclerosis was considered highly improbable. The fact that treating high cholesterol with cholesterol-lowering drugs was becoming enormously profitable threw in another stumbling block to the acceptance of his theory.

"When these results were presented at a national meeting," recalls McCully, "nobody made a comment; the audience maintained a stony silence...This response to what I thought was an extraordinary experiment confirming my conclusions about the atherosclerotic effect of an amino acid was very disappointing. Investigators interested in the traditional approach of feeding cholesterol and fat to animals totally ignored our results and went back to studying cholesterol and lipoproteins."[10]

McCully had difficulty relating his new theory with the prevailing ideas on cholesterol. Children with homocystinuria had normal blood cholesterol levels and no

cholesterol deposits in the plaque of their arteries. Rinehart's monkeys with vitamin B-6 deficiency that developed atherosclerosis also had normal cholesterol levels and only after prolonged periods of intermittent deficiency did some fatty deposits develop. The failure to find cholesterol or fat deposits in these arteries and the absence of elevated blood cholesterol in children with homocystinuria made it especially troublesome for many scientists to accept his discovery as relevant to atherosclerosis as it is seen in the general population.

Commenting on this McCully states: "The controversy over acceptance of the homocysteine theory of atherosclerosis is partly related to misinterpretation of the significance of fat and cholesterol deposits in plaques and their role in the development of plaques. The idea that plaques are filled with or obstructed only by greasy fat deposits is incorrect for the vast majority of plaques...Typically arteriosclerotic plaques are tough, inelastic, thickened and heavily encrusted with calcium deposits, making them difficult to dissect with scalpel or scissors. In advanced plaques, their complex structure also includes cholesterol crystals, fatty deposits, areas of degeneration or death of tissue, blood clots, protein deposits, the growth of small blood vessels into the artery wall and areas of bleeding that predispose to complete blockage by formation of blood clots."[11]

The suggestion that an amino acid, homocysteine, rather than cholesterol or fat, could be the cause of atherosclerotic plaques was difficult for many experts to accept.

Whole Fish Versus Processed Oils

Omega-3 fatty acids have been credited with lowering risk of heart attack. Another explanation why people who eat fish seem to gain protection from heart disease is that fish is a good source of the B vitamins including folic acid and B-6. This may be why studies have shown a greater degree of protection against heart disease among those who eat whole fish over those who only take fish oil or flaxseed oil supplements. The B vitamins are are vary likely the unknown substance in whole fish that some researchers have speculated are present that provide heart protective properties beyond its oil content.

The prostaglandins derived from Omega-3 oils do not heal or reverse atherosclerotic disease. The effects these oils have are only temporary and, like drugs, must be taken regularly to have any effect at slowing down the disease process. On the other hand, vitamin B-6 and folic acid not only protect the arteries from damage, but help to reverse the atherosclerotic process.

Some of those in the medical community denounced the new homocysteine theory because it threatened to undermine the conventional view. The vast majority, however, simply ignored it.

At first there was almost a complete refusal by others in the medical community to acknowledge the significance of McCully's work. Another curious thing happened which didn't help matters. One group of investigators offered to collaborate with McCully and repeat his experiments in their laboratory. At the conclusion of their tests they sent him slides from the arteries of their rabbits to examine independently. These arteries also showed early atherosclerotic plaques in rabbits, just as McCully found earlier. However, when their study was published in 1974 they contradicted McCully's findings, claiming the plaques were "spontaneous and of no significance." They illustrated their report not with the slides they had sent McCully, but with a photograph of a normal artery![12]

"I felt totally betrayed by this," says McCully. "Because of what they did, the whole idea of homocysteine causing vascular disease was called into question—by this one paper. In retrospect, I realize what I should have done was to photograph the lesions and publish an illustrated rebuttal. But I was too busy doing other things, and I was too naive to think they would pull a trick like that."[13] Subsequently, the investigators refused further collaboration and returned to their own studies.

Later, scientists in Japan also repeated McCully experiments. Their results confirmed those of McCully's showing atherosclerotic plaque and blood clot formation.[14] They also repeated the experiments of Rinehart with vitamin B-6 deficiency in monkeys, observing atherosclerosis after prolonged periods of partial deficiency of the vitamin. They went on to show that vitamin B-6 therapy caused reversal and regression of the atherosclerosis that had been induced by vitamin B-6 deficiency. Because their report was published in Japanese in a Japanese journal, most medical researchers in other parts of the world were totally unaware of it.

In 1978 as a result of his "radical" views, McCully was dismissed from the Harvard faculty and the hospital where he worked informed him he would have to find a position elsewhere.

Although he possessed excellent credentials, he found that no other medical school, hospital, or research institution would hire him. It was as if no one wanted a scientist who threatened to rock the established cholesterol theory. Cholesterol research by this time had become big business. Pharmaceutical companies were pouring millions into research to promote the use of blood pressure medications and cholesterol-lowering drugs.

After two years and with the help of a colleague, he finally secured a job at the Veterans Administration Medical Center in Providence, R.I. Here, under less than ideal conditions, he was able to continue his homocysteine work. Studies by McCully and others over the next 20 years slowly, but surely, confirmed the homocysteine theory, despite continuous objections from cholesterol proponents.

Homocysteine Comes of Age

By the 1990s the evidence supporting the homocysteine theory had become so overwhelming that the medical community was forced to acknowledge it.

Studies showed that human subjects fed oral doses of methionine developed high levels of blood homocysteine.[15,16] Epidemiological studies of human populations compared the blood levels of homocysteine in patients with coronary heart disease, stroke, peripheral vascular disease, and kidney failure with the blood homocysteine levels of normal subjects. The results of these studies showed a strong relationship of elevated homocysteine levels with atherosclerotic disease.[17,18] A study of over 1,000 subjects from the Framingham Heart Study showed that the higher the level of blood homocysteine, the greater the degree of narrowing of carotid arteries to the brain.[19] A homocysteine reading greater than 14 micromoles per liter was established as a recognized risk factor for atherosclerosis, and the higher the homocysteine level, the higher the risk.

One of the problems with the cholesterol theory is that elevated cholesterol is only one of several risk factors associated with atherosclerosis, and it isn't a very significant factor at that. Gender, age, smoking status, high blood pressure, thyroid disease, and diabetes are risk factors that are better predictors of atherosclerosis than cholesterol levels. And many people who suffer heart attacks don't have any of these risk factors. So there are other more important factors involved that have not been recognized. Another problem is the absence of a explanation that could tie all the known risk factors together. What common element is there among all these risk factors? They appear to be totally unrelated. The cholesterol theory has failed to provide a cohesive explanation.

The homocysteine theory, however, provides the missing correlation between the risk factors. All of these factors affect blood homocysteine levels in ways predicted by the theory.[20] Elevated homocysteine levels have become the most accurate indicator in identifying risk of atherosclerosis.

In comparison with traditional risk factors, elevation of blood homocysteine was found to be a greater risk factor (22 to 40-fold) than elevated blood cholesterol (1.2 to 3.1-fold), high blood pressure (8 to 18-fold), or cigarette smoking (3.5-fold) in patients with early-onset atherosclerosis.[21] After a review of 209 published studies on homocysteine it was the consensus of these studies that homocysteine has emerged as the most significant independent risk factor for atherosclerosis. A detailed study of coronary arteries by X-ray angiography in 163 males with angina pectoris concluded that the degree of narrowing of the coronary artery by atherosclerotic plaques correlated better with blood levels of homocysteine than with blood levels of cholesterol.[22]

These conclusive studies were published in 1991, but even now most people have never heard of homocysteine or using B vitamins to reduce heart disease risk. The emphasis is still on the outdated, but enormously profitable, cholesterol approach. You can get your cholesterol level tested just about anywhere, but no one ever talks about getting a homocysteine test. It's a simple test, but the emphasis is still on cholesterol. Recently headlines in the newspapers and television loudly proclaimed: "Heart drugs not prescribed to 20 million needing them!" The news reports went on the say that "at least 20 million Americans at risk of heart attacks aren't getting cholesterol-lowering drugs that could save their lives." These scare tactics are totally untrue, but publicity efforts by drug companies and other supporters of the cholesterol theory continue to loudly proclaim the myth, and will continue to do so as long as there is a profit to be made. Their strategy is to continue to brainwash the public into thinking cholesterol is the sole cause of heart disease and the only way to prevent it is by the aggressive use of drugs. In so doing, knowledge of and acceptance of the homocysteine theory will be overshadowed by the cholesterol mantra.

The homocysteine theory has faced resistance by those who embrace the cholesterol theory because it provided an explanation for atherosclerosis that does not rely on cholesterol, fats, or lipoproteins. Many researchers have built their entire careers on the study of these substances; they are not about to accept a new theory that makes their research inconsequential. So there has been and still is heavy resistance to the homocysteine theory even though a mountain of evidence strongly supports it. In time, the evidence supporting homocysteine will become so prevalent that even the cholesterol supporters will have to accept it. But this may still be some years in the future.

ENIGMA SOLVED

Despite a decades-long effort by thousands of medical researchers, the cholesterol theory fails to adequately explain many observed facts while heart disease remains our number one killer. The homocysteine theory, however, has provided a cohesive explanation for observations that have baffled cholesterol adherents, and treatment based on this theory has proven to be far safer and more effective than cholesterol-lowering drugs.

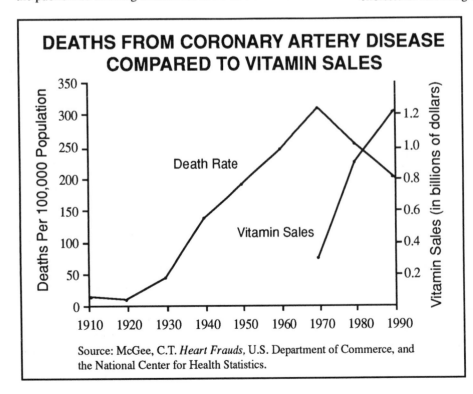

DEATHS FROM CORONARY ARTERY DISEASE COMPARED TO VITAMIN SALES

Source: McGee, C.T. *Heart Frauds*, U.S. Department of Commerce, and the National Center for Health Statistics.

Deaths from heart attack reached a peak in the late 1960s and then began to fall. The decline does not correlate to changing cholesterol levels, saturated fat intake, heart bypass or other surgical procedures, or even drug therapy. The Medical community, in general, has been at a loss to explain the decline. Many now believe the fall in fatal heart attacks is due to the increasing use of vitamin supplements. Since the late 1960s vitamin sales have skyrocketed. During this same time period heart disease deaths have declined.

There are two historical enigmas that have completely baffled cholesterol researchers. The first one is the cholesterol theory's complete failure to explain the rapid escalation of atherosclerosis, heart disease, and stroke that occurred during the mid-20th century. Detailed studies of the composition of the diet have failed to reveal a correlation between cholesterol and fat content of the food and the occurrence of atherosclerotic disease.[23] If excessive fat and cholesterol consumption were the cause, there should be a direct correlation, but there isn't.

The second enigma was the dramatic decline of heart disease deaths in the United States beginning in 1968. Since that time, heart disease deaths have continued to fall. In many other countries, however, heart disease continues to climb. The reason for this has remained a mystery. In 1979 a conference was held at the National Institutes of Health. Experts gathered from all over the country to try to discover the reason for this decline. They found that it was *not* due to changes in blood cholesterol levels or dietary fats and cholesterol. Fat consumption had remained relatively constant. Other factors, including changes in lifestyle, smoking, and exercise could not explain it either. There was discussion about the effect of coronary care units, bypass surgery, and other medical procedures, but none of these provided the answer why the incidence of atherosclerotic disease had declined.

It wasn't until McCully introduced the homocysteine theory that an explanation for both the rapid rise in heart disease in the early part of the 20th century and the subsequent dramatic decline in the late 1960s was found. During the 1930s, 40s, and 50s the processed-food revolution completely changed the way we eat. The diet in most industrialized countries changed from one of primarily fresh produce and meat to one dominated by highly processed, packaged, convenience foods. People in less developed countries who continued to eat their native diets suffered little from heart disease, or any other degenerative disease for that matter. According to McCully's theory, the lack of B vitamins in processed foods created a situation of subclinical malnutrition. We continued to eat large quantities of meat and dairy, rich in the amino acid methionine which raises homocysteine levels. These levels remain elevated because the processed foods commonly eaten are deficient in vitamins B-6, B-12, and folic acid which are necessary to metabolize homocysteine. These vitamins are sensitive to heat and so are quickly destroyed during processing. As the population began to rely more and more on nutrient-deficient processed foods, heart disease increased. Studies have shown a widespread deficiency of vitamin B-6 in the population, as well as deficiency of B-6, folic acid and B-12 in the elderly and in cardiac patients.[24, 25, 26]

The decline in heart disease can be directly related to a growing awareness to good nutrition and the increased consumption of vitamin supplements. Beginning in the mid-1960s vitamin consumption greatly increased with a direct inverse relationship with the decline in heart disease. Another factor is that over the past few decades, improved transportation and food distribution methods have made more fresh fruits and vegetables available all year long. As people began getting the B vitamins they needed, homocysteine levels dropped and heart disease deaths declined.

Vitamin sales began to jump in the late 1960s. During this time period the death rate from coronary artery disease began to fall for the first time. Consumption of vitamins has continued to increase. According to the U.S. Department of Commerce, vitamin sales at the wholesale level increased from $268 million to $1,193 million between 1970 and 1990. At the same time, the death rate from coronary artery disease fell by 35 percent. In 1986, 169,000,000 Americans were using vitamins and minerals, or 67 percent of the population. By contrast, only 15 percent of physicians admit to taking vitamins.

The United States is the only industrialized nation in the world that has experienced a significant drop in the heart attack death rate. It is also the only country that has experienced such an increase in vitamin sales. In countries where foods are not fortified and vitamin supplements not routinely used, heart disease continues to climb. Although only an association, it appears highly likely a cause-effect relationship is at work.

THE B VITAMINS
Vitamin B-6

The three B vitamins that are directly associated with homocysteine are B-6, B-12, and folic acid. Of the three, vitamin B-6 seems to be the most important indicator of homocysteine. Low levels of vitamin B-6 correlate with elevation of blood homocysteine. The results of many studies show that the amount of dietary vitamin B-6 necessary to prevent abnormal elevation of blood homocysteine and reduce risk of atherosclerosis is 300 to 350 mcg per day. The current Recommended Dietary Allowance (RDA) for this vitamin is only 200 mcg (2.0 mg) for adult men and 160 mcg (1.6 mg) for adult women.

The RDA for vitamin B-6 was set without consideration of the fact that homocysteine can cause vascular disease. The current RDA of 160 to 200 mcg is too low. A Tufts University study showed clearly that we actually require 350 to 400 mcg per day to prevent accumulation of homocysteine—nearly twice the RDA.

Folic Acid

The RDA for folic acid is 200 mcg per day. To prevent elevated homocysteine, the amount required is 350 to 400 mcg, nearly twice that amount. Folic acid is also known as folate. Folate is a B vitamin naturally found in leafy green vegetables, citrus fruits, and other foods. It is called folic acid when manufactured synthetically.

Folic acid has also received publicity in recent years because of its role in preventing spina bifida and other spinal and brain problems known as neural tube defects. According to the Centers for Disease Control and Prevention, some 4,000 pregnancies in the United States every year are affected by neural tube defects. Roughly 2,400 babies are born with major defects such as spina bifida, which can cause paralysis, mental retardation and a fatal condition called anencephaly (incomplete formation of the brain). Most all of these defects could be prevented if women consumed adequate daily amounts of folic acid in their diet or through vitamin supplements, the CDC states.

In an effort to reduce birth defects, the Food and Drug Administration began requiring folic acid additives in a wide variety of processed foods beginning in 1998. Flour, bread, rolls, pasta, rice and cereal are among the fortified foods. However, women of childbearing age still may not getting enough folate when they need it most—during the first weeks of pregnancy. The spinal cord of a fetus forms 16 to 25 days after conception. That's why doctors recommend that all women capable of getting pregnant be getting adequate folic acid all the time. The damage may have already been done by the time most women realize they are pregnant.

Vitamin B-12

Our body's requirement for vitamin B-12 is very small. The RDA is only 3 mcg per day for adults. But unlike most other vitamins which are found in a wide variety of foods, vitamin B-12 is formed only by microorganisms. We get almost all of our vitamin B-12 from foods of animal origin such as meat and dairy products. Most normal adults who eat foods of animal origin consume about 5 to 8 mcg per day of vitamin B-12, more than an adequate intake to meet RDA requirements. Most of us eat enough animal products to get plenty of this vitamin. Some people have genetic problems that hamper their body's ability to absorb vitamin B-12 and in these cases supplements would be helpful.

Strict vegetarians who eat no animal products what so ever are at greatest risk of suffering a vitamin B-12 deficiency. Some vitamin B-12 is synthesized by the bacteria in our intestines, so deficiencies may take 20 or 30 years to develop. Those who are vegetarians can avoid a vitamin B-12 deficiency by taking supplements or by eating cultured or fermented foods such as miso, yogurt, or apple cider vinegar.

B Vitamin Complex

The B vitamins consist of thiamin (B1), riboflavin (B2), niacin (B3), folic acid (folate), vitamin B-6, Vitamin B-12, pantothenic acid, biotin, choline, inositol, and PABA. Together they make up the vitamin B complex. These vitamins are not isolated from each other but for the most part are present together in a wide variety of foods.

The B vitamins are utilized as coenzymes in almost all parts of the body. They are essential to the health of nearly every organ and system in the body, including the immune system, and in maintaining normal mental function. The B vitamins are necessary for the metabolism of carbohydrates, fats, and proteins and the generation of energy.

The B vitamins are water-soluble so the body can tolerate a large amount without serious complications. As with all water-soluble vitamins, excesses above that which the body requires are simply excreted in the urine. The RDA for the B vitamins are generally low—around 200 mcg (2.0 mg) or so. Physical and emotional stress as well as illness and exposure to environmental toxins places a heavy burden on our vitamin reserves and more than the RDA may be needed.

A deficiency of a single B vitamin is rare. People tend to have multiple deficiencies. Foods normally contain a mixture of these vitamins and, if the diet is lacking one B vitamin, it is more than likely lacking in others as well. So, if a person is deficient (or getting a less than optimal amount) of vitamin B-6 or folic acid then he or she is probably deficient in the other B vitamins as well.

Often people will read an article about one of the B vitamins and feel they have a deficiency or need to take more of that vitamin to prevent a problem in the future. So they take mega doses of one or two B vitamins. This is a big mistake. You should never take high doses of a single B vitamin without increasing the amount you take of all the others. The reason for this is because the B vitamins all work together and depend on each other. If you don't have all four wheels on your car you're not going to go very far. The same is true with the B Vitamins. They depend on each other for numerous metabolic processes. For example, folic acid assists in thiamin absorption. A folic acid deficiency, therefore, can cause a thiamin deficiency (i.e., beriberi), and even thiamin supplements don't correct the thiamin deficiency until after the folic acid deficiency has been corrected. The enzymes involved in the metabolism of many other nutrients, including vitamin B-6, folic acid, and niacin require riboflavin. Thus a riboflavin deficiency invariably causes deficiencies of other nutrients. If a deficiency of one vitamin exists then it is apparent there is a multiple deficiency, as rarely is there ever just a deficiency of one.

Another reason you should not take large doses of any one or two of these vitamins is because all of the B vitamins compete in the intestines for absorption into the body. If you consume an enormous amount of B-6, for example, you might decrease the amount of niacin absorbed and end up with a niacin deficiency.

The RDA for most vitamins is set at the point where consumption equals excretion. This is the point where tissues are considered saturated and any additional consumed will just be excreted. The RDA is set to satisfy the needs of most *healthy* individuals. If you supply the body with enough to theoretically saturate the tissues (RDA) then you can add a little more of a select few to suit your particular needs. But keep in mind if you are under a lot of stress (a common situation in our hectic society) or are exposed to a lot of environmental toxins and germs (as most of us are),

you should take more of all of them. In general, it is safe to take up to about two to three times the amount of the other B vitamins you are taking. For instance if you take 100 mg of the entire B complex, you can then safely take a total of up to 200-300 mg of vitamin B-6.

Heat and irradiation destroy vitamin B-6, folate, and other vitamins. So all processed, canned, and even frozen foods are depleted of these vitamins. Up to 50 percent of these vitamins are lost during the processing of canned and packaged foods. So they are only half as nutritious as the fresh product.

Frozen produce is better but still not as good as fresh. Produce must be blanched before freezing. This requires vegetables to be immersed in boiling water or heated to a high temperature for a few minutes to inactivate enzymes. Without blanching, frozen foods slowly deteriorate because the enzymes remain active even at freezing temperatures. Blanching destroys about 10 to 15 percent of vitamin B-6 and folic acid as well as other heat-sensitive nutrients.

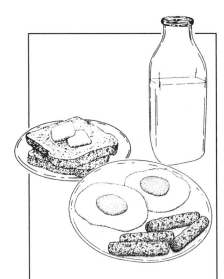

Chapter 13

MEAT, EGGS AND DAIRY

"A frequent complaint of patients who consult me is lack of energy. If I can convince them to cut down on the amount of protein they eat, increase their intake of starch and vegetables, and do more aerobic exercise, most of them find that they feel better and have more energy."

—Andrew Weil, M.D.,
*Natural Health,
Natural Medicine*

What did you have for lunch? For dinner last night? What about the night before? If you are like most of us, your meals included some type of animal product—meat, eggs, or dairy—with meat being the most popular. Our modern diet is based around meat. Meat is the most important part of the meal and anything else is just an accompaniment. When we go to a restaurant we order steak, chicken, or fish. The side dishes are of little importance. At home, meals always contain meat in one form or another and, if they don't, they are loaded with milk, cream, or cheese instead. We have become so accustomed to eating meat and dairy that we don't know how to fix a meal without them.

If asked why we eat so much meat, the answer might be because it tastes good and besides, how else are we going to get all the protein we need? Thanks to the meat and dairy industries, we have been brainwashed into thinking that meat and dairy are our only sources of protein. This is simply not true. All plant foods contain protein. You can get all the protein you need from a strict vegetarian diet. The cow, for example, gets all the protein it needs to grow from a 50-pound calf into an 800-pound steer from the grass it eats. It doesn't need to eat cheeseburgers or chicken fried steak to get its protein. We do not need to eat meat or dairy products every day to get protein, and most of us eat far too much animal protein.

Excess animal protein can create some serious health problems. When we eat meat in place of other foods, like vegetables, we are depriving ourselves of vital nutrients plant foods provide. Protein, and especially animal protein, puts a heavy strain on the kidneys, and too much can cause kidney damage. Protein also pulls minerals out of our bones, contributing to osteoporosis. Homocysteine, which is derived from protein, is a major cause for atherosclerosis and related diseases. It appears that the protein in meat is more harmful than the fat. Studies show that a low-fat diet that is high in protein can and does promote the formation of coronary artery blockages.[1]

Protein is an important part of the diet and animal products do supply the richest source of this nutrient. Meat, eggs, and dairy products, like most other foods, are fine in moderation, but can become serious health problems if eaten in excess.

THE DANGERS OF HIGH PROTEIN CONSUMPTION
The Acid Body

If you dropped an old penny into a glass of cola and left it there overnight, the phosphoric acid in the soda would eat through the surface of the coin, turning it from a dark brown into a shinny light copper color. If you put a few drops of hydrochloric acid on a chunk of limestone, it would bubble and fizz as it ate its way through the rock. Acid from you car battery would eat holes through a piece of cloth in no time. All of these are examples of what acids can do to a variety of materials.

We have acids in our bodies as well. Our stomach secretes chemicals that form hydrochloric acid to help in breaking down and digesting food. It normally does no harm to the stomach lining because it is protected by a thick layer of mucus. The moment food covered in acid leaves the stomach and enters the intestinal tract, it is drenched in alkalizing fluids that neutralize the acids. If there were no alkalizing fluids or not enough to neutralize these acids, the tissues in our intestines would be damaged like the penny or cloth described above.

Our bodies are dynamic systems that continually make adjustments to environmental and internal stimuli in an effort to maintain homeostasis—a chemical balance in which the body works best. One of the requirements for homeostasis and good health is the maintenance or quick restoration of the acid-base balance of its fluids. What this means is keeping the concentration of hydrogen ions in body fluids relatively constant or in balance. This is of vial importance. If the hydrogen ion concentration deviates even slightly, normal chemical reactions are disrupted and health is compromised. The acidity or alkalinity of a solution is expressed numerically on a scale which ranges from 0 to 14. A pH of 7 is neutral. The lower the pH, the stronger the

acid. A pH of 6 is slightly acidic while 1 is very acidic. In contrast, a pH of 8 is slightly alkaline (basic) and 13 very alkaline.

By nature our bodies are primarily alkaline (basic). Most all body fluids (blood, saliva, interstitial fluid, cytoplasm, etc.) are slightly alkaline. Stomach juices are an exception. In the stomach, fluids are acidic, a necessity for proper digestion. If the stomach acid is not strong enough, even by a very small degree, certain nutrients could not be digested or assimilated into the body.

Blood must be kept at a very narrow range of between 7.35 to 7.45 to function properly. When it deviates from these values even slightly, chemical processes are disrupted and disease develops. When pH goes higher than 7.45, a condition called alkalosis develops, meaning the blood is too alkaline. When pH dips below 7.35, acidosis and physical degeneration begin to develop. Both can become fatal. Because of the importance of maintaining pH at normal levels, the body constantly works to keep the acid-alkaline levels within optimal range.

Our diet affects the pH of the body. Some foods have an acidifying effect and some an alkalizing effect. A few are neutral. The pH balance of our bodies and consequently our health, depends greatly on the types of foods we eat.

When food is completely metabolized in the body, it leaves an ash-like residue. This ash is what is left over after most of the usable nutrients have been removed. The elements comprising the ash are either absorbed into the body or eliminated. Most all food leaves an ash residue. This ash

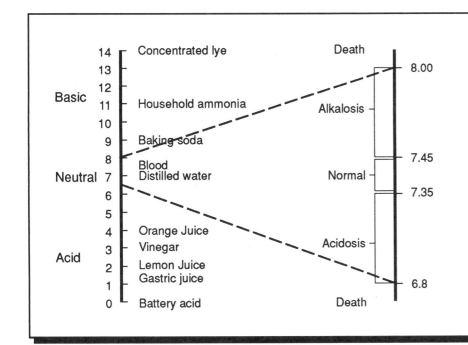

THE pH SCALE

The lower the pH the stronger the acid. A pH of 0 is a very strong acid. A pH of 7 is neutral. A pH of 14 is a very strong alkaline or basic. Human blood can only function normally between a pH of 7.45 and 7.35. Outside of this range degeneration and disease occur. Cancer, heart disease, and most other common degenerative conditions occur in people whose body chemistry is overly acidic (acidosis or subclinical acidosis). An over acid condition creates excess free radicals.

can have an acidic, alkaline, or neutral effect on the body's chemistry. Alkaline ash leaves alkalizing minerals which the body can use to neutralize excess dietary acid. Alkaline ash is good because our bodies are supposed to be slightly alkaline. Acid ash, on the other hand, leaves minerals that must be neutralized before the body can dispose of them. Foods high in sulfur, chloride, nitrogen, and phosphorus have an acidifying effect. The residue contains strong acids, such as sulfuric acid and phosphoric acid, that must be neutralized and eliminated by the kidneys. Nitrogen intake beyond the body's needs is converted to uric acid and removed by the kidneys as urine or by the skin as sweat. Some foods have a higher percentage of acidifying minerals than others. Protein, especially animal protein, is high in acidifying elements.

Acidifying elements must be neutralized in order to maintain the acid-base balance. Alkaline minerals such as sodium, calcium, potassium, and magnesium serve this function. These elements are found most abundantly in plant foods. The body will store these minerals to maintain pH balance. Besides holding our bodies up, bones serve as our primary storage site for alkalizing minerals, particularly calcium. Magnesium, one of our most important alkalizing minerals, is also found in the bones as well as inside all of our cells.

The body is capable of handling acidifying foods as long as alkalizing foods are eaten in equal amounts. However, if most of the foods we eat leave an acid ash, the body will be continually pulling alkalizing elements from its reserves, depleting itself of vital minerals. If the body is constantly struggling to neutralize acid, health will suffer. Cellular reactions become less efficient, causing tissues and organs to lose their ability to function properly. As the body becomes more acidic, free-radical production also increases, leading to cellular degeneration.

A great many people suffer from subclinical or mild chronic acidosis. They don't notice any symptoms immediately, but hang on the edge, suffering gradual degeneration. Acidosis even in its mildest form leads to loss of calcium and weakening of the bones (osteoporosis), increasing blood pressure (hypertension), degeneration of joints (arthritis), precipitation of calcium in body tissues (kidney stones, gout, atherosclerosis), and development of painful bone spurs. Body chemistry is constantly pushed to its limits, which creates tremendous stress and encourages the breakdown and degeneration of tissues, weakening the immune system, increasing susceptibility to disease, and further depressing normal bodily functions. Combined with massive free-radical destruction, the body ages at an accelerated rate.

In general, foods which have a high protein content leave an acid ash residue (see chart on following page).

Foods which have the greatest acidifying effect are meat, fish, poultry, dairy, and eggs—animal products. Most grains, nuts and legumes, which are good sources of plant protein, also leave an acid ash residue but to a much lesser degree. With few exceptions, fruits and vegetables leave an alkaline ash residue. Eating a diet consisting primarily of animal products and flour (bread, crackers, pasta, etc.) will lead to acidosis. This is yet another reason why vegetarians or near vegetarians are so much more healthy then nonvegetarians.

High meat consumption can create a deficiency of calcium and magnesium because these minerals are used to neutralize the acidic effects of protein. High protein diets, whether from meat, protein drinks, or other sources, can lead to serious health problems.

Harrison's *Principles of Internal Medicine* states: "Another factor which some have implicated in bone loss is the possibility that excessive acid intake, particularly in the form of high-protein diets, results in 'dissolution' of bone in an attempt to buffer the extra acid." (8th ed. vol II. page 2029).

The body, in order to maintain acid-alkaline balance for thousands of chemical functions, must neutralize this excess acid, and does so by buffering with calcium from the bones. But in this process, calcium is mobilized out of the bone and excreted in the urine. It is a disease of calcium loss, not a calcium deficiency. As Harrison's book states, "There is no difference in the calcium intake of [the] osteoporotic compared with control subjects of similar age and sex."

While this disease is widespread in affluent Western society, osteoporosis is virtually nonexistent in millions of people in Africa and Asia where animal products are rarely eaten and dairy products are virtually unknown. For example, the Chinese eat mainly rice, beans, corn, wheat, barley, oats, fruits, and vegetables. Their babies are breast fed and then weaned to this diet. The bones and teeth of children and adults are strong and healthy.

The average American eats 2-5 times as much protein as he or she needs. The daily protein intake of Americans is 90-120 grams and represent about 25% of total calories. The ideal protein intake is 20-40 grams per day. This represents about 10% of total calories. The World Health Organization recommends 37 grams of protein per day.

The protein requirement varies for size and gender. The RDA for protein is 63 grams per day for adult men and 50 grams for day for adult women. Some experts suggest the optimal amount is closer to 25-30 grams. Most people eat much more than this. The RDA of protein can be obtained easily without even realizing it. If you started breakfast with one egg and a glass of milk, at lunch you had a garden salad with a little cheese sprinkled on top, and for dinner you ate

ALKALINE ASH AND ACID ASH FOODS

Alkaline Ash Foods		Acid Ash Foods		Neutral Ash Foods
Almonds	Lettuce	Bacon	Peanuts	Sugar
Apples	Lima beans	Barley	Peas, dried	Corn oil
Apricots	Limes	Beef	Pike	Olive oil
Avocados	Millet	Blueberries	Plums*	Coconut oil
Bananas	Molasses	Butter	Pork	
Beans, dried	Mushrooms	Carob	Prunes*	In general, fruits and vegetables
Beets	Muskmelon	Cheese	Rice	leave an alkaline ash residue while
Blackberries	Onions	Chicken	Salmon	meat, dairy, grains, and nuts leave an
Broccoli	Oranges	Codfish	Sardines	acid ash residue.
Brussels sprouts	Parsnips	Corn	Sausage	Although citrus fruits such as
Cabbage	Peaches	Cranberries*	Scallops	oranges and lemons contain citric acid
Carrots	Pears	Currants	Shrimp	and may have an acid taste, thy are not
Cauliflower	Pineapple	Eggs	Squash, winter	acid forming when metabolized. The
Celery	Potatoes	Haddock	Sunflower seeds	acid-forming potential of a food is
Chard	Radishes	Honey	Turkey	determined largely by the chloride,
Cherries, sour	Raisins	Lamb	Walnuts	sulfur, and phosphorus elements found
Cucumbers	Raspberries	Lintels, dried	Wheat	in the noncombustible mineral residue
Dates, dried	Rutabagas	Lobster	Yogurt	or ash after metabolism of the food has
Figs, dried	Sauerkraut	Milk*		occurred. Acids such as those found in
Grapefruit	Soy beans, green	Macaroni		citrus fruits are normally fully oxidized
Grapes	Spinach, raw	Oatmeal		by the cells during metabolism and
Green beans	Strawberries	Oysters		leave no mineral residue.
Green peas	Tangerines			
Lemons	Tomatoes	*Leaves an alkaline ash but has an		Source: M. Ted Morter, Jr., *Your Health*
	Watermelon	acidifying effect on the body.		*Your Choice*, pgs 85-86.

one chicken leg with another glass of milk, you would have far more than 50 grams of protein just from the dairy and meat. Any bread, vegetables, or other foods would provide additional protein.

How many people eat just one egg for breakfast? Or one chicken leg for dinner? Or just a sprinkle of cheese on a lunch salad? Ordinarily people eat two or more eggs along with bread or pancakes (also good sources of protein). At dinner one small piece of chicken isn't going to satisfy anyone except a small child. Often, people will devour three, four, and even more pieces of chicken as well as rolls, potatoes, and other side dishes, all of which also contain protein. The protein intake soars to two and three times more than what is necessary. In affluent societies, our diets are based on meat and dairy products. That is the way we were raised and the only way most of us know how to eat.

You don't need to give up eating meat, but it would be advisable to cut down on the amount you consume. Eat smaller portions and eat more meatless meals. Look at meat more as an accompaniment or flavoring rather than as the main course. Eat fewer steaks and more stews or casseroles

that contain less meat. Try to limit your meat consumption to no more than one meat meal a day.

Calcium

Ninety-nine percent of the body's calcium is stored in the bones. The other 1 percent is in the blood and body fluids. Besides being the primary mineral in bone, it is also involved in normal muscle contraction and relaxation (including heart muscle), proper nerve functioning, blood clotting, blood pressure, and immune defenses. Principal sources are milk and milk products, soybeans, green vegetables, and legumes.

Calcium is one of the principal minerals used by the body to counter the acidifying effects of protein. For this reason, protein exerts a significant effect on the calcium status of our bodies.[2] In the United States the recommend daily amount of calcium for adults is 800 mg and 1,200 mg for pregnant and lactating women. The World Health Organization recommends only 400 to 500 mg per day for adults. The reason for the difference is that in North America protein intakes are often twice that in other countries. The more protein that is eaten, the more calcium is lost and more must be eaten to compensate.

One might think that taking calcium supplements will prevent osteoporosis and other complications of eating too much acidifying foods. But that is not necessarily true. A study on calcium reported in *The American Journal of Clinical Nutrition* showed that eating too much protein depletes calcium reserves even when taking supplements.[3] In this study, subjects who were given 1,400 mg of calcium (the RDA is only 800 mg) along with 142 grams of protein, suffered a mean calcium *loss* of 84 mg. Even though they consumed 1,400 mg of calcium they lost 84 mg more than they ate. When their protein consumption was reduced to 47 grams, the subjects retained 10 mg of calcium. The conclusion that can be drawn from this study is that even if you take calcium supplements, if you eat a high-protein diet you may still have a net loss of calcium.

Magnesium

Another mineral that is used to balance excess body acid is magnesium. Magnesium is found most abundantly in the bones and teeth. It is an important constituent in all the cells of the soft tissues where it is involved in protein synthesis and energy production. It serves as a catalyst for several hundred intracellular enzymes and is necessary for proper muscle function and transmission of nerve impulses. Magnesium has attracted so much attention that an international conference is held yearly to discuss new studies on this single mineral.

The most significant sources of magnesium are nuts, legumes, whole grains and dark green vegetables. A deficiency can be caused by excess protein consumption; inadequate magnesium in the diet; consumption of excessive amounts of calcium; use of medications such as antibiotics, antacids, diuretics, estrogen, and oral contraceptives; regular use of caffeinated beverages (coffee, tea, and soda pop); alcoholism; and prolonged stress.

Magnesium deficiency can contribute to such health problems as osteoporosis, cardiovascular disease, kidney stones, diabetes, hypoglycemia, migraine headaches, morning sickness, excessive menstrual cramping, premenstrual syndrome, asthma, chronic fatigue syndrome, muscle weakness, and mental confusion.[4]

Magnesium has become recognized as an important factor in maintaining a healthy heart and circulatory system. It has been noted that in areas where water is low in natural magnesium, people experience higher rates of coronary artery disease.[5]

Many studies have shown that people who suffer from a variety of cardiovascular diseases have lower magnesium levels as compared to the general population.[6, 7] Giving patients with cardiovascular problems magnesium supplements has increased their survival rate. Magnesium supplementaion is now commonly prescribed as an aid against coronary heart disease.[8, 9, 10, 11, 12] Magnesium has proven useful in reducing destructive effects of heart disease and prolonging life.

Because of the many factors that can deplete magnesium stores in our bodies, deficiencies, particularly subclinical deficiencies, are much more common than we realize. Dr. M.A. Brodsky reported in the *Journal of the American College of Nutrition* that as much as 80 percent of the population may be magnesium deficient.[13]

People nowadays aren't getting as much magnesium in their diet as they used to. According to Dr. Heikki Karppanen of the University of Helsinki, the dietary intake of magnesium in developed countries has fallen by two thirds in the past 50 years. He cites the use of white flour as one of the primary reasons for the reduction of magnesium in our bodies. People who eat baked goods made of white flour consume only 18 percent of the magnesium they would receive if they ate whole wheat bread. Losses from the conversion of brown rice to white rice are similar. Another big drop in consumption occurs when people eat commercially processed foods. Up to 50 percent of the minerals may leach out during soaking and cooking. Certain chemical additives used to keep frozen vegetables a bright shade of green pull out essential minerals, including magnesium.

The Recommended Dietary Allowance (RDA) of magnesium is 350 mg for men and 280 mg for women. Many mineral researchers think we should be getting about 420-475 mg of magnesium a day to make up for losses and to help protect us from developing cardiovascular problems as we age.

Excessive protein consumption and the use of medications drain the body of magnesium. Magnesium is not distributed evenly between cells and fluids of the body. The level of magnesium inside our cells is about 10,000 times higher than outside of cells (such as in the blood and interstitial fluid). Magnesium in the blood and other fluids is used to buffer the acidifying effects of protein. As the body attempts to maintain blood pH, magnesium levels in the blood become depleted. The body makes a serious effort to maintain normal magnesium levels in the blood by shifting it out of the cells. Magnesium levels in the cells may be depleted by as much as 30 percent before blood levels begin to fall below their normal range. This is important because as magnesium shifts from the cells into the blood, the cells of the body become more acidic. As a consequence, cellular functions slow down and become more susceptible to disease and degradation. If your cells are operating at a depressed level, then the tissues composed of those cells will also be depressed, which in turn will affect the function of the entire body.

A diet high in meat, eggs, dairy, and soda pop (which contains phosphoric acid) cause acid levels of the body to increase. Magnesium is drawn out of cells to neutralize this acid and is eventually excreted in the urine. The result is a continual drain of magnesium, and when the diet is also deficient in this mineral, reserves are constantly being depleted. The result is the gradual loss of normal cellular function and the development of disease.

With the growing awareness of the importance of calcium in the prevention of osteoporosis many people are taking large quantities of this mineral in supplemental form. This could be counterproductive. Calcium competes with magnesium for absorption and, therefore, supplementation with large amounts of calcium may decrease the amount of magnesium that is absorbed. A magnesium deficiency can also lead to osteoporosis. But, too much magnesium can interfere with calcium absorption. The consensus among researchers is that the calcium-to-magnesium ratio should be about 2:1.[14] We hear a lot about calcium supplementation, and so people consume a lot of calcium and in the process can help create a magnesium deficiency which can promote osteoporosis, kidney stones, heart disease, PMS, chronic fatigue, and other problems.

ANIMAL PROTEIN

You've heard the ads "drink milk—it does a body good" or "eat pork—the other white meat" we hear such slogans all the time. For years the meat and dairy industries have flooded our minds with the idea that we must eat their products in order to get all the protein we need to be healthy. Protein is, after all, a necessary nutrient.

The resulting emphasis on protein has created the idea that the *only* source of protein is from animal products. In our society meals are centered around meat. We've become a meat society. Meat and dairy have become such important parts of our diet that many people don't have any idea how to make a meal without them. A tossed salad is the only meatless meal they have ever eaten. Our obsession with getting enough protein and our habit of eating animal products at every meal has created a situation of protein intoxication. We often consume two to three times the amount of protein our bodies actually need.

Excessive consumption of protein, especially animal protein, puts an enormous burden on the kidneys. Harry Newburgh's studies back in the 1920s provided evidence that excess animal protein consumption could be harmful. The sulfur-containing amino acids cystine, lysine, histidine, tyrosine, tryptophan, and methionine can all cause kidney damage when eaten in excess. In the 1970s when high-protein drinks became popular among body builders numerous people suffered kidney failure and many died from drinking too much of these powdered beverages.

Food of animal origin, such as meat, eggs, milk, and cheese, generally contain more protein than most plant foods. In addition, the protein of animal foods contains two to three times as much methionine as the protein of plant foods. Methionine is metabolized into the amino acid homocysteine. A deficiency in B vitamins allows homocysteine to build up, leading to atherosclerosis, heart disease, and stroke.

Meat is our primary source of iron. Although necessary in small amounts, this mineral promotes destructive free-radical chain reactions and in excess can increase the risk of heart disease. In experiments involving animals, the feeding of excess homocysteine causes increased uptake and storage of iron in the liver and other tissues.[15] This will accelerate free-radical formation. In this way homocysteine contributes to a host of degenerative conditions caused by free radicals.

In Europe during World War II, meat and milk products were in short supply and people were encouraged to plant gardens. People began eating more produce. At the same time the death rate from heart disease dropped. When the war was over and meat and milk consumption resumed, heart disease quickly rose back to prewar levels.[16] Those who believe in the cholesterol hypothesis assumed that this phenomenon was due to the fat content of the meat and milk rather than the protein. We know this is not true because lowering the cholesterol and saturated fat content of the diet in other populations has not shown to lower the heart attack death rate. However, now that we understand homocysteine's role in heart disease, we know that excess consumption of animal protein, rich in the amino acid methionine and the highly oxidative mineral iron, and the lack of fresh produce were the real factors involved. It has been noted that populations that are mainly vegetarian have much fewer health problems. Even vegetarians within our own society generally are healthier and live longer.

Saturated fat and cholesterol are guilty only by association. If we reduce our meat and dairy consumption, we will reduce risk for a multitude of protein-caused illnesses as well as reduce saturated fat and cholesterol. Removing the fat from animal products and leaving the protein will reduce calories, but it won't make the food any healthier nor will it reduce your risk of developing degenerative disease.

Studies show that meat eaters are almost twice as likely to die from heart disease, 60 percent more likely to die from cancer, and 30 percent more likely to die from other diseases.

ANIMAL FAT

In this book I have stressed the point that saturated fat is less harmful to health than polyunsaturated fat. Our ancestors ate a good deal of animal fat without suffering any apparent health problems. I don't necessarily recommend that you start eating a lot of animal fat. The saturated fat generally available to us nowadays is not the same as it was a generation or two ago. I wouldn't recommend using bacon drippings or beef tallow in cooking, or even butter. The reason I wouldn't is that all these fats are contaminated. They're filled with pesticides, artificial hormones, antibiotics, and other drugs.

Most animals raised for human consumption are fed foods full of pesticides. They're routinely given artificial hormones and antibiotics. These chemicals are fat-soluble, which means that once they are eaten they tend to collect in the fatty tissues of the animals. A cow that has been fed all its life on feed loaded with pesticides will have a high amount of these contaminants stored in its fatty tissues. Cutting out the fat won't eliminate it. The fatty tissues permeate the meat. Animals collect so much of these chemicals in their tissues that some 95 percent of the pesticides we are exposed to in our diet come from meat and milk and not from fruits and vegetables. Although the fruits and vegetables may have been sprayed several times and still retain pesticide residue, meat will have more.

Most all commercially raised meat, dairy, and eggs are contaminated with chemical residue. In my opinion this makes them unfit to eat. Dairy products include anything made with milk—cheese, cottage cheese, cream, butter, etc. The only safe animal products are those that have been raised without antibiotics and hormones on an open range where their food has not been adulterated by pesticides. These products are labeled as "free range" or "organic." This is equivalent to the type of food eaten by our ancestors, free from chemical pollutants.

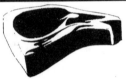 # HOW MUCH PROTEIN DO YOU EAT?

Dietary guidelines generally recommend that our protein intake contribute about 12 percent of the total calories consumed. Sixty percent of calories should come from carbohydrate, and 30 percent or less from fat (1 gram of protein = 4 calories, 1 gram of carbohydrate = 4 calories, 1 gram of fat = 9 calories, so 1 gram of fat contributes more than twice as much energy as 1 gram of either protein or carbohydrate). Most people in affluent cultures eat much more protein than 12 percent. Protein need depends on a person's muscle mass and bone structure. Larger people (not fatter) need more protein than smaller people. On average 50 grams a day is recommended as ample protein for most people of average size. Some health authorities believe this figure is far too high and should be closer to 20-30 grams a day. 50 grams a day is very easy to obtain even on a strict vegetarian diet. In fact, most people eat far more than 50 grams of protein a day. A single meal with protein-rich foods such as meat and dairy products can easily supply all the protein a person needs for an entire day. If you eat meat and/or dairy two or more times a day, you are running the risk of protein overload. A diet like this day after day leads to acidosis and all of its accompanying health risks. Because some vegetable foods, such as soy, dried beans, rice, and pasta, are good sources of protein, even vegetarians can get too much protein in their diets. This is one reason why fruits and vegetables are so important.

The Committee on Dietary Allowances of the Food and Nutrition Board of the National Academy of Sciences states the RDA in grams of protein per kilogram of body weight per day. They consider that a generous protein allowance for a healthy adult would be 0.8 grams per kilogram of *appropriate* body weight per day.

Most adults need between 2,000 and 3,000 Calories a day to fuel metabolism and daily activities. These figures vary depending on muscle mass and bone structure. A larger more muscular person requires more calories. Men generally require 500 to 800 more calories than woman. An average-sized woman would need 2,100 and average sized man about 2,900 calories.

The following chart lists the amount of grams in common foods. Use this list to determine your daily protein intake. What was your protein consumption yesterday? Write down all the foods you ate and the approximate serving size, include all meals and snacks. For foods not listed on the chart make an estimated guess. For example, if you ate two handfuls of potato chips you could approximate that as being equivalent to $^1/_2$ potato which would amount to $2^1/_2$ grams of protein.

Continued on next page

Another source of highly saturated fat that is free from contamination and is of vegetable origin are the tropical oils made from coconuts and palm kernels. These are oils high in a type of saturated fat that has no bad health effects, but does provide many healthful benefits.

By replacing the polyunsaturated vegetable oils in your diet with uncontaminated saturated oils, particularly coconut oil, you can eliminate much of the damage that goes on inside your body from free-radical destruction as well as save yourself from prostaglandin overload and all the health consequences it creates. In this respect, eating saturated fat in place of refined vegetable oil may very well save your life.

MILK AND DAIRY PRODUCTS

Does raw milk rich in saturated fat and cholesterol contribute to heart disease? According to the lipid hypothesis it does. Consider one interesting example: The nomadic Masai of Kenya and Tanzania consume a diet of milk and meat with twice the fat and cholesterol content of Americans, yet were found to have low serum cholesterol levels and to be essentially free of heart disease, notes George V. Mann of Vanderbilt University. If fat is the cause of high cholesterol and heart disease, Mann explains, "then people who habitually consume large amounts of animal fat should have hypercholesteremia (high blood cholesterol), atherosclerosis, and coronary heart disease."

Mann and a number of researchers have recently called for the cholesterol hypothesis to be discarded. They are concerned that continued emphasis on saturated fat and cholesterol to the exclusion of other important risks may actually lead people toward more unhealthy food choices.[17]

Milk is a highly nutritious food packed with essential vitamins and minerals. After all, it was specifically designed to be a complete and nourishing food for humans and other

---

A cup of fruit juice would be approximately equivalent to 1 cup fruit or 1 gram protein. One apple would also be equivalent to about 1 cup fruit. A hamburger patty is about 3 ounces (21 grams). You can estimate meat portions using the chart below as a guide.

Food	Amount	Protein Content
Wheat bread	1 slice	3 (grams)
White bread	1 slice	2
Pasta (white)	1 cup cooked	7
Pasta (wheat)	1 cup cooked	8
Cornmeal	1 cup dry	10
Rice (brown)	1 cup cooked	5
Rice (white)	1 cup cooked	6
Rice (instant)	1 cup cooked	3
Dried beans	1 cup cooked	15
Tofu	1/2 cup	10
Meat (all types)[1]	1 oz	7
Egg	1 egg	6
Vegetables[2]	1/2 cup	2
Fresh fruit	1 cup/each	1
Potato (without skin)	1 potato or 1 cup	3
Potato (with skin)	1 potato or 1 cup	5
Milk[3]	1 cup	8
Yogurt (plain)	1 cup	12
Cheese	1 oz/slice	6
Nuts	1 oz	3
Fat	1 teaspoon	0
Sugar	1 tablespoon	0

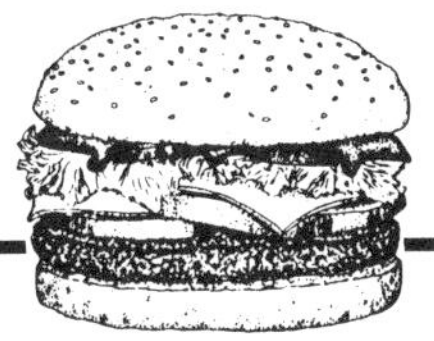

(1) Includes fish and fowl, lean or high fat. (2) Except potatoes. (3) Nonfat, low-fat, or whole.

Using this list you can determine the amount of protein in a typical fast food meal consisting of a cheeseburger, fries, and milkshake. One 3-ounce ground beef patty provides 21 grams of protein; one bun (two sides) has 4 grams of protein; condiments, including dressing, tomato, lettuce, pickle, etc. equal about 1 gram. A single 1-ounce slice of cheese adds 6 grams. The total amount of protein in just the cheeseburger comes to 32 grams. Combine that with a 16-ounce milkshake (16 grams) and fries (4 grams) and you have a grand total of 52 grams of protein, enough for the body for an entire day.

The serving sizes used here are average, not the large portions typically ordered. Two regular cheeseburgers, one large order of fries, and milkshake would provide 84 grams of protein, far in excess of dietary needs for most individuals, including large physically active people. It is very easy to get too much protein by eating fast foods.

Below are protein figures for some common fast foods:
Arby's regular roast beef sandwich 22g
Burger King Whopper 27g, Whopper w/cheese 31g
Long John Silver's fish and fries, 3 pce 43g
KFC chicken breast 1 piece 24g, thigh 18g
McDonald's Big Mac 25g
Taco Bell beef burrito 22g, bean burrito 13g, regular taco 10g

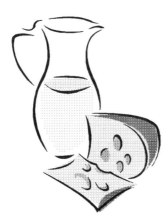

mammals. For thousands of years people have consumed dairy products and thrived, existing without degenerative disease as we see it now. But if you drink milk nowadays you're risking your life. This isn't because of the saturated fat or cholesterol content, but what we do to it.

The milk we drink nowadays is far different from the milk the African tribesmen drink or that even our grandparent and great grandparents drank. Modern milk isn't the natural food it once was, but is now a man-made version of the original. Milk contains contaminants just like meat, so it is full of antibiotics, hormones, and pesticides. If that wasn't bad enough, it is chemically altered into a substance unfit to drink.

When you go to the store you can buy whole milk, low fat (2%), skim (1%), or nonfat. How are these varieties produced? You don't get whole milk from a whole cow and nonfat from a lean one. There are no nonfat cows. All milk comes from the same source and is highly processed, involving heating, fractionalization, reconstitution, and homogenization. In the process, nutrients are lost and toxic byproducts produced.

All milk is heated or pasteurized to kill any bacteria that may have contaminated it. This is done by law to prevent illness and in the United States and some other countries you can't buy milk unless it's been pasteurized.

Fresh raw milk is full of fat which tends to float to the top. The milk at the top is richer and creamier than the milk at the bottom. You never see this in milk anymore because, for one reason, all milk is fractionalized and reconstituted to produce a product with a precise amount of fat. This involves removing all the fat from the milk. This fat can be used to make butter or cream. Some fat is added back to the watery fluid from which it came to make low-fat and a little less to make skim. In this way milk producers can create a variety of milks that are exactly alike.

According to the late Henry Schroeder, M.D., a prominent researcher at Dartmouth, when dairies "fractionalize" milk to remove fat, the skimmed or low-fat milk loses many essential nutrients. The only way to restore all the nutrients

is to reintroduce the original butter. Nutritionists unanimously recommend whole milk for weaned toddlers, because of the essential fatty acids, vitamins, and energy not contained in skim or low-fat milk. Whole milk is also better tolerated by those who are lactose intolerant.[18]

While fresh raw milk does *not* contribute to heart disease, modern pasteurized and homogenized milk may. When whole milk is dehydrated, its fat content becomes oxidized, including the cholesterol. Powdered whole milk containing oxidized cholesterol is added back to nonfat milk to make low-fat and skim milk.[19] When you drink low-fat and skim milk, you are consuming dangerous oxidized fat, and this isn't heart healthy. All varieties of milk have been homogenized and this too contributes to heart disease.

Homogenization

When you look at a container of milk, it proudly says its been "homogenized" as if this were something that is of benefit to the consumer. But what is homogenization and why is it done?

Milk is primarily water with various nutrients, proteins, and fats floating in it. If allowed to stand quietly for any length of time, the fat being lighter than other constituents of the milk would float to the top. To some people having the richest or creamiest part of the milk at the top is undesirable. So to make the texture of the milk uniform it is homogenized.

Homogenization was introduced in the United States in 1932. This process involves forcing the milk though tiny screens to break the fat down into minute particles. These fat particles are so small they remain suspended in the milk without floating to the top. The result is a product that has a uniform or homogenous texture. This may sound desirable but in the process an enzyme is affected that can have a significant influence on our health.

According to Dr. Kurt A. Oster, Chief of Cardiology at Bridgeport's Park City Hospital, homogenization releases an enzyme known as xanthine oxidase which is normally locked in the fat globule. When milk is *not* homogenized, both the fat and the xanthine oxidase are completely inactivated by our stomach acids and digestive enzymes and pose no threat. Dr. Oster and colleagues found that the homogenization process causes xanthine oxidase to become trapped within the tiny fat globules. This forms a protective layer of fat around the xanthine oxidase so it passes through the stomach and into the intestinal tract unharmed. Here it is readily absorbed through the intestinal wall and into the bloodstream where it acts as a free radical attacking the arterial wall, causing injury and contributing to the atherosclerotic process. Dr. Oster feels that this rogue enzyme is a principal player in initiating atherosclerosis and heart disease.

In 1973 Dr. Oster proposed his theory of atherosclerosis in the publication *Medical Counterpoint*. In contrast to the prevailing lipid hypothesis, his theory didn't set well with funding institutions, and may have been the reason why he used his own funds to finance much of his research.

In support of his theory, he notes that those countries that have the highest homogenized milk consumption also have the highest atherosclerosis death rate. He noted that Finland (at the time he conducted the study, 1967) had the highest death rate, 244.7 per 100,000, and consumed 534 pounds of homogenized milk per person.[20] Sweden, Finland's next door neighbor who shares similar genetic roots, consumes a total of 374 pounds of milk, but only 7 pounds per person is homogenized. Their death rate is only 75.9 per 100,000. They consumed lower amounts of homogenized milk and had a lower atherosclerosis death rate.

In the United States, the death rate at the time was 211.8 per 100,000, and consumed 259 pounds of homogenized milk per person. The Sweeds consumed 162 pounds more milk per person than those in the U.S., but had a death rate only one third as much. But their homogenized milk consumption was far lower that Finland or the U.S. Japan, which consumed only 2 pounds of homogenized milk per person, had a death rate of only 39 per 100,000.

Organic Milk

One of the problems of eating any animal product is the presence of contaminants such as residual antibiotics, hormones, and pesticides found in all meats, eggs, and dairy products which have been produced by conventional methods. These substances are toxic and some produce free radicals. Organic dairy products are much safer to use and the only ones I would recommend.

Raw, unpasteurized, unhomogenized milk is a healthy nutritious food, but is unavailable to most people. Just about the only way to get this kind of milk is to have your own cow. Even *organic* milk available at the store has been pasteurized and homogenized and, therefore, isn't fit to drink.

Only products that are made out of homogenized milk would contain biologically active xanthine oxidase which can pass intact through the intestinal wall into the bloodstream. Butter contains no biologically active xanthine oxidase. According to Dr. Oster, butter has no potential for triggering circulatory disease.[21] Organic butter and cultured dairy products such as yogurt, cheese, and cottage cheese are generally safe, to use as they are usually made from unhomogenized milk.

Milk is often recommended as one of the best sources of calcium. Because we lose calcium as we age, if we don't get enough of this mineral we might suffer from osteoporosis. So, if you don't drink milk, where can you get the calcium you need? You can get calcium from cheese and cultured dairy products. One pound of Swiss cheese, for example, contains the calcium equivalent of 3.5 quarts of milk. Other excellent sources of calcium are green leafy vegetables. Keep in mind that protein, especially animal protein, leaches calcium from our bones. So a low-meat diet will help you retain your calcium reserves.

OXIDIZED DAIRY AND MEAT PRODUCTS

Arteriosclerosis can develop without eating cholesterol, because it is caused primarily by injury from free radicals and other stresses, combined with an unbalanced diet which lacks protective nutrients. Any oxidized cholesterol (or oxidized polyunsaturated fat) in the body is attracted to arterial plaque like a magnet and contributes to the clogging of the arteries. Oxidized fat generates free radicals that can injure arterial walls.

Food processing can oxidize the cholesterol and unsaturated fat in animal products. There are a few foods that are extremely high in oxidized cholesterol and fat and, therefore, highly dangerous to health. They constitute some of the worst foods you could possibly eat in regards to cardiovascular health. If you want to die from a heart attack or stroke, the foods that will contribute the most toward this end are: deep fried foods; powdered eggs; powdered milk; dehydrated cheddar, blue, parmesan and romano cheese powders, as well as sour cream and butter powders; and freeze-dried and cured meats.[22] All of these foods contain variable but significant quantities of oxidized products capable of ripping free-radical holes through your cells, disintegrate DNA, and quickly age your skin, liver, kidneys, and brain. No organ is immune.

Out of this list, the most troublesome are deep fried foods. Heated oils are quickly oxidized and the more often they are heated and the higher the temperature, the worse they become. Deep fried foods cooked in vegetable oil are perhaps the worst foods on the planet to eat. Foods cooked this way constitute some of the most popular restaurant and snack foods we eat, such as French fries, onion rings, chicken and fish nuggets, donuts, potato chips, corn chips, egg rolls, fried wan ton, etc.

The cholesterol in fresh milk, eggs, and meat is *not* oxidized and is utilized in the body to strengthen cell membranes, synthesize vital hormones, and build brain and nerve tissue. The drying process in making powdered milk, cheese, and eggs fully oxidizes the cholesterol in these products. Once oxidized it cannot be utilized in the normal fashion to build and strengthen body tissues, but is packed away into the plaque of injured arteries. Eating such foods will surely clog your arteries faster than any other substance known on the face of the earth.

MEAT-BASED DIET

Some health experts say eating lots of protein is beneficial, while others warn us that eating too much can lead to serious health problems. Who are we to believe? Those who promote eating large amounts of protein claim that primitive man subsisted on a diet predominantly of protein, so genetically we are better suited to this type of diet. They also point out that in more recent times people such as the Eskimos lived and thrived on a meat-based diet. It was when they switch to a plant-based diet that the Eskimo began to develop the degenerative diseases of modern civilization. If eating too much meat is detrimental to good health, why didn't the Eskimos and other meat eaters suffer?

The answer is simple. The animal protein eaten nowadays is a far cry different from that which was eaten by our ancestors and by the Eskimo. Few of us would even consider eating the type of meat they ate. When we talk about a high-protein diet we think of eggs, dairy, and lean cuts of meat—the protein foods typically sold in grocery stores. Primitive societies ate very little of these foods. When an Eskimo killed a caribou he didn't eat just the muscle meat and throw away the rest like we would do, he ate everything that was possibly edible—the heart, brain, tongue, kidneys, intestines—everything! Nothing went to waste. The organ meats are rich in vitamins and minerals, much more so than muscle tissue. Furthermore, these meats were usually eaten raw or dried. Few of us would eat a raw steak, let alone raw entrails. Cooking destroys many nutrients making meat less nutritious. Modern food processing also introduces many chemical and biological toxins into our meats.

Primitive societies were able to live on meat-based diets because they ate all of the animal and, consequently, obtained all of the vitamins and minerals they needed to not only survive, but thrive without deficiency disease. The same is true with carnivorous animals. They don't eat just the muscle, but they eat all of their prey and usually prefer the vitamin-rich organ meats.

Simply put, muscle meats do not provide all of the vitamins and minerals necessary to maintain good health. Eating a lot of meat also reduces the intake of vitamin-rich fruits, vegetables, and gains. As a consequence, diets high in muscle meats can lead to nutrient deficiencies.

Cholesterol from fresh meat is harmless for the most part. Even when cooked intact, beef muscle contains little or no cholesterol oxides.[23] But when meat is cut, molded, cured, mixed with spices and preservatives and rendered into hot dogs, ham, bacon, pepperoni, bologna, and other luncheon meats, it has had ample opportunity for the cholesterol and other fats to oxidize. Things that cause more oxidation in fresh meat are cutting and grinding (more fat exposed to oxygen), overcooking (heat oxidizes fat), age (the longer the meat hangs around, the more oxidation occurs), and the addition of nitrates and nitrites (used in curing meats) intensifies free-radical potential.

Dried eggs and powdered milk contains high levels of oxidized cholesterol.[24] Powdered eggs are often used as a source of oxidized cholesterol in laboratory experiments to test its detrimental effects on animals.

You may be thinking to yourself, "I don't have to worry about these foods I don't drink powdered milk and I never eat powdered eggs. Who eats powdered eggs anyway?" Chances are you do. If you eat packaged convenience foods, you eat them all the time. Look at the ingredient labels of the foods in the stores and you will be surprised how many items have powdered milk, cheese, or eggs. They don't always say "powdered" or "dehydrated," but it is obvious that a cake mix, for example, that lists eggs in the ingredients uses powdered eggs. They can't very well put fresh eggs into the mix can they?

Powdered eggs and milk are widely used in boxed cake, pancake, and muffin mixes, and by commercial bakeries to make all types of baked goods. The breads you buy at the store are often made with them. Boxed meals that contain cheese, such as macaroni and cheese, use dried cheese that comes in little packets. You would be surprised at how many packaged foods contain these powdered items. Even many frozen foods use them because it is more convenient and economical for the manufacturer to store and use dried dairy products than fresh. Food producers don't always tell you the dairy products they use are dried or powdered. But if you see eggs, milk, or cheese listed on a boxed item stored on a shelf, you know they are powdered because these items when fresh are highly perishable.

If that isn't enough, you can buy these items in powdered form yourself to add even more free radicals to your foods in the form of instant milk, grated romano and parmesan cheese, and powdered eggs.

Restaurants use lots of powdered dairy products. One particularly dangerous item found in most fast food outlets as well as many other types of restaurants is soft-serve ice cream. This is the soft ice cream you get out of self-serve machines or that fast food chains use for ice cream cones and milk shakes. This stuff is made from powdered milk and sugar. It's not fresh ice cream and often has hydrogenated vegetable oil added to it. So you get both oxidized cholesterol and hydrogenated oil at the same time—two of the worst oils you can put in your mouth! A single soft-serve ice cream cone probably has more artery-clogging oxidized cholesterol in it than 100 pounds of cooked beefsteak. If you eat soft ice cream, you're begging for a heart attack. If you want to eat ice cream, stick to the real thing.

DEGENERATIVE DISEASE: THE RESULT OF BOTH EXCESS AND DEFICIENCY

The combination of too much meat and dairy, the overprocessing of foods with the addition of harmful additives, and the lack of fresh fruits and vegetables and whole grains has led us down the path of subclinical malnutrition and into the realm of degenerative disease.

The major factor affecting the poor state of health in industrialized countries is our reliance on refined and overly processed foods. Nutrients are lost and contaminants (including chemical additives and vegetable oils) are added. Our bodies use up vitamins and minerals at an accelerated rate in order to process and eliminate these contaminants. Nutrient-poor foods such as white flour products and sugar require more nutrients to metabolize than what they supply, depleting nutrient stores even more. Whenever nutrient-poor foods are eaten, fewer nutrient-rich foods are eaten.

The reliance on processed nutrient-deficient plant foods has created a situation where excess protein, especially animal protein, becomes harmful. Without the necessary vitamins and minerals needed to properly process and metabolize protein, the body spirals toward greater deficiency. Protein pulls alkalizing minerals out of our bodies. As these minerals are removed the body slowly becomes more acidic. This acidic environment encourages free-radical generation which, in turn, depletes antioxidant reserves which can create a deficiency in antioxidant vitamins and minerals. The result of is chronic or intermittent nutrient deficiency and degeneration. Most all the degenerative disease that plagues mankind today can be traced to nutrient deficiencies.

Heart disease caused by a vitamin deficiency, is it possible? In North America, Western Europe, and other industrialized areas of the world where food is plentiful, it is hard for many to imagine a disease as widespread as atherosclerosis to be attributed to a vitamin deficiency. The simple fact of the matter is: our foods are killing us!

The idea that vitamin/nutrient deficiencies could be responsible for or participate in the cause of the most common diseases in industrialized countries has not, until recently, been taken seriously by the medical community. The homocysteine theory combined with our knowledge of the effects of free radicals on human tissue has provided a comprehensive explanation for the generation of atherosclerosis, heart disease, cancer, and numerous other degenerative diseases that have plagued the modern world for the past century.

Researchers have long noted that eating fresh fruits and vegetables provides protection against many of the degenerative diseases common in modern industrialized societies. We now understand why eating nutrient-deficient processed foods high in empty calories, such as sugar and fat, and low in fresh fruits, vegetables and whole grains can lead to disease.

Foods that will protect us from atherosclerosis, cancer, and other degenerative diseases are readily available, but not enough of us eat them, and children are the worst offenders. The food industry relentlessly promotes products which are profitable to them but deleterious to our children. If we engage in nutritional abuse, we will pay the price as we get older.

As we age we need to pay even more attention to our diet. What we were able to eat in our youth may kill us later in life. The reason for this is that our organs and tissues become less efficient. Years of free-radical abuse and the simple processes of aging take their toll. Homocysteine levels rise as enzyme production slows down. Nutrient reserves become depleted more quickly.

A classic study by Hultberg from Sweden measured vitamin B-6 and folic acid in fetuses, infants, young children, teenagers, and adults. It showed a very dramatic decline in these vitamins with aging.[25] Most older adults do not get enough vitamins and minerals. If you start now you can protect yourself against the degenerative consequences of nutrient deficiencies. In the next chapter I outline a program designed to reduce your exposure, protect you from destructive food and food components, and provide you with the nutrients you need to live a full, vibrant life.

Chapter 14

HOW TO STOP PREMATURE AGING AND DEGENERATIVE DISEASE

"The natural force within each one of us is the greatest healer of disease."
—Hippocrates

"All would live long, but none would be old."
—Benjamin Franklin, *Poor Richard* (1749)

"The object of preventive medicine is to enable people to die young as old as possible."
—Ernst L. Wynder, M.D.

We are currently in a sorry plight. There are 155,000 new cases of colon and rectal cancer each year, and more than 60,000 of their victims die annually. Breast cancer has increased 24 percent in six years, and one out of every eight women alive today will develop breast cancer. One out of every nine men will develop prostate cancer. Approximately 30,000 American men die of prostate cancer each year. Pancreatic cancer is the fifth leading cause of cancer death, claiming 25,000 Americans each year. Lung cancer has increased from about 10 deaths per 100,000 people in 1939 to nearly 110 per 100,000 today. This has happened even though per capita fewer people smoke. Despite an effort to reduce fat consumption, heart disease is still our number one killer. The disease and death rates in Canada, Great Britain, and other Western countries are similar. Wherever people eat a diet composed primarily of refined processed foods, degenerative disease is rampant.

My goal in life is to die healthy. This is a goal we can all strive for. My grandfather did it. He died peacefully at the age of 94. Although he wasn't as mentally sharp and didn't have the strength and vigor that he had in his youth, he did not suffer with any crippling or painful degenerative disease either. He remained physically active and continued to work full-time until the day he died. He liked to keep busy and be mentally active. This is the way it should be, the way it can be if we take care of ourselves and eat the right types of foods. In this chapter I outline a program designed to help you live healthy all your life without the pain and suffering that has become so common among the aged in our society.

THE EXPERIMENT THAT CHANGED MY LIFE

To never be sick again—that's my goal. I plan on living a long healthy life, free from most of the chronic pain and degenerative disease that so commonly afflicts most people at some point in their lives. My grandfather lived into his nineties without experiencing degenerative disease. My parents weren't so lucky. Both died much younger after suffering years with diabetes, heart disease, Alzheimer's, gallbladder disease, and other degenerative conditions. I don't plan to follow in my parents' footsteps.

Chronic illness and degenerative disease are most prevalent among those with weak or overworked immune systems. Many scientists believe that the key to a long, healthy life is determined by our immune system. In other words, if your immune system remains young and vital, the odds of living longer and healthier are greatly enhanced. One clue to the level of health of our immune system and, consequently, our future health, is how often we become sick with colds and flu. The more often we come down with seasonal illnesses, the less efficient our immune system.

Several years ago I tried a little experiment. In my 20s I considered myself relatively healthy. I rarely missed a day from work due to illness, although I would go to the office when I wasn't feeling in the best of health. If the illness wasn't too severe, I usually headed off to work. Don't you do the same?

If someone asked me how often I was sick each year, I would think back to how many days I missed work. It seemed like only two or three. Somehow, I lost track of all the many days I went to work knowing I was battling some infection. So I decided to run an experiment.

I kept a detailed record of every illness I had, whether or not I went to work. If I knew I was fighting an infection, I recorded the symptoms, when they started, and when they subsided. At the end of the year I was shocked. It had been a normal year for me healthwise, but I recorded 74 days of illness of one sort or another. This was not simply aches and pains from everyday life or stress, but definite sickness. I continued this record for six years!

In that time I found that I was sick, on average, for 54.5 days each year!* This was surprising because I was still young and considered myself far healthier than most people. I ate a so-called "balanced" diet that included plenty of fruits and vegetables, exercised faithfully an average of four days a week, did not eat many sweets or junk foods. So why was I sick so often?

I had always believed in natural health and tried to live healthfully. But I found out that what most people consider a healthy diet is not necessarily one that will prevent illness or stop degenerative disease from developing later in life. My father was an M.D., yet he died from the effects of atherosclerosis and Alzheimer's. His knowledge about health and medicine didn't save him.

Over the years I've found that free radicals and not saturated fat or cholesterol are our worst enemies. These two fats in themselves aren't that bad. The real culprit is our modern processed and refined foods and the additives in them, particularly vegetable oils. All polyunsaturated oils, including the so called "healthy" ones like flaxseed oil, de-

press the immune system and, therefore, greatly contribute to premature aging and the development of disease.

I've changed my diet from the one I thought was healthy years ago. The only fats I eat now are saturated and monounsaturated fat and cholesterol (i.e., coconut oil, butter, animal fat, and olive oil). I eat only whole natural foods and avoid nutrient-deficient packaged products. As a result, since I've been on this new program, I've had no sick days...zero...no colds, no flus, no stomach aches, no sore throats, no fevers, nothing! I haven't been sick for even a single day in years and I've been around some very sick and contagious people.

I've even reversed the effects of failing eyesight and glaucoma—a degenerative disease that has no medical cure—and I'm totally free from all other chronic degenerative disease. I'm now in my late 40s and enjoy better health now than at any time in my life. I fully expect to live a long healthy life without suffering with the pain and financial burden brought on by degenerative disease.

Aging does not cause disease. This was proven to me by my grandfather who lived for nearly a century and suffered none of the degenerative conditions so common today. I'm not the only one who has experienced improved health. The following sections provide a few additional examples.

THE BEAST

The following true story is an account of one person's own discovery about the health consequences of dietary oils.

"I've been troubled with a severe case of psoriasis for over twenty years. It covered my face from my eyebrows to my chin with inflamed, red, flaky, itchy skin. At times it would become so bad it oozed fluids and even bled. I also had a horrible case of dandruff that had plagued me at least since I was in high school. My dandruff was so bad skin would seem to come off in sheets rather than just tiny flakes. I looked like I had just come in from a snowstorm. Fortunately, strong medicated shampoo kept my dandruff problem pretty much under control. Only when I used nonmedicated shampoos did the dandruff return. And when it did, it came with a vengeance within a few days.

"I first noticed the problem with my skin in my early 20s. Patches on my face would become inflamed, dry, and itchy, and peal off. At first it wasn't too serious; it would flair up for two or three days and disappear. Was it something I was eating? The thought did not cross my mind.

"As each year passed, the psoriasis came more frequently and persisted longer. It spread to my chest, creating small flaky patches over my body. By the time I reached

*Studies by The Centers for Disease Control and Prevention have shown that the average number of sick days each person experiences per year is about 65. This includes major illness as well as minor sniffles, upset stomachs, etc. which we all ignore and quickly forget about. If you kept a detailed diary you would be surprised how often you feel "under the weather."

my mid 30s, it had gotten so bad that the skin on my face was inflamed virtually all the time, and dry itchy skin continually flaked off. Cracks would form that penetrated deep into my skin, causing it to ooze and bleed. People who saw me at first thought I had a severe sunburn. Splotches appeared on other parts of my body, particularly my chest. I got to the point where I was embarrassed to be seen in public.

"I had gone to doctors and dermatologists to see what could be done, but they didn't regard it as anything serious and gave me medicated creams and told me it was just a type of dandruff. But dandruff shampoo did not help my psoriasis and the prescription creams they recommended were expensive and of little use. I continued to suffer.

"As I was approaching 40, I began to become more conscious of diet and health. I had suspected that the skin problem was an allergic reaction of some sort and kept detailed records of all the foods I ate to discover which ones might be causing this reaction. I did this for months, but there was no correlation that I could detect. The doctors I saw made no indication that diet would have any affect on my condition.

"I began to eat more healthfully. For a couple of years I was nearly a pure vegetarian, eating almost no meat, dairy or eggs. I removed all hydrogenated oils, including margarine and shortening from my diet. The only oils I used were the 'healthy' ones—olive and canola oils. During this time my psoriasis improved by about 50 percent! I now had days when the inflammation was gone and my skin was free of flakes. But some dryness always lingered and some days were better than others. Although it wasn't cracking and bleeding as it was before, my face still became very itchy and flaky at times.

"I eventually stopped using medicated shampoo. My dandruff came back, but not nearly as severe as it had in the past. On my new healthy diet my skin had made significant improvement, but it still was not normal.

"Then I learned about the health benefits of coconut oil and about the health-destroying effects of polyunsaturated oils. I was using canola and olive oils in all of my cooking. Although both of these are high in unsaturated fatty acids, they were not as bad as other vegetable oils. I stopped using them completely. Instead I used coconut oil and organic butter. Since many of the packaged foods I buy, even at health foods stores, are made using vegetable oils, I began taking vitamin E and other antioxidants every day.

"It was then that a miracle happened. The psoriases on my face and chest gradually began to clear up. It didn't happen overnight. It took several weeks. The skin on my face became smooth and soft, inflammation was gone, dryness was gone, flakiness gone. The dandruff problem I'd had

since I was a teenager cleared up too. I felt that the ugly beast that had attacked my health and destroyed my skin was now gone. What was this beast? I believe it was vegetable oils—including canola. It wasn't until I eliminated them all from my diet and began using coconut oil and organic butter that my skin problems were finally healed. I still have some redness on occasion, but I would say I've improved by 90 percent."

WHERE'S THE PROOF?

I've told you about the good oils and bad, about antioxidants, and subclinical malnutrition and how they all tie together to contribute to the decaying health of our society. Although I've used many references to scientific studies, historical facts, and simple logic, some people will still be unconvinced. One of the problems is that the ideas I express in this book are new to most people and are contrary to what you see and hear every day. If you are told a lie often enough and long enough you will begin to believe it. That is what has happened to us. Most people still believe the cholesterol theory of heart disease even though it has been soundly disproved.

If what I have stated in this book is true, you might expect that there would be some people who have gained benefit from changing their diets. Although anecdotal evidence is not absolute proof, it does help to validate the facts that have been presented. Here are a few things others have said:

"I'm sold on this program. I've had pain in my knees from arthritis for several years. I could only walk short distances and climbing stairs was nearly impossible. After taking the recommended amount of antioxidants and watching my diet, the pain was gone within three weeks. I can go up and down stairs with relative ease now."

"I've been bothered with chronic fatigue for several years. I love to play golf, but it tires me so much that by the time I finish nine holes I'm ready to call it quits. I could hardly continue. I was getting to the point where I wasn't even bothering to play any more. After going on this program, I began feeling so good I went out and played a full 18 holes and felt great afterwards. I had just as much energy after the 18th hole as I did when I started."

"I used to come down with the flu and get colds at least five or six times a year. I worked for a fast food restaurant and ate burgers, fries, and soda all the time. After changing jobs and changing my diet, avoiding fried foods and all vegetable oils, eating more fruits and vegetables and supplementing my diet with antioxidants, I stopped getting sick. I was amazed how a simple dietary change affected my health. An acne problem that had plagued me since high school also cleared up. I was amazed! I used to wash my face daily with antibiotic soaps and use acne creams with only limited results. It's made such a big difference in how I look and how I feel that I'm staying on this program for the rest of my life."

"For the past two years I'd been experiencing increasing arthritic-like pain in the joints of the fingers in my left hand. I had either broken or sprained these fingers in my youth several times, and now at the age of 46 they were beginning to give me problems. At times the pain would be so bad I couldn't use them at all.

"Like most men my age, I also was experiencing symptoms of prostate enlargement which had me getting up two and three times or more a night to relieve myself. I figured these symptoms were all part of the aging process that we all pass through as we get older.

"When I heard about this health plan and how it has helped others with prostate problems, I was anxious to try it out. After only a few weeks on the program, I was sleeping through the night. This is something I hadn't done in years. Since I started the program mainly because of my prostate problem, I didn't pay much attention to other symptoms. About a month passed when I realized that I didn't have any pain in my left hand. I also noticed an increase in my energy level. I used to be exhausted by 8:00 p.m., but now I stay up to 10:30 p.m. and sometimes later without feeling the least bit sleepy, yet when I go to bed I sleep soundly and without having to get up every few hours. I feel great!"

"I hated to wear skirts or shorts because of varicose veins in my legs. They looked ugly and it was embarrassing. This bothered me because at 36 I felt I was still relatively young. When I discovered lumps in my breasts, I really began to think seriously about my health. I dreaded the thought of subjecting myself to medical treatment and especially wanted to avoid a mastectomy. My sister introduced me to this health program and said it had helped others with cancer. After three months, the lumps in my breast were totally gone. Not only that, but the varicose veins in my legs were almost unnoticeable. I can now wear shorts again without feeling self-conscious. It's made me feel like a new woman."

"I didn't get into this program as a means to lose weight, but I did. I'd tried dieting before without success

and came to the realization that I would never lose my excess baggage. I didn't like dieting and I didn't have the will power to stick to those weight-loss programs. So I was surprised that after six months on this program I'd lost 20 pounds. And I've kept them off for over two years now. What's unbelievable to me is that I eat just as much now as I did before, and I eat more saturated fat that I ever did. This diet has truly been a blessing for me."

"I was excited, yet somewhat skeptical when I learned that this program was good at relieving allergy symptoms. I'd suffered for years with allergies, and nothing I'd tried in the past seemed to work. To be honest, I didn't expect this to work either. But I figured I didn't have anything to lose and just maybe, it could help. At that point I'd have been grateful to find anything that could bring some relief. I began the program in the fall when my allergy symptoms weren't much of a problem. When spring came I was amazed. While those around me were suffering from allergy symptoms, the same ones I used to fight with, I was doing fine. I had some minor sniffles at times but the overall improvement was astounding."

THE ANTIOXIDANT HEALTH PLAN

The center of this program is the diet. Whenever we hear the word "diet," most of us shudder, conjuring up visions of calorie restriction, lettuce salads, hunger, and discomfort. For most of us, dieting is misery. This program is different. There is no calorie counting. You can eat as much as you like. And you are allowed to eat butter, meat, and fat, including saturated fat. In fact, saturated fat is the preferred fat in this plan. It can almost be called the undiet diet.

On this program you will lose unwanted weight and gain better health. This sounds unreal because all our lives we have been told to reduce our fat intake. Saturated fat and cholesterol have been unjustly pegged as our most villainous foods, and they are the ones people eliminate first. Many people have lost weight on a variety of low-fat, calorie-restricted diets. But how many of these people have kept the weight off permanently? Very, very few. Surveys show that somewhere around 90 percent of the people who go on weight-loss diets, regain the weight after a couple of years. Many of them gain back more than they lost. Such diets do more harm than good.

Unlike most other diets, this program is meant to bring about a permanent change in eating habits along with a change for the better in body weight and overall health. This is a program that is meant to be followed for life. I prefer not to call it a diet, but rather an eating plan or health plan.

It isn't a diet to lose weight or to overcome any particular illness, but is a health-enhancing plan that can do these things as your body becomes stronger and healthier. Because the basic concept behind this eating plan is to counter cellular destruction and premature aging caused by free radicals, I call it the Antioxidant Health Plan.

Most diets don't work for long because people get tired of feeling hungry and deprived. In this plan, instead of limiting the amount of food you eat and counting calories, you just watch the type of food you eat and eat as much as you like. Another difference between this eating plan and most other diets is in the type of fat you can eat. In this plan you can eat saturated fat in the form of butter, coconut oil, and animal fat or lard. And believe it or not, you will lose weight and you will feel better. In many cases you will be able to break free from the chains of pain and premature degeneration. You can reverse the direction your health is headed now and lift yourself to higher levels of mental and physical well-being.

The Antioxidant Health Plan is broken down into three sections: (1) dietary oils, (2) wholesome foods, and (3) dietary supplements. Each of these is described below.

Dietary Oils

The most unique feature about this health plan is the type of fat used. The oils permitted include coconut oil, organic butter, and organic animal fat (lard and beef tallow). A limited amount of extra virgin olive oil is also permitted.

Use of any of the polyunsaturated vegetable oils is completely discouraged. This includes safflower, sunflower, cottonseed, soybean, peanut, corn, canola (rapeseed), walnut, almond, sesame, and all other vegetable oils. It doesn't matter if these oils are heat processed or cold pressed. Virgin and light olive oils are also in the "do not use" category. Flaxseed, evening primrose, borage, cod liver, and other oils used as dietary supplements are also discouraged.

All oils contain many more calories than other foods, so it is still a good idea to refrain from eating too much oil of any type.

Coconut Oil

The title of this book, *Saturated Fat May Save Your Life*, comes from the concept that by replacing the vegetable oils that you now eat with saturated fat, primarily from coconut oil, you can bring about a dramatic change in your health.

Among all the dietary oils in the world, coconut oil is a most precious gem. It is composed predominantely of saturated fatty acids and, therefore, is highly resistant to oxidation and free-radical formation. Because it is not susceptible to oxidation like monounsaturated and polyunsaturated fats, it does not cause free-radical damage that contributes to cancer and other degenerative conditions.

Coconut oil is heart healthy. Most of the saturated fatty acids in coconut oil are of the medium-chain variety. Unlike the more common long-chain fatty acids found in most meats and plants, these fatty acids are not absorbed directly into the bloodstream and, therefore, do not directly raise blood fat levels or contribute to cardiovascular disease. The medium-chain fatty acids in coconut oil are absorbed straight into the portal vein and sent directly to the liver. In the liver they are metabolized like carbohydrates, yielding energy and, as an added benefit, they *stimulate metabolism*. Because the medium-chain fatty acids in coconut oil increase the body's metabolism, more calories are consumed, thus reducing the number of calories that could be packaged in the body as fat. Coconut oil yields slightly fewer calories than other fats. Also because it has a stimulatory effect on the body's metabolic rate, more total calories are burned up. The over-all effect is like eating a fat that has fewer calories than any other dietary fat on the planet. It can be called a low-fat fat if there ever could be such a creature. If you want to add fat to your diet and still lose weight, coconut oil is your best choice.

In this health plan, you replace all cooking oils with coconut oil. Coconut oil has a very mild, almost undetectable, flavor so it can be used to cook any type of food. Because it is primarily a saturated fat, the heat of cooking does not create a free-radical soup like it does with polyunsaturated vegetable oils. You can feel safe when you eat it knowing that you aren't damaging your health. Coconut oil, however, has a low smoking point when used on the stove, so you need to keep the temperature down to about 325° F (160° C). If you don't have a temperature gauge on your stove, you can tell when it goes over this point because the oil will begin to smoke. This is a moderate cooking temperature, but you can cook anything at this heat, even stir fry vegetables. When used to grease pans or in baked goods, coconut oil can be cooked in the oven at higher temperatures. All your cooking that requires oil should be done with coconut oil. Although stable under moderate temperatures, coconut oil should not be used for deep frying. The high temperatures used in deep frying are destructive to any oil.

Coconut oil melts at 78° F (26° C) becoming a clear liquid that looks like most any other vegetable oil. Below this temperature, it solidifies and takes on a creamy white appearance. At moderate room temperatures it has a soft buttery texture and is sometimes called coconut butter. Because it has a buttery consistency at normal room temperature, it isn't used much as a salad dressing.

Coconut oil can be spread on bread as a healthier replacement for butter or margarine. But there isn't much flavor to it. If you like the taste of real butter, you can make a more flavorful spread using half butter and half coconut oil whipped together.

Use coconut oil in place of other oils in recipes that call for butter, shortening, margarine, or vegetable oil. Try it in cookies, cakes, muffins, pie crusts, and pancake batter. Use a melted coconut-butter mixture with seasonings over rice, pasta, or vegetables instead of butter or cream sauce.

Not all coconut oils are the same. Check the label to make sure it's pure unrefined coconut oil, without additives. Coconut oil is commonly sold as a body cream. Do not use this type in your food! It is not food quality and is often hydrogenated. You don't want to eat any oil that has been hydrogenated. Because this type of coconut oil is not sold to be eaten, but used on the skin, it may not state that it is hydrogenated and it may not state that it is a body cream. It may only say "Coconut Oil." The way to tell is when the temperature is above 78° F (26° C), it will be liquid. If it is

not completely liquid above this temperature, it's been hydrogenated—don't use it. I've had oil like this in our bathroom on hot summer days with the temperature in the 90s and only about a third of the oil turned into liquid. Unadulterated coconut oil would be totally liquid after a couple hours in temperatures above 80° F (27° C).

Because of the negative campaign launched by the soybean industry, coconut oil has been replaced by vegetable oils in restaurants and stores. At the present, it is still difficult to find in some areas. The best places to look for it is in health food stores. If you can't find any in your area, write to HealthWise Publications, P.O. Box 25203, Colorado Springs, CO 80936 for information for obtaining organic coconut oil.

Animal Fats

Animal fats can be divided into two categories: (1) fats from animal tissue like lard or tallow and (2) milk fat. Butter made from milk fat is the healthier of the two. Both are predominately saturated fat and, therefore, not vulnerable to free-radical formation like vegetable oils. Butter has a significant amount of short- and medium-chain saturated fatty acids (the good guys) like coconut oil. For this reason, I consider it the second best oil to use. It can be used for any cooking purpose, but like coconut oil, it has a low smoking point and should not be heated above 325° F (160° C).

Both butter and tissue fat are better for your health than vegetable oils. If you have a choice between a food cooked in corn oil or lard, your best choice would be the one cooked in lard. All animal fats are better than polyunsaturated vegetable oils.

I prefer eating only organically raised or free-range meat and dairy products. Organic meat and dairy products, including butter, are available at most health food stores. Many supermarkets are now beginning to stock these items as well. If your local store doesn't have these items in stock, ask them to start carrying some. As awareness of the contamination in animal products grows, demand for "clean" food will increase.

I don't recommend milk even if it is from organically raised cows because most milk is homogenized. Homogenization breaks the fat molecules into microscopically tiny particles that can increase free-radical reactions in the body. Dairy products that are not homogenized, such as yogurt and cheese, are better as long as they are organic.

Olive Oil

Olive oil is predominately a monounsaturated fat. Monounsaturated fats are not as susceptible to free-radical formation as polyunsaturated fats, but are more susceptible than saturated fats.

BODY MASS INDEX

Body weight influences our health. As weight increases, risk of developing numerous diseases increase and life expectancy decreases. Health risks associated with weight can be determined using a measurement known as the body mass index (BMI). The higher the BMI the greater the health risks. BMI is based on your weight and height. In kilograms and meters the formula is: BMI = weight (kg)/height^2 (m)

To determine your BMI using pounds and inches first, multiply your weight in pounds by .45 to get kilograms. Next, convert your height to inches. Multiply this number by .0254 to get meters. Multiply that number by itself. Then divide this into your weight in kilograms.

$$BMI = \frac{weight\ (lb) \times .45}{[height\ (inches) \times .0254]^2}$$

Your answer will probably be a number in the 20s or 30s. It is your BMI. A man with an BMI greater than 27.7 or a woman greater than 27.2 is considered too fat. Ideal weight is 20.7 to 24, for men and 19.1 to 23.5 for women.

	Men	Women
Underweight	< 20.7	<19.1
Acceptable weight	20.7 to 27.7	19.1 to 27.2
Overweight	>27.7	>27.2
Severe overweight	>31.0	>32.2
Morbid obesity	>45.3	>44.7

Extra virgin olive oil is the preferred type to use. The more processing it has undergone, the greater degree of free-radical damage it has encountered and the more contaminantes it may contain. Extra virgin, being simply pressed from the olives without heat or chemical additives, is relatively safe. Other types of olive oil have been subjected to solvents and heat-damaging processes.

Olive oil is safe to use in moderation. Do not use it for cooking because it will oxidize. It is best used raw in salad dressing or as a flavoring.

Polyunsaturated Vegetable Oil

The use of polyunsaturated vegetable oils is one of the greatest tragedies of our modern food industry. The increasing use of vegetable oils over the past several decades parallels the rising incidence of numerous degenerative diseases. Pointing the blame of many of these diseases at saturated fat and cholesterol has thrown us off the track and given the vegetable oil a cloak of protection to hide behind.

One of the basic premises of this book is that free radicals are a major cause or at least a contributing factor in most all types of disease, particularly those of a degenerative nature. Highly processed, fractionated foods are lacking in essential nutrients (including important antioxidants). These foods are often contaminated with chemical additives that expose us to an elevated number of free radicals. We have limited control over the air we breath, but we have a great deal of control over the food we eat. One of the most destructive components added to our food is vegetable oil. One of the basic steps in this diet is to eliminate *all* polyunsaturated vegetable oils from the diet. It doesn't matter if they are heat processed or cold pressed, they still cause free radicals. Even after you've eaten them and they are circulating around in your blood, they can churn out destructive free-radical terrorists by the millions.

Polyunsaturated oils are known to inhibit the immune system. They do it so well that they are purposely given to patients who have received organ or tissue transplants taken from other people. The patient's immune system must be compromised or it will reject the foreign tissue. If the immune system is damaged or depressed, it can not function optimally and foreign substances such as transplanted organs, as well as cancer and viruses, are able to survive. Remember, the health of your immune system is a measure of your ability to ward off disease and remain healthy. When you eat polyunsaturated oils you are just shortening your life by providing a doorway for disease.

Hydrogenation of vegetable oils creates a toxic molecule known as a trans fatty acid. You should never eat anything that is made with hydrogenated or partially hydrogenated vegetable oil. The most common hydrogenated oils are margarine and shortening. These oils are used in almost all packed and frozen prepared foods. Read the ingredient labels of every packaged food you buy. If it contains these oils, put it back. Your health is more important.

Essential Fatty Acids

Contrary to popular belief, essential fatty acids could be detrimental to your health—especially if taken in supplemental form—because it is easy to overdo it. A little may be good in certain circumstances, but it is far too easy to get too much.

Most of us will do just fine without supplementing our diet with the essential fatty acids. Adding supplements is in-

Homemade Mayonnaise

Mayonnaise is a favorite ingredient for a variety of foods. However, one of the major ingredients in commercially prepared mayonnaise is vegetable oil. Here is a recipe that you can use made with either olive or coconut oil. If you use olive oil choose one with a delicate taste and aroma, as a strongly flavored oil can be overpowering.

This recipe makes 1/2 pint (300 ml). Reduce the ingredients for smaller quantities. *Use all ingredients at room temperature.*

2 egg yolks
Salt
1/2 teaspoon dry mustard
1 tablespoon white wine vinegar or lemon juice
1/2 pint (300 ml) extra virgin olive oil or liquid coconut oil.
Ground black pepper
1 tablespoon boiling water (optional)

Put the egg yolks into a large mixing bowl and whisk for about two minutes. This should produce a smooth paste. Add in a pinch or two of salt, mustard, and a tablespoon of wine vinegar or lemon juice. Beat for another minute. Keep beating while you add the oil, drop by drop, until half has been absorbed. Add the remainder a tablespoonful at a time, beating it in each time. If the mayonnaise is too thick at this stage you may add more vinegar or lemon juice and beat it in. Add pepper and additional salt to taste.

If the mayonnaise is not going to be used immediately, beat in a tablespoon of boiling water to stop it from curdling. Cover and store in the refrigerator. It should last about a week.

viting toxicity and rancidity reactions. After all, linoleic (omega-6) and alpha-linolenic (omega-3) acids are polyunsaturated oils and are, therefore, very vulnerable to oxidation and free-radical formation just as other unsaturated oils are. Just because the liquid oil is in an air tight jar or even sealed in gel caps, doesn't mean they're free from free-radical damage. And once they are eaten, they can still become oxidized and still initiate destructive free-radical chain reactions. Flaxseed oil (omega-3), sold as a liquid in bottles, is particularly dangerous even if stored in the refrigerator. People often let the oil sit for weeks, even months, before finishing it. This is far too long. By then all they are doing is consuming a free-radical cocktail.

The best way to get your omega-3 and omega-6 fatty acids is in foods, as nature intended. We can and should get our essential fatty acids from our foods and not rely on supplements. The best natural sources for omega-3 fatty acids are from fish, seaweed, and green leafy vegetables (i.e., beet greens, mustard greens, kale, spinach, chard, bok choy, collards, etc.). Almost all foods contain omega-6 fatty acids and a true deficiency is nearly impossible.

Researchers state that as little as one or two fish meals a week can provide significant protection from heart disease. You might extend this to saying also that a few meals a week of green leafy vegetables would also provide a similar degree of protection. This is especially true if you eliminate refined vegetable oils from your diet.

Coconut oil contains only 2 percent of the essential fatty acids which can still contribute to our body's need for this oil without overdoing it. Coconut oil also contains 15 percent caprylic and capric acids and, according to Kaunitz,[1] the presence of these two MCFA diminishes the need of EFAs in human nutrition.

Naturally occurring omega-3 fatty acids, that are eaten in fish or vegetables, are always protected from free-radical damage by vitamin E and other antioxidants. Supplements often have vitamin E added to retard spoilage, but they are never completely free from oxidative damage. You never know how old the supplements are or what conditions they have been subjected to. They are just not safe to take. Getting your omega-3 from foods greatly reduces your chance of free-radical damage.

Fresh flaxseed oil has a mild nutty aroma and flavor. Flaxseed oil spoils very quickly when exposed to light, oxygen, and heat. Many health food store brands are highly refined and often completely spoiled before they are even purchased. You can tell when flaxseed oil is going rancid by its bitter, musty flavor, kind of like turpentine or paint thinner. If it has gone this far, don't eat it!

Omega-6 fatty acids found in most vegetable oils compete with alpha-linolenic acid (omega-3) for the enzymes required for its metabolic conversion to EPA and PGE3.[2] If you consume omega-6 fatty acids as supplements (evening primrose oil, borage oil, black currant oil, etc.) or eat a lot of vegetable oils, less alpha-linolenic acid is converted into PGE3. You can actually cancel the beneficial effects that you were trying to get from both by taking them together. How many people take both at the same time? You are wasting your money. For the life of me I can't understand why someone would want to take a toxic free-radical-producing supplement anyway.

The foods in our diet—the meat, produce, seeds, and grains—provide us with *all* the omega-3 and omega-6 fatty acids we need. We don't need vegetable oils and in most cases we don't need dietary oil supplements. The human race has survived for thousands of years without resorting to flaxseed supplements. Fatty acid deficiencies are a modern phenomena that have risen as we have consumed more refined vegetable oils. The healthiest peoples throughout the world live on traditional diets which supply them with all the essential fatty acids they need. We can do the same. Primitive man did not need to add flaxseed oil to his diet to be healthy, nor do the villagers of Africa or Polynesia, so why should you?

The positive side of omega-3 supplementation is that it can be used to counterbalance the heart disease promoting effects caused by omega-6 and PGE2. But the downside is that both omega-6 and omega-3 generate free radicals that promote cancer, autoimmune and inflammatory illnesses, and other degenerative conditions.

Using omega-3 oils, such as that found in flaxseed oil, is a temporary quick fix that eliminates the symptoms, but does not cure the problem. The problem is overconsumption of omega-6 fatty acids from vegetable oils. The solution is simple—stop eating vegetable oils. If you do this, you wouldn't need omega-3 supplements and you would be saved from the free-radical destruction both omega-3 and omega-6 oils cause.

Wholesome Foods

Foods provide our bodies with all the nutrients we need for growth and development and to maintain health. The quality of the food we eat determines the quality of our health. Our bodies must have a certain amount of a variety of nutrients in order to function at an optimal level. If these nutrients are not supplied on a regular basis, the body suffers and health declines.

The most nutritious foods are the ones our ancestors ate—straight from the source with minimal processing. Modern food practices, in an attempt to make foods more enticing in appearance, taste, and texture, and to extend their shelf life, have greatly altered their chemical makeup. Processing has stripped foods of much of their nutrient value and added harmful chemicals and substances devoid of essential vitamins and minerals. The result is a nutrient-deficient, contaminated blend of flavors, chemicals, and empty calories. It's no wonder wherever modern foods go in this world degenerative disease follows closely behind.

Our most commonly eaten foods are white flour, white rice, sugar, and vegetable oils of one type or another. These foods are essentially all empty calories. They provide calories, but lack nutritive value—little or no vitamins, minerals, or phytochemicals. They also lack fiber, which is an essential food component. Look on the ingredient labels of packaged foods, and these items compose the main ingredients along with assorted chemical flavorings, preservatives, emulsifiers, thickening agents, and the like.

Meat and dairy products can be another problem. Most people eat far too much of them. Excess animal protein can have detrimental effects on health. These effects are greatly magnified when the diet is deficient, even if only marginally, in vitamins and minerals. No one who eats a typical western diet gets even the minimum recommended dietary allowance (RDA) of all the nutrients. Studies have shown this to be the case. Our actual requirement for some nutrients is much higher than the RDA; this has become evident with the discovery of the importance of homocysteine and the B vitamins. You can't get all the nutrients your body needs by eating the typical western diet. It isn't possible. Even the fortification of foods and the taking of vitamin supplements can't make up completely for what is lost in processing.

Deep fried foods are the worst types of foods you can eat. They are fried in heat-damaged vegetable oil reeking with free radicals. Sautéing or stir frying are much better alternatives if the oil used is coconut oil. Even butter or lard would be better than vegetable oil.

Think of all the foods you eat that are made primarily of white flour, white rice, and sugar: bread, rolls, tortillas, crackers, cookies, donuts, cake, pie, pancake mix, pasta/noodles, cold cereal, etc. Think of the foods rich in vegetable oil: margarine, shortening, baked goods, canned meals (beef stew, refried beans, spaghetti), frozen dinners (pizza, TV dinners), boxed meals (macaroni and cheese), frosting, mayonnaise, salad dressing, cookies, crackers, etc. If these are the types of foods you eat every day —watch out, you are a prime candidate for atherosclerosis, cancer, arthritis, or any number of other degenerative diseases that plague modern society.

Replace those items above with wholesome foods— fresh fruit, vegetables, beans, and whole grain products that have undergone minimal processing. Most of your favorite foods can be made using wholesome ingredients. Perhaps the most important change would be to use whole grain products in place of those made with white flour. Whole wheat goods are available in an amazing variety of products. You can buy whole wheat bread, rolls, tortillas, pasta, etc. Pasta can be found made from brown rice and corn.

With modern food distribution, nowadays fresh fruits and vegetables are available all year long. Eat a mixture of both raw and cooked foods. Frozen fruits and vegetables can be eaten, but because they may have lost 10-15 percent of their nutrient value, it isn't wise to eat only frozen produce.

Fiber is essential to good health because it aids in the movement of food through the digestive tract; slows down absorption of sugars (which puts less strain on our blood sugar-regulating system); absorbs and removes certain fats, heavy metals, and other toxins from the foods we eat; and gives us a feeling of fullness which keeps us from eating too much. Our bodies prefer high-fiber foods.

The highest fiber foods are whole grains and legumes. These foods should constitute the bulk of our diet just as they did in our great-gradnparent's day. Wheat has been known as the "staff of life" for centuries because it has been the primary food for much of the Western and Near Eastern world. Rice holds that same status in the Far East. Whole grains and legumes should be supplemented by fruits and vegetables (most of which contain only moderate amounts of fiber).

High-fiber foods add bulk to meals without adding calories. When you fill up on fiber-rich foods, you have less room for calorie-rich foods. Fiber also gives a feeling of fullness and slows down digestion so you don't get hungry as quickly. White bread and white rice have much of their fiber removed, so they are digested quickly, leaving you hungry sooner. You then eat more often and end up consuming more calories and, consequently, gaining weight. When you eat high-fiber foods, your calorie consumption is automatically reduced, so you don't need to worry about counting calories. You can eat as much as you like so long as the food is wholesome and natural. An apple is natural; apple strudel is not. Whole wheat bread is natural; white bread is not. A baked potato is natural; potato chips are not.

You can eat as much of the wholesome foods as you like, as long as they don't contain sugar or vegetable oil, and you won't need to worry about your weight. Excess pounds will melt away and your body will adjust to a weight that is right for your height and bone structure.

Fresh fruits, vegetables, beans, and whole grain breads can be found in most grocery stores. Health food stores, however, carry the widest variety of such goods. Many of their products are made without sugar, white flour, vegetable oil, and chemical additives, and make much better selections than the typical foods found in most food stores.

I need to briefly discuss sugar. An entire book can be written on the health aspects of sugar, indeed many have. Although sugar isn't the main topic of this book, it is important enough to mention. A little sugar isn't likely to do much harm, however, most of us eat far too much. We consume an average of 140 pounds of sugar per person per year. This amounts to 41 teaspoons per day! We also get an additional 40 to 50 pounds per year in fruits. Sugar contains no vitamins, and no minerals, but is loaded with calories. Our body must use up its vitamin and mineral reserves in order to process the sugar. When we eat sugary, white flour products—like a donut—it actually lowers our bodies' nutrient reserves. Eating such foods also lowers the amount of healthy foods we might otherwise consume. In addition, sugar has detrimental effects on our health.

Several sugars, including glucose, oxidize very slowly to produce free radicals. Thus, it has been suggested that decades of exposure of body tissues to elevated blood glucose can result in diabetic patients suffering "oxidative stress" that may contribute to the side effects of hyperglycemia.[3] This may be the reason why diabetics are prone to atherosclerosis and heart disease. Free radicals generated from high blood-glucose levels damage arterial walls initiating plaque formation. John Yudkin, of the University of London, found the association of heart disease was stronger with sugar than it was with cholesterol.

Natural sugars such as raw honey, molasses, and maple syrup contain some vitamins and minerals and in that respect are better for you than table sugar. It is a good idea to *reduce total sugar intake* and in place of white sugar eat more natural sugars.

Dietary Supplements

Dietary changes alone are usually not enough to bring about significant changes in health when chronic conditions exist. The next part of the Antioxidant Health Plan is to reverse years of dietary imbalance and subclinical malnutrition by taking dietary supplements. Switching to wholesome foods will not supply you with all the nutrients you need to overcome years of dietary abuse. Most of us have eaten polyunsaturated oils, margarines, and shortening for years and the fatty acids in these products have been incorporated into the structure of every cell in our bodies.

Your cells are composed from the foods you eat. The more polyunsaturated oil you have eaten in your life, the greater the concentration of it in your cells. The bad thing about having a high concentration of these oils in your body is that they are highly susceptible to free-radical formation. This puts a heavy demand on your antioxidant reserves. A body filled with polyunsaturated fatty acids will need more antioxidant nutrients to keep free-radical reactions in check.

Eating more saturated and monounsaturated oils will gradually replace many of these polyunsaturated fats in the body, thus reducing your antioxidant requirements. The process of replacing a less healthy fat with a healthier one takes time. So transforming a polyunsaturated body into a more natural monounsaturated and saturated body will take a few years. In the meantime, you can get the protection you need by taking vitamin and mineral supplements until dietary changes have time to make significant changes in cellular structure and reestablish nutrient reserves.

Dietary changes must be accompanied by vitamin and mineral supplements at first. Studies show, for example, that supplements lower homocysteine more effectively than just eating more fruits and vegetables. B vitamin supplementation showed a more consistent and stronger effect in lowering blood homocysteine than just increasing the consumption of vegetables and fruits.[4]

The minimum amount of vitamins needed to prevent deficiency disease may not be enough to prevent degenerative disease. Folic acid and vitamin B-6 are prime examples of that. The amount set as the RDA will not prevent elevated homocysteine levels which damage our arteries. And the more meat we eat, the more of these vitamins we need to remove the homocysteine. Similarly, the amount of vitamins C and E to prevent deficiency symptoms and the amount to prevent free-radical damage are not the same. A person can get the daily requirement and not suffer deficiency symptoms, but he may age like a prune. Studies have shown how free radicals can cause aging. In one, for example, mice were fed diets containing either saturated or polyunsaturated fat. Each was given more than enough vitamin E to prevent a deficiency. The mice on the polyunsaturated fat diet required more vitamin E. As the years went by, it became very apparent that the mice being fed the polyunsaturated oils were dying sooner of old age then the mice on the saturated fat diet. Though none of the mice developed signs of vitamin E deficiency, the ones on the polyunsaturated fat were aging and dying more rapidly.[5]

Why can't we just get our vitamins and minerals from the foods we eat? After all, that's how the human race did it in the past. A century or two ago we probably could have gotten all the vitamins and minerals we needed from our foods, just as the animals do. But we live in a different environment now. We are exposed to an enormous amount of chemical pollution in the air we breathe, the water we drink, and the food we eat. These chemicals are like foreign invaders that wear down our immune system, tax enzyme production, and deplete antioxidant reserves. Stress of modern life also burns up vitamins at an accelerated rate. It is very difficult to get all the nutrients we need nowadays to fight off the continual assault to our health.

Table 18-1 lists the maintenance and therapeutic amounts for several vitamins and minerals suitable for adults. The maintenance level is similar to the RDA and should supply you with enough, if you eat a wholesome diet. Start the program by taking the therapeutic amount. You need this to overcome years of dietary abuse. Continue to take the therapeutic amount for 6-12 months. After that, if you're eating as directed above, you can drop back to a maintenance level. You may remain at the maintenance level indefinitely.

When taking supplements, it is best to divide them so that you take half in the morning with breakfast and half in the evening with dinner. So, if you are taking 1,000 mg of vitamin C, divide it into two 500 mg doses. Taking them with meals combines them with the nutrients in your foods for improved absorption and utilization.

If you are male or a postmenopausal female, avoid all supplements containing iron unless there is a clearly iden- tified medical need monitored by laboratory tests. Also avoid foods that contain added iron. Most processed flour prod- ucts are fortified with iron and a few vitamins. When flour is processed, many nutrients are removed. Iron is always added back in larger quantities than what was originally present.

The problem with recommending dietary supplements is that some people believe if they eat the supplements they don't need to worry about their diet so much. This is *not* true! Supplements are not foods and are not meant to re- place wholesome foods and will not erase the negative ef- fects of eating poor-quality packaged foods. You take supplements to enhance the effects of wholesome foods. They are *supplements* not replacements.

Supplements do not contain all the nutrients our bod- ies need to maintain or obtain optimal health. Scientists have identified over a dozen vitamins that are recognized as be- ing necessary for health, but there are hundreds of thousands

Table 18-1   DIETARY SUPPLEMENTS

Supplement	Maintenance Dose	Therapeutic Dose
Vitamin B complex(a)		
Thiamin	1.0-1.5 mg	1.5 mg
Riboflavin	1.3-1.8 mg	1.8 mg
Niacin	15-20 mg	20 mg
Biotin	30-100 mcg	100 mcg
Pantothenic Acid	4-7 mg	7 mg
Vitamin B-6	2.0-4.0 mg	4.0-8.0 mg
Folate (folic acid)	200-400 mcg	400-800 mcg
Vitamin B-12	2.0 mcg	2.0 mcg
Beta-carotene		
with mixed carotenoids(b)	10,000 IU	25,000 IU
Citrus or rutin bioflavonoids	500 mg	1,000-2,000 mg
Proanthocyanidins(c)	50 mg	100-200 mg
Vitamin C	500 mg	1,000 to 2,000 mg
Vitamin E		
with mixed tocopherols	200-400 IU	400-800 IU
Magnesium(d)	300-500 mg	1,000-1,200 mg
Calcium	600-1,000 mg	1,000-1,200 mg
Selenium	70-100 mcg	200-300 mcg
Zinc	15 mg	30-50 mg

This table does not list all the vi- tamins, only those discussed in this book. Other major vitamins and min- erals include vitamin D, vitamin K, manganese, copper, chromium, mo- lybdenum, phosphorous, and iodine. While not listed, they are important and should be taken in at least the RDA level when taking these other vitamins. Most complete vitamin and mineral supplement formulas will in- clude all of these. Make sure that whatever multi-vitamin supplements you use contain at least those listed in this table. Units of measure may be different on some supplements: 1 gram = 1000 mg, 1 mg = 100 mcg.

(a) The B vitamins should always be taken as a group. Not all of them are listed here, but any complete B-complex supplement will include those not listed. For the therapeutic level, you should add more vitamin B-6 and folic acid than what will be available in a typical B-complex supplement.
(b) Since beta-carotene is converted into vitamin A, it satisfies the requirement for this vitamin.
(c) Other terms used for this bioflavonoid are: grape seed or grape skin extract, Pycnogenol, or procyanidolic oligomers (PCOs). You can use any of these forms.
(d) Calcium and magnesium should always be taken together. On the therapeutic level, use a ratio of 1:1. At the maintenance level use a ratio of calcium to magnesium of about 2:1

of phytochemicals (plant chemicals), most of which are yet to be discovered and only a few have been extensively studied. The carotenoids, for example, are not classified as necessary nutrients because we don't produce any recognizable deficiency symptoms if they are not in our diet, but they protect us from cancer and heart disease. I would consider them important nutrients. The vast majority of these nutrients are not available in tablet form; we can only get them in our foods. Therefore, we need to eat wholesome foods to get a wide selection of these phytochemicals.

When you take supplements, you need to take a variety and not just one or two. Folic acid in large doses has been reported to lower zinc concentrations in the blood, which may cause zinc deficiency.[6] If you add zinc to compensate for the added B-6, you could create a copper deficiency. Adding zinc up to two or three times the RDA can deplete copper reserves. Also, the B vitamins compete with each other for absorption, and too much of one may cause a deficiency in another. All the vitamins work synergistically with each other, and you gain greater benefit by taking a complete mix than you do from large quantities of any one or two. This is another reason why you need to eat good nutritious foods with the vitamins to supply phytochemicals not contained in the supplements.

One concern that always comes up is: you can carefully watch what you eat and avoid all the foods with vegetable oils and white flour, but when you're away from home and eating out at a restaurant or friend's house, you have

---

DIETARY RECOMMENDATIONS

• **Foods You Should Eat Daily:**
Whole grain cereals and breads, fresh fruits, vegetables, nuts, seeds, herbs, spices, and water.

• **Recommended Edible Oils:**
Coconut oil, organic butter, extra virgin olive oil.

• **Foods That Should Be Eaten in Moderation:**
Red meat, fowl, fish, eggs, dairy (preferably organic or free range), and sugar.

• **Food You Should Avoid Completely:**
Vegetable oil, hydrogenated and partially hydrogenated oils, artificial fats, refined flour and bread products, white rice, fortified foods containing iron, powdered dairy or egg products or foods that contain them, milk, freeze-dried meat, cured meats, and deep fried foods of all types.

---

little control over how the food is prepared. What do you do? The best thing to do is not to eat it. This is difficult for most people to follow. The second best thing to do is to make wise food choices with the selection you're offered. For example, if you have a choice between margarine and butter, choose butter. Choose a baked potato over fries, baked fish or chicken over fried, whole wheat over white bread, and vinegar and water over an oily salad dressing. No matter how careful you are, when you eat out, you will consume some vegetable oil. All restaurant foods have it and the typical foods in most homes have it. So to offset the added oil you are going to eat, take an extra 100-200 IU of vitamin E before eating. This isn't a perfect solution, but it will provide you with some extra protection.

Keep in mind that taking extra vitamin E will help to keep fats we have eaten from oxidizing inside of us. If the fats were oxidized before we eat them, vitamin E will do little for us. Deep fried foods and heat-damaged oils are heavily oxidized. Powdered milk (and soft-serve ice cream), cheese, and eggs are all oxidized. These oils go directly into your arteries regardless of how many antioxidants you take.

THE ANTIOXIDANT HEALTH PLAN IN A NUTSHELL

In order to completely describe which foods you should eat and which ones you should avoid would really require a full book on nutrition and food processing. To avoid getting too complicated, I have distilled down the Antioxidant Health Plan into a few basic guidelines that are relatively easy to follow and will make a dramatic difference in your life if you stick closely to them.

My guidelines are to eat only *whole grain* breads and bread products. Eat more fruits, vegetables, and beans. Eat meat and dairy products sparingly.* Use coconut oil for most of your cooking needs. Organic butter and extra virgin olive oil are all right to use sparingly.

Avoid all white flour and white rice products, and reduce sugar consumption. *Do not eat anything that contains hydrogenated or partially hydrogenated oil, shortening, margarine, or vegetable oil.* Avoid all artificial fats such as olestra (Olean) and salatrim (Benefat). Also, avoid anything that contains *powdered* cheese, milk, or eggs. Even if it only contains a tiny amount, don't touch it! Products that

---

*In this context "sparingly" is defined as about 3 to 6 ounces of meat, cheese, or dairy a day. Three ounces of meat is the size of one hamburger patty. A good way to limit meat consumption is to use it as a flavoring rather than as the main course. Use it in soups, casseroles, and other dishes with lots of vegetables and whole grains.

have these things in them almost always contain sugar and chemical additives and are lacking in nutritive value. Whole, low-fat, skim, and nonfat milk are also off the list, but yogurt, cheese, butter and other dairy products are allowed. So avoiding any foods containing vegetable oils and powdered dairy and egg products will help steer you away from the foods that are your worst enemies. Get into the habit of reading ingredient labels on everything you buy. Make a commitment to never eat these oils again. If you do that, you will see dramatic improvement in your health.

Don't worry about saturated fat and cholesterol. Eat meat, eggs, and dairy in moderation and you don't need to think about getting too much of these fats. Do be concerned about the amount of polyunsaturated fats and trans fatty acids you consume. The fewer the better. Remember you always get polyunsaturated fats in your foods from fruits, vegetables, nuts, grains and even meats. Foods supply all the polyunsaturated fats your body needs, so supplementation is unnecessary. If you want more polyunsaturated fats, eat fish, not oil.

There are many other things you can do to improve the quality and nutritive value of your diet. I'm not going discuss those, but leave it up to you to research further if you are interested in taking this diet to a higher level. There are many excellent books available on the subject. I would recommend any of the macrobiotic diet books or my own book *The Detox Book*. This book also discusses other important factors in health such as exercise and stress reduction.

It is important that you accompany the dietary changes I suggest with vitamin and mineral supplements. Therapeutic doses are needed until dietary changes have time to make changes in your body. Take the therapeutic dose for 6-12 months, then cut back to a maintenance dose for however long you feel is necessary. Because of the pollution we are exposed to daily, I would suggest taking the maintenance dose of antioxidants indefinitely.

EXERCISE

Exercise is such an important factor in health and weight control that I can't leave it out of the Antioxidant Health Plan. Numerous studies have demonstrated the health benefits of regular exercise. However, many people are intimidated by the thought of strenuous exercise, conjuring up visions of jogging miles every day or straining away on weights or struggling with complicated fitness machines. The truth of the matter is, strenuous exercise is not necessary; a simple exercise like walking can provide enough of a workout to significantly affect health in a positive way. Several studies have demonstrated this fact.

Dr. Arthur S. Leon and colleagues as part of the Multiple Risk Factor Intervention Trial (MRFIT) discovered an interesting relationship between exercise and health. In their study, 12,138 middle-aged men were divided into three groups based on their level of exercise. During seven years of follow-up, those who exercised moderately had one-third *fewer* deaths from all causes, including heart disease, than those who were sedentary. Walking, or its equivalent, for at least thirty minutes a day was defined as moderate exercise. The mortality rates of those with high levels of exercise were *not* significantly different from those with moderate levels of exercise.[7]

Another study performed at the Institute for Aerobic Research lasted eight years and included 10,224 men and 3,120 women, all of whom were apparently healthy. They were divide into five categories depending on their level of physical activity. Category 1 was the least fit, and Category 5 was the most fit. After eight years the death rates of the five groups were compared. The ones with the lowest overall fitness had three times the death rate when compared with the most fit group. But the greatest difference was between categories 1 and 2—no exercise and moderate exercise; again showing that a little exercise can make a dramatic difference, and that a lot of exercise is only a little better in terms of longevity.

Since oxygen is the main element involved in the oxidization of fats and the creation of free radicals, some people have questioned the benefits of exercise. When we exercise we consume more oxygen which increases the oxygen content in the blood. Theoretically, this greater concentration of oxygen would lead to an increase in lipid peroxidation. Lipid or fat peroxidation is believed to play a significant role in the development of atherosclerosis. But studies indicated that exercise protects against oxidation rather than encourages it. Researchers took blood samples from 39 male and female athletes before and after a triathlon. Competing in the triathlon significantly reduced the susceptibility of blood fats to oxidation. This was true even in those who did not take antioxidants prior to the competition.[8] So exercise can reduce the tendency of fat in the body to oxidize which, in turn, slows down the aging process.

Exercise not only strengthens our muscles, but strengthens our antioxidant system as well. As long as we eat enough of the nutrients necessary for the body to manufacture superoxide dismutase catalase, glutathione peroxidase, and other vital antioxidants it will do so. When we exercise, we increase our oxygen consumption. The body responds or adapts to this increase of oxygen by producing more antioxidant bodyguards to protect the cells and tissues. This elevated number of antioxidants remains even after exercise has stopped. In time, they are slowly depleted as they fight off a continual attack from free radicals. During this time, which may last a couple of days, you've had the benefit of the added protection and thus experience less oxidative deterioration. Exercise will again elevate antioxidant reserves and the process continues. So, with regular exercise a person can continually maintain an increased level of antioxidants. This may be one reason why those who are physically active look and feel so much younger than those who don't.

As you exercise, keep in mind that the body builds its antioxidant reserves in response to an increase in oxygen consumption. This means, in order to get the most benefit you need to do something vigorous enough to get your heart pumping and increase your respiration rate. When you are exercising you should be breathing heavier than you normally do. A *leisurely* walk won't do much for most people because this level of activity puts little demand on the body's need for oxygen. Walking at a moderate or quick pace will significantly increase respiration and is simple enough that most anybody can do it.

If you're not used to exercising, start slowly. A ten-minute walk every day is a good start. A leisurely walk may be all you can manage at first. That's okay. As your body

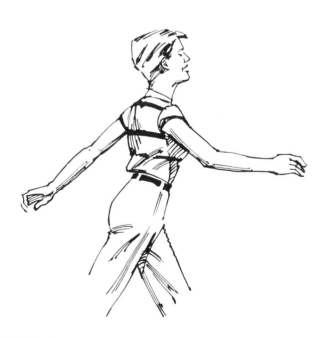

Individuals with sedentary lifestyles have the highest risk of death from all causes. Even a small degree of activity such as walking or moderate cycling several times a week corresponds to a decrease in the risk of mortality. Greater levels of fitness are associated with only slightly more reduction in risk.

adjusts to this level of activity you can gradually increase the time. A good goal to shoot for is 30 minutes a day—every day. However, even if you can only squeeze in 10 minutes a day, that's better than nothing.

The key here is to get *regular* exercise that will be vigorous enough to have you breathing harder than normal. Regular, means every day or as close to it as possible. The more days you miss the less benefit you get. Three days a week is generally recommended as the *minimum* amount necessary to gain any benefit from a regular exercise program. If you exercise only once or twice a week you may actually do more harm than good. Why? When we exercise we increase oxygen consumption which increases the potential for free-radical reactions. If the body is accustomed to exercise it will already have an elevated antioxidant level to handle the demand. If not, exercise could increase oxidative stress. It takes time for the body to adjust to our level of physical activity. Just as it takes time for a weight lifters muscles to build up strength, it takes time to build up antioxidant reserves. Exercising one or two days a week isn't enough to do this. So someone who exercises infrequently will increase free radicals without significantly increasing antioxidants to fight them. This is one reason why weekend athletes—those who sit at desk all week then play a vigorous game of basketball on the weekend—come away feeling sore and fatigued. When you start an exercise program you need to do it regularly.

The most common obstacles people mention as to why they don't get regular exercise are that its boring, it hurts, they don't have enough time, they don't have enough energy, and it's not convenient. While walking is one of the easiest and most convenient forms of exercise, it doesn't overcome all these obstacles. Another form of exercise that is even better than walking and does overcome all these objections is rebound exercise. Rebound exercise is simply jumping on a rebounder or mini-trampoline. Rebounding has been described as the "most efficient, most effective form of exercise yet devised by man." It is unique in that you can exercise at your own level of fitness. Professional athletes have used it in their training, so have people crippled so severely with arthritis they needed assistance to walk. Even people who use walkers or need wheelchairs to get around can rebound. This is such a dynamic form of exercise that I have produced an audio tape titled *Rebound to Better Health*. In this tape I explain why rebound exercise is the most efficient, most effective exercise in existence and how it is used therapeutically to stimulate better health and reverse degenerante conditions. It is one exercise that can be done by anyone at any fitness level and does not require a lot of time. NASA scientists studied rebound exercise and concluded that it was 68% more effective as a form of exercise than jogging. In other words, you can get more benefit in less time rebounding than you can jogging. Also, the mat and springs absorb nearly 90 percent of the force of impact so there is virtually no threat of injury like those you would experience with other aerobic activities.

A BETTER LIFE

The Antioxidant Health Plan works at a cellular level. That is, as old diseased cells die and are replaced, new healthier cells will take their place. It takes as long as seven years for every cell in your body to be replaced. This doesn't mean that you have to wait that long to see dramatic improvement. Many people notice changes after only a few weeks. Some see significant changes in only a few months. But for others it may take a year or two for noticeable improvement to become manifest.

Since it is a cellular rebuilding process, change is very gradual and often imperceptible. You may not even notice the changes taking place until one day you find yourself doing something you hadn't done in years. For example, a person who suffers from arthritis may twist open a jar and suddenly realize that she hadn't been able to do that without pain for years. The loss of pain wasn't because the pain was masked by drugs, it happens because the body has repaired itself and reversed the diseased condition. Drugs work quickly because they deaden nerves and alter chemistry. Natural processes are slower because they don't harm the nerves or alter normal chemistry, but fix the imbalance that causes the problem.

Many health benefits you will receive will be unnoticeable at first because our health can be destroyed without our realizing it. Heart disease, for example, gives little warning. For many people, the first symptom they have of heart disease is a full blown heart attack. Heart disease doesn't just happen all of the sudden. It's a slow process that takes years to develop. Atherosclerosis, the condition that leads to heart disease, can start while we're still young. Nowadays even teenagers are developing it at an alarming rate and setting up the conditions for a heart attack in the future when they are 40 or 50 years old.

One of the benefits you will notice from this program over time is an increase in energy and productivity. Mental capacity will improve and you will have a heightened sense of well-being. When the body is not stressed by nutrient deficiencies or burdened by sick cells, it works better, feels better, and is more resistant to disease. Since I started this program, my immune system is much more efficient than it used to be. I haven't had a single viral or bacterial infection in years.

You have control over your own health. If you want to be healthy, you can be by following this simple health plan. Keep in mind that the better you adhere to this plan, the quicker the results. One of the keys to the speed and degree of improved health is how faithfully you follow the program. Some people may think that just taking vitamins or antioxidants will be enough, and they can continue with their health-destroying habits. Some people will undoubtedly see improvement if they do this. But they must continue with therapeutic doses every day of their lives to keep disease at bay. As they get older, however, and organs and cells lose youthful vitality, it will become harder and harder to maintain good health while doing things that are harmful to the body.

Those who takes antioxidants, but continue to consume processed vegetable oils, will not experience the benefits they would desire. The reverse is also true, avoiding vegetable oils is not enough, especially if you have abused your body with years of poor eating habits. Some improvement may be achieved, but the best results can only come by following the entire program.

In his travels around the world, Dr. Weston Price found that when people introduced even a little sugary, vegetable-oil-laden, vitamin-deficient processed foods into their diets, their level of health was significantly affected. Dental cavities, weight problems, and degenerative disease was the result.

Often, people think that adding one serving of vegetables at dinner time will offset their diet of white bread, sugar, and other nutrient deficient foods. This is not true. Sugar and white bread are mostly empty calories and displace or replace the consumption of nutrient- and fiber-rich foods. Eating a raw carrot will not protect you against the effects of eating three donuts, two cups of coffee, a hamburger, and French fries. These types of foods do not supply adequate antioxidants and are loaded with free-radical-causing additives and oils. Eating them may keep you alive, but not healthy. You have the choice to live a healthy vibrant life, or to live inside a degenerating body that will eventually succumb to sickness, pain, and dysfunction.

You can have better health. All it takes is replacing health-destroying foods with wholesome natural foods. There is no other way. There will never be a cure for cancer or heart disease. The cure is in the foods we eat. Free radicals tear cells apart and no drug will ever be able to repair and revive damaged cells and tissues. And no drug can ever compensate for a lack of vitamins and minerals.

PROVE IT TO YOURSELF

The false idea that saturated fat and cholesterol are the cause of cardiovascular disease is so pervasive that many people will find the message in this book difficult to accept. Hundreds of "health" books have been written warning against these fats, calling them deadly. Many of these sources recommend using polyunsaturated oils in the diet in place of these. They are perpetuating a myth and leading people into disease. I don't advocate eating more foods high in saturated fat and cholesterol, as we eat far too much of them already. My message is to avoid the real trouble maker—polyunsaturated oil—and substitute coconut oil for all cooking needs.

Many people will refuse to accept these facts because they are brainwashed by proponents of the cholesterol theory—most of which have a heavy financial investment at stake. I believe that in time the facts I have presented will be widely recognized and the cholesterol hypothesis will fade into the background. You don't have to wait 10 or 20 years for that to happen. You can test out these ideas right now, today, for yourself. Seeing the changes you can make in your own health is believing. If you have an open mind, you will see changes in your health as you follow the program outlined in this chapter. All I say is try it, and you will prove it to yourself.

I know many closed-minded people will refuse to even test it. They will argue and belittle the facts and conclusions I present here. But the true test of anything is if it works.

Keep in mind this program is not a cure for any specific disease and should not replace the counsel of your doctor. But it will improve your health no matter what condition you are in presently. If you follow this program, and stick with it, you will gain better health, have more energy, and feel better. For some people it has been the means by which they have been able to completely overcome crippling disease. For others it has given them the strength to better cope with serious health problems.

I would like to hear from you. Give this program a try. It may take several months, a year, or perhaps more to notice significant improvement. Write to me and tell me what the program has done for you. You can reach me c/o HealthWise Publications, P.O. Box 25203, Colorado Springs, CO 80936.

Appendix

FATTY ACIDS

Our bodies are fatty acid organisms, that is, these substances comprise the vast majority of our fatty tissues. The membranes of the cells in your skin, muscles, heart, brain and other organs are composed predominantly of fatty acids.

The huge majority of the fatty acids in our bodies are packaged as triglyceride molecules and stored as body fat. Three fatty acids joined together by a glycerol molecule make a triglyceride. Another important, but far less abundant, fat molecule is the phospholipid. Phospholipids are structurally similar to triglycerides. Like the triglyceride, the phospholipid has a glycerol "backbone," but holds only two fatty acids. In place of the third fatty acid is a phosphate group. Most of the fatty acids in our cell membranes are in the form of phospholipids.

There are three basic classifications of fatty acids—saturated, monounsaturated, and polyunsaturated. Any combination of these three fatty acids can be found in triglycerides and phospholipids.

A fatty acid molecule consists of an acid group (COOH) attached to a chain of carbon atoms with accompanying hydrogen atoms. Fatty acids can vary in the length of their carbon chain and degree of unsaturation. Acetic acid, found in vinegar, has a chain only two carbon atoms long. A longer acid chain may have four, six, eight, or more carbon atoms. Naturally occurring fatty acids usually occur in even numbers. Butyric acid, one type of fatty acid commonly found in butter, consists of a four-carbon chain. The

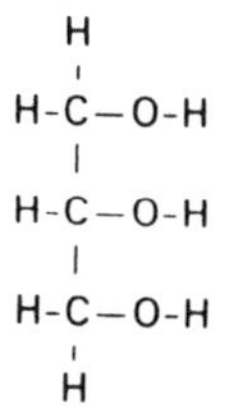

Glycerol

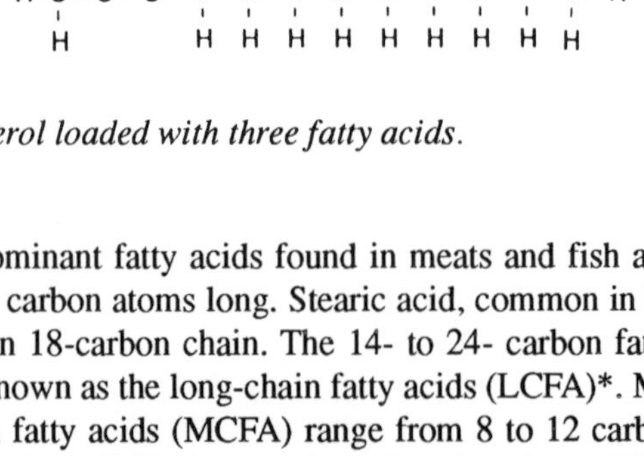

Glycerol loaded with three fatty acids.

predominant fatty acids found in meats and fish are 14 or more carbon atoms long. Stearic acid, common in beef fat, has an 18-carbon chain. The 14- to 24- carbon fatty acids are known as the long-chain fatty acids (LCFA)*. Medium-chain fatty acids (MCFA) range from 8 to 12 carbons and short-chain (SCFA) range from 2 to 8 carbons. The length of the carbon chain is a key factor in the way dietary fat is digested and metabolized.

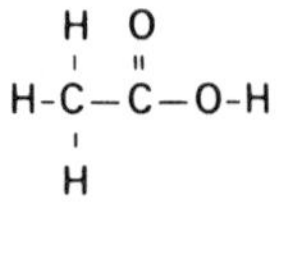

---

*When three fatty acids of similar length are joined together by a glycerol molecule, the resulting molecule is referred to as long-chain triglyceride (LCT), medium-chain triglyceride (MCT), or short-chain triglyceride (SCT).

Acetic acid

192

Saturated fats are loaded, or saturated, with all the hydrogen (H) atoms they can carry. The fatty acid shown in the illustration below is a saturated fat.

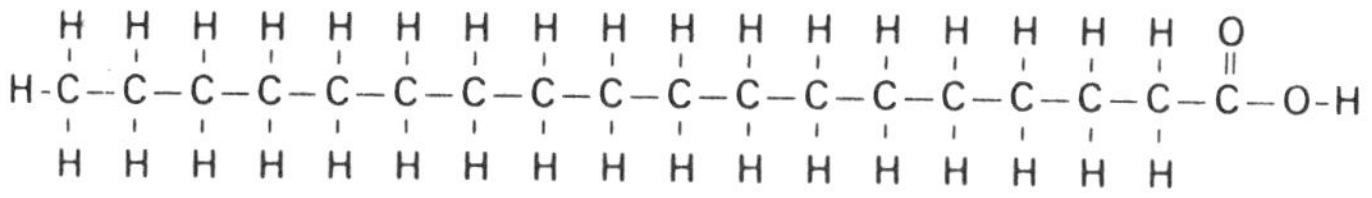

```
 H  H  H  H  H  H  H  H  H  H  H  H  H  H  H  H  H  H  O
 |  |  |  |  |  |  |  |  |  |  |  |  |  |  |  |  |  |  ‖
H-C--C--C--C--C--C--C--C--C--C--C--C--C--C--C--C--C--C--O-H
 |  |  |  |  |  |  |  |  |  |  |  |  |  |  |  |  |  |
 H  H  H  H  H  H  H  H  H  H  H  H  H  H  H  H  H  H
```

Stearic acid

If hydrogens were to be removed, the carbon atoms would form double bonds with one another in order to satisfy their bonding requirements. The result would be an unsaturated fat. If two hydrogen atoms were removed, one double bond would be created between two carbons. This would form a monounsaturated fatty acid (see example below). In this case, oleic acid, the monounsaturated fatty acid which is found predominantly in olive oil.

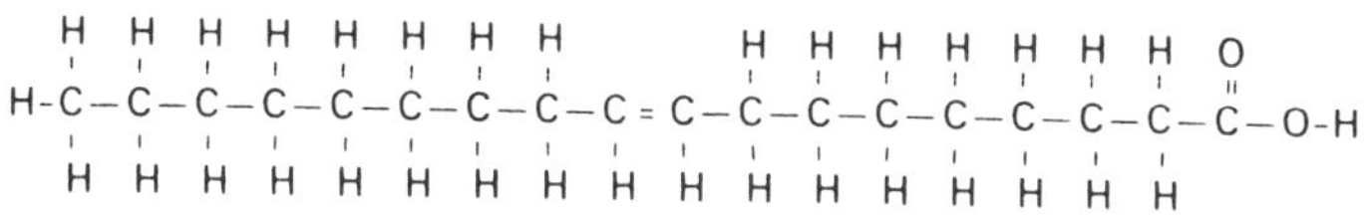

```
 H  H  H  H  H  H  H            H  H  H  H  H  H  H  O
 |  |  |  |  |  |  |            |  |  |  |  |  |  |  ‖
H-C--C--C--C--C--C--C--C=C--C--C--C--C--C--C--C--C--O-H
 |  |  |  |  |  |  |  |            |  |  |  |  |  |  |
 H  H  H  H  H  H  H  H            H  H  H  H  H  H  H
```

Oleic acid

If two or more pairs of hydrogen atoms are missing and more than one double carbon bond is present, it is referred to as a polyunsaturated oil.

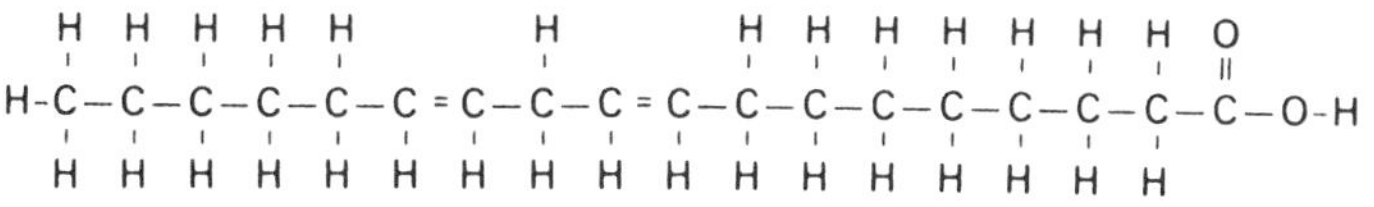

```
 H  H  H  H  H            H            H  H  H  H  H  H  O
 |  |  |  |  |            |            |  |  |  |  |  |  ‖
H-C--C--C--C--C=C--C--C--C=C--C--C--C--C--C--C--C--O-H
 |  |  |  |  |  |  |  |  |  |  |  |  |  |  |  |  |
 H  H  H  H  H  H  H  H  H  H  H  H  H  H  H  H
```

Linoleic acid

Table A-1 SATURATED FATTY ACIDS

Fatty Acid	Carbons	Common Source
Acetic	2	Vinegar
Butyric	4	Butterfat
Caproic	6	Butterfat
Caprylic	8	Coconut oil
Capric	10	Palm oil
Lauric	12	Coconut oil
Myristic	14	Nutmeg oil, butterfat
Palmitic	16	Animal and vegetable oil
Stearic	18	Animal and vegetable oil
Arachidic	20	Peanut oil

In summary, the fats and oils in our diet are predominately triglycerides, comprised of three fatty acids. Those fatty acids that are fully loaded with hydrogen atoms and have no double carbon bonds are the saturated fats; those that have one or more double bonds are unsaturated fats.

The body's cells are equipped with many enzymes that can convert one compound or molecule to another. To make triglycerides, all the enzymes need is a usable food source containing the atoms (building blocks) that triglycerides are composed of: carbon, hydrogen, and oxygen. Glucose, derived primarily from carbohydrate foods, can easily be converted to fat. In fact, given an excess of blood glucose, this is precisely what the cells do. Enzymes cleave the glucose to make 2-carbon fragments, and then combine these fragments with the appropriate alterations, to make long-chain fatty acids. Regardless of the source, all of the fat stored in our bodies is converted into fatty acids, predominantly of the long-chain variety.

The physiological function of most of the fat in our bodies is to serve as fuel for cellular metabolism. It is an economical way of storing fuel since the fat molecule consists almost entirely of carbon and hydrogen atoms with no incombustible nitrogen as is present in protein molecules. A gram of fat, upon oxidation in the body, yields 9 calories, over twice that of protein or carbohydrate.

Table A-2 UNSATURATED FATTY ACIDS

Fatty Acid	Carbons	No. of Double Bonds	Common Source
Palmitoleic	16	1	Butterfat
Oleic	18	1	Olive oil
Linoleic	18	2	Linseed and vegetable oil
Alpha-Linolenic	18	3	Linseed oil
Arachidonic	20	4	Lecithin
Eicosapentanoic (EPA)	20	5	Fish oils
Docosahexaenoic (DHA)	22	6	Fish oils

Linoleic and arachidonic acids belong to the omega-6 family. Alpha-linolenic, eicosapentanoic, docosahexaenoic acids belong to the omega-3 family. Palmitoleic and Oleic acids belong to the omega-9 family.

CARBON CHAINS

The fats found in animal tissue, as well as our own bodies, are mainly the triglycerides of stearic, palmitic, and oleic acids. Oleic acid is a monounsaturated fat. Stearic and palmitic acids are saturated fats.

The saturated fat found in food consists of a mixture of the different types. Milk, for example, contains palmitic, myristic, stearic, lauric, butyric, caproic, caprylic, and capric acids. Each of these fatty acids has different effects on the body which are governed by the length of the carbon chain.

Saturated fatty acids with up to 26 carbon atoms (C26) and as little as 2 (C2) carbon in the chain have been identified as constituents of fats. Of these, palmitic acid (C16) is the most common, occurring in almost all fats. Myristic (C14) and stearic (C18) acids are other common saturated fatty acids.

The melting points of the saturated fatty acids increases with carbon chain length. Esters of fatty acids with more than 18 carbon atoms are characteristic constituents of waxes. Fatty acids less than 10 or greater than 22 carbons long are not generally abundant in nature. Tables A-1 and A-2 list fatty acids and their primary sources.

Saturated fats have received a lot of criticism for their role in raising blood cholesterol. While some saturated fats do raise blood cholesterol, others do not. To say that all saturated fats raise cholesterol is simply not true. Myristic (C14) and palmitic (C16) acids exert the greatest cholesterol raising effect. Stearic (C18) and most of the shorter chain saturated fatty acids (less than 12 carbons) do *not* raise blood cholesterol.

REFERENCES

Introduction—A New Look at Health
1. Gutteridge, J.M.C. and Halliwell, B. *Antioxidants in Nutrition, Health, and Disease* 1994. Oxford: Oxford University Press. pg 23

Chapter 1—Dietary Fats and Oils
1. *Science News*, 1990. Trans fats: worse than saturated? 138(8):126
2. Mensink, R. P. and Katan, M.B. 1990. Effect of dietary trans fatty acids on high-density and low-density lipoprotein cholesterol levels in healthy subjects. *N. Eng. J. Med.* 323(7):439
3. Raloff, J. 1996. Unusual fats lose heart-friendly image. *Science News* 150(6):87
4. Kummerow, F.A. 1975. *Federation Proceedings* 33:235
5. Mensink, R. P. and Katan, M.B. 1990. Effect of dietary trans fatty acids on high-density and low-density lipoprotein cholesterol levels in healthy subjects. *N. Eng. J. Med.* 323(7):439
6. *Science News*, 1990. Trans fats: worse than saturated? 138(8):126
7. Willett, W. C., et al. 1993. Intake of trans fatty acids and risk of coronary heart disease among women. *Lancet* 341(8845):581.
8. Thampan, P.K. 1994. *Facts and Fallacies About Coconut Oil.* Jakarta: Asian and Pacific Coconut Community, pg 20
9. Booyens, J. and Louwrens, C.C. 1986. The Eskimo diet. Prophylactic effects ascribed to the balanced presence of natural cis unsaturated fatty acids and to the absence of unnatural trans and cis isomers of unsaturated fatty acids. *Med. Hypoth.* 21:387
10. Kritchevsky, D., et al, 1967. *Journal of Atherosclerosis Research* 7:643
11. Schell, O. 1985. *Modern Meat.* New York: Vintage Books. pg 254-268
12. Cornellussen, P.E. 1969. Pesticide residues in total diet. *Pesticides Monitoring Journal* 2:140-152
13. Regenstein, L. 1982. *How to Survive in America the Poisoned.* Herndon, VA: Acropolis Books, pg 273
14. Cornellussen, P.E. 1969. Pesticide residues in total diet. *Pesticides Monitoring Journal* 2:140-152

Chapter 2— Oxidation and Free Radicals
1. Gutteridge, J.M.C., and Halliwell , B. 1994. *Antioxidants in Nutrition, Health, and Disase.* Oxford: Oxford University Press, pg 7
2. Passwater, R. A. 1985. *The Antioxidants.* New Canaan, CT: Keats Publishing
3. Passwater, R. A. 1992. *The New Superantioxidant—Plus.* New Canaan, CT: Keats Publishing, pg 15
4. Gutteridge, J.M.C. and Halliwell, B. 1994. *Antioxidants in Nutrition, Health, and Disease.* Oxford: Oxford University Press, pg 38
5. Ibid. pg 10
6. Ibid pg 112
7. Breimer, L.H. 1988. *British Journal of Cancer* 57:6
8. Gutteridge, J.M.C. and Halliwell, B. 1994. *Antioxidants in Nutrition, Health, and Disease.* Oxford: Oxford University Press, pg 13
9. Aruoma, O.I. and Halliwell, B. eds. 1991. *Free Radicals and Food Additives.* London: Taylor and Francis
10. Kaur, H. and Perkins, M.J.1991. *Free Radicals and Food Additives.* Aruoma, O.I. and Halliwell, B. eds. London: Taylor and Francis, pg 31-33
11. Halliwell, B.1991. *Free Radicals and Food Additives.* Aruoma, O.I. and Halliwell, B. eds. London: Taylor and Francis, pg 38
12. Gutteridge, J.M.C. and Halliwell, B. 1994. *Antioxidants in Nutrition, Health, and Disease.* Oxford: Oxford University Press, pg 113
13. Reddy, K. K. 1994. Serum lipid peroxides and lipids in urban and rural Indian men. *Archives of Environmental Health.* 49(2):123
14. Gutteridge, J.M.C. and Halliwell, B. 1994. *Antioxidants in Nutrition, Health, and Disease.* Oxford: Oxford University Press, pg 115
15. Ibid. pg 117
16. Cheraskin, D. 1993. *Vitamin C: Who Needs It.* Birmingham, Al: Arlington Press, pg 2, 9
17. Ames, B.N. 1983. *Science.* 221:1256
18. Alexander, J.C. et al. 1987 *Journal of Toxicology and Environmental Health* 21:295
19. Passwater, R. A. 1985. *The Antioxidants.* New Canaan, CT: Keats Publishing
20. Meffert, H. and Lohrisch, I. 1971. Inhibition of respiration byproducts of lipid peroxidation. *Derm. Mschr.* 157:793
21. Gutteridge, J.M.C. and Halliwell, B. 1994. *Antioxidants in Nutrition, Health, and Disease.* Oxford: Oxford University Press, pg 14
22. Walford, R.L. 1986. *The 120 Year Diet: How to Double Your Vital Years.* New York: Simon & Schuster
23. Wilson, R. B. 1976. *CRC Critical Reviews in Food Science and Nutrition* 8:325
24. Alexander, J.C. 1983. *Xenobiotics in Foods and Feeds*, Finley, J.W. and Schwass, D.E. eds. ACS Symposium Series 234 pg 129-148, Washington, DC. American Chemical Society
25. Carew, T.E., et al. 1987. *Proceedings of the National Academy of Sciences of the USA*, 84:7725
26. McGee, C. T. 1993. *Heart Frauds: The Misapplication of High Technology in Heart Disease*, Coeur d'Alene, ID: MediPress, pg 162
27. Ross, R. 1993. The pathogenesis of arherosclerosis: A perspective for the 1990s. *Nature* 362:801
28. Warburg, O. 1956. On the Origin of Cancer Cells, *Science* 123:309
29. Goldblatt, H. 1953. Induced malignancy in cells from rat myocardium subjected to intermittent anaerobiosis during long propagation in vitro. *J. Exp. Med.* 97:525

Chapter 3—Vegetable Oils
1. Peat, R. *Ray Peat's Newsletter.* 1997 Issue, pg 3
2. Wallach, J. and Lan, M. 1994. *Rare Earths.* Bonita, CA: Double Happiness Publishing
3. Addis, P.B. and Warner, G. J. 1991. *Free Radicals and Food Additives.* Aruoma, O.I. and Halliwell, B. eds. London: Taylor and Francis, pg 77
4. Begin, M.E. 1990. Fatty acids, lipid peroxidation and diseases. *Proc. Nutr. Soc.* 49:261
5. Loliger, J. 1991. *Free Radicals and Food Additives.* Aruoma, O.I. and Halliwell, B. eds. London: Taylor and Francis, pg 121
6. Liebman, B. and Hurley, J. 1993. The heart of the matter. *Nutrition Action Healthletter.* 20(8), pg 1
7. Carroll, K.K. and Khor, H.T. 1971. *Lipids*, 6:415
8. Mascioli, E.A., et al. 1987. *Lipids.* 22 (6) 421
9. C.J. Meade and J. Martin. 1978. *Adv. Lipd. Res.* 127. Cited by Ray Peat, *Ray Peat's Newsletter.* 1997 Issue, pg 3
10. Ip, C., et al.1985. *Cancer Res.* 45
11. Naji and French. 1989. *Life Sciences.* 44
12. Kramer, J.K.G., et al. 1983. *Lipids.* 17:372. Cited by Ray Peat, *Ray Peat's Newsletter*, 1997 Issue, pg 3
13. Davis, G. P. and Park, E. 1984. *The Heart: The Living Pump.* New York: Torstar Books, pg 81
14. Raloff, J. 1993. Saturated fats may foster lung cancer. *Science News.* 144(23):373
15. Carroll, K.K. and Khor, H.T. 1971. Effects of level and type of dietary fat on incidence of mammary tumors induced in female sprague-dawley rats by 7, 12-dimethylbenzanthracene. *Lipids* 6:415
16. Wilson, R.B., et al. 1977. Dimethylhydrazine-induced colon tumors in rats fed diets containing beef fat or corn oil with and without wheat bran. *Amer. J. Clin. Nutr.* 30:176
17. Kramer, J.K.G., et al. 1983. *Lipids.* 17:372. Cited by Ray Peat, *Ray Peat's Newsletter*, 1997 Issue, pg 3
18. Harman, D., et al. 1976. Free radical theory of aging: effect of dietary fat on central nervous system function. *Journal of the American Geriatrics Society* 24(7): 301
19. Lea, C.H. 1962. The oxidative deterioration of food lipids, in *Symposium on Foods: Lipids and Their Oxidation*, ed. by H.W. Schultz, E.A. Day and R.O. Sinnhuber. Westport, CT: Avi Publ. Co., pg 3-28

20. Harman, D. et al. 1976. Free radical theory of aging: effect of dietary fat on central nervous system function. *Journal of the American Geriatrics Society.* 24(7): 301

21. Rizek, R.L., et al. 1974. Fat in today's food supply: level of use and sources. *J. Amer. Oil Chem. Soc.* 51:244

22. Sirtori, C.R., et al. 1986. Controlled Evaluation of fat intake in the Mediterranean Diet. *Am. J. Clin. Nutr.* 44(5):635

23. Belitz, H.D. and Grosch, W. 1987. *Food Chemistry,* 2nd Ed. Translated by D. Hadziyev, Berlin: Springer-Verlag, pg 480

24. *Atherosclerosis, Thrombosis and Vascular Biology.* November, 1997. Cited in High fat indulgence invites strokes and clots. *Energy Times* March, 1998

Chapter 4—Essential Fatty Acids

1. Burr, G.O. and Burr, M.M. 1929. A new deficiency disease produced by the rigid exclusion of fat from the diet. *J. Biol. Chem.* 82:345

2. Zamula, E. 1986. The Greenland Diet: can fish oils prevent heart disease? *FDA Consumer* 20:6

3. Cunnane, S.C. 1996. The Canadian Society for Nutritional Sciences 1995 Young Scientist Award Lecture: Recent studies on the synthesis, beta-oxidation, and deficiency of linoleate and alpha-linolenate: are essential fatty acids more aptly named indispensable or conditionally dispensable fatty acids? *Can. J. Physiol. Pharmacol.* 74:629

4. Whitney, E.N., et al. 1991.*Understanding Normal and Clinical Nutrition,* 3rd Ed. St. Paul, MN: West Publishing Co. pg 112

5. Peat, R. *Ray Peat's Newsletter,* Membrane Issue. pg 1

6. W.H.O./F.A.O. 1977. Dietary fats and oils in human nutrition, Report of an Expert Consultation U.N. Food and Agriculture Organization Rome

7. Zamula, Evelyn 1986. The greenland diet: can fish oils prevent heart disease? *FDA Consumer* 20:6

8. Kromhout. D, 1985. *New England Journal of Medicine.* 312:1206

9. Lindner, L. 1990. FDA cracks down on fishy ads: those oil pills aren't a cure-all. *American Health* 9(9):91

10. *Annals of Internal Medicine.* May 1988. pg 663. Cited in *Harvard Medical School Health Letter,* 1989. 14(10):5

11. *Atherosclerosis.* March 1988. pg 73. Cited in *Harvard Medical School Health Letter,* 1989, 14(10):5

12. Simon, H. 1990. The scales of evidence: eating fish cuts heart attacks, but fish oils may not. *American Health* 9(6):91

13. Ibid

14. Burr, M.L., et al. 1989. Effects of changs in fat, fish, and fibre intakes on death and myocardial infarction. *Lancet* 2:757

15. Christine, M. A. et al. 1998. Fish consumption and risk of sudden cardiac death. *JAMA* 279(1):23

16. Shekelle, R.B., et al. 1985. Fish consumption and mortality from coronary heart disease. *N. Engl. J. Med.* 313:820

17. Daviglus, M.L., et al. 1997. Fish consumpiton and the 30-year risk of fatal myocardial infarction. *N. Engl. J. Med.* 336:1046

18. Kromhout, D. et al. 1995. The protective effect of a small amount of fish on coronary heart disease mortality in an elderly population. *Int. J. Epidemiol.* 24:340

19. Ascherio, A., et al. 1995. Dietary intake of marine n-3 fatty acids, fish intake, and the risk of coronary disease among men. *N. Engl J. Med.* 332:978

20. Morris, M.C., et al. 1995. Fish consumption and cardiovascular disease in the Physicians' Health Study: A prospective study. *Am. J. Epidemiol.* 142:166

21. Curb, J.D. 1985. Fish consumption and mortality from coronary heart disease. *N. Engl. J. Med.* 313:821

22. Vollset, S.E., et al. 1985. Fish consumption and mortality from coronary heart disease. *N. Engl J. Med.* 313:820

23. Kremmer, J., et al. 1987. Fish-oil acid supplementation in active rheumatoid arthritis. *Ann. Intern. Med.* 106(4):497

24. Van der Tempel, et al. 1990. Effects of fish oil supplementation in rheumatoid arthritis. *Ann. Rheum. Dis.* 49(2):76

25. Kremer, J.M., et al. 1990. Dietary fish oil and olive oil supplementation in patients with rheumatoid arthritis. *Arthritis Rheum.* 33(6):810

26. *Tufts University Diet and Nutrition Letter.* Should you begin taking fish oil supplements? January 1987, pg 2

27. Albers, C. M., et al. 1998. Fish consumption and risk of sudden cardiac death. *JAMA* 279(1):23

28. Siscovick, D.S., et al. 1995. Dietary intake and cell membrane levels of long-chain n-3 polyunsaturated fatty acids and the risk of primary cardiac arrest. *JAMA* 274:1363

29. deKoning, A.J. and Milkovitch, S. 1989. The storage behavior of a number of fish oil health capsules at ambient temperature. *S.A.J. Food Sci. Nutr.* 1:7

30. Aruoma, O.I. and Halliwell, B. eds. 1991. *Free Radicals and Food Additives.* London: Taylor and Francis

31. Marwick, C. 1989. What to do about dietary saturated fats? *JAMA* 262 (4):453

32. Rivers, J.P.W. and Hassam, A.G. 1975. Defective essential fatty acid metabolism in cystic fibrosis. *Lancet* 2:642

33. Horrobin, D.F. 1980. The regulation of prostaglandin biosynthesis; negative feedback mechanisms and the selective control of formation of 1 and 2 series prostaglandins: relevance to inflammation and immunity. *Medical Hypotheses* 6:687

34. Horrobin, D.F. 1980. Prostaglandins and schizophrenia. *Lancet* 1:706

35. Whealan, J. 1997. Polyunsaturated fatty acids: Signalling agents for intestinal cancer. *Nutr. Today* 32(5):213

36. Craig-Schmidt, M., et al. 1993. Menhaden, coconut, and corn oils and mammary tumor incidence in BALB/c virgin female mice treated with DMBA. *Nutrition & Cancer* 20 (2):99

37. Carroll, K.K. and Khor, H.T. 1971. Effects of level and type of dietary fat on incidence of mammary tumors induced in female sprague-dawley rats by 7, 12-dimethylbenzanthracene. *Lipids* 6:415

38. Boorman, G.A., et al. 1987. *Toxicol. pathol.* 15(4):451

39. Sakai, K. and Okuyama, H. 1994. Fatty acid compositions of plasma lipids in atopic dermatitis/asthma patients. *Jap. J. Allergol.* 43:37

40. Murry, M.J. 1995. Select dietary fatty acids attenuate cardiopulmonary dysfunction during acute lung injury in pigs. *Am. J. Physiol.* 269:2090

41. Ziboh, V.A. and Fletcher, M.P. 1992. Dose-response effects of dietary gamma-linolenic acid-enriched oils on human polymorphonuclear-neutrophil biosynthesis of leukotriene B4. *Am. J. Clin. Nutr.* 55:39

42. Jeffery, N.M., et al. 1996. The ratio of n-6 to n-3 polyunsaturated fatty acids in the rat diet alters serum lipid levels and lymphocyte function. *Lipids* 31(7):737

43. Ikemoto, S., et al. 1996. High-fat diet-induced hyperglycemia and obesity in mice: differential effects of dietary oils. *Metabolism* 45(12):1539

44. Bjerve, K.S., et al. 1987. Alpha-Linolenic Acid Deficiency in patients on long-term gastric-tube feeding: Estimation of linolenic acid and long-chain unsaturated n-3 fatty acid requirement in man. *Amer. J. Clin. Nutr.* 45:66

45. Wagner, W. and Nootbaar-Wagner, U. 1997. Prophylactic treatment of migraine with gamma-linolenic and alpha-linolenic acids. *Cephalalgia.* 17(2):127

46. Caughey, G.E., et al. 1996. The effect on human tumour necrosis factor alpha and interleukin 1-beta production of diets enriched in n-3 fatty acids from vegetable oil or fish oil. *Amer. J. Clin. Nutr.* 63(1):116

47. Jeffery, N.M., et al. 1996. The ratio of n-6 to n-3 polyunsaturated fatty acids in the rat diet alters serum lipid levels and lymphocyte function. *Lipids* 31(7):737

48. Inui, K., et al. 1996. The effect of alpha-linolenic acid-rich emulsion on fatty acid metabolism and leukotriene generation of the colon in a rat model with inflammatory bowel disease. *Ann. Nutr. Metab.* 40(3):175

49. Jeffery, N.M., et al. 1996. The ratio of n-6 to n-3 polyunsaturated fatty acids in the rat diet alters serum lipid levels and lymphocyte function. *Lipids* 31(7):737

50. Clark, W.F., et al. 1995. Flaxseed: A Potential Treatment for Lupus Nephritis. *Kidney Inter.* 48:475

51. Parbtani, A. and Klark, W.F. 1995. Flaxseed and its components in renal disease. In: *Flaxseed in Human Nutrition.* ed. S.C. Cunnane and L.U. Thompson. Champaign, IL: AOCS Press, pg 245-260

52. Frances, H. et al. 1996. Effect of dietary alpha linolenic acid deficiency on habituation. *Life Sci.* 58(21):1805

53. Delion, S., et al. 1994. Chronic dietary alpha-linolenic acid deficiency alters dopaminergic and serotoninergic neurotransmission in rats. *J. Nutr.* 124(12):2466

54. Stordy, B.J. 1995. Benefit of docosahexaenoic acid supplements to dark adaptation in adult dyslexics. *Lancet* P385, 346:8971

55. Stevens, L.J., et al. 1995. Essential fatty acid metabolism in boys with attention-deficiet hyperactivity disorder. *Am. J. Clin. Nutr.*1995:761

56. Carroll, K.K. and Khor, H.T. 1971. Effects of level and type of dietary fat on incidence of mammary tumors induced in female sprague-dawley rats by 7, 12-dimethylbenzanthracene. *Lipids* 6:415

57. Purasiri, P., et al. 1994. Modulation of cytokine production in vivo by dietary essential fatty acids in patients with colorectal cancer. *Clin. Sci.* 87:711

58. Kinsella, J.E., Effects of polyunsaturated fatty acids on factors related to cardiovascular disease. *Am J Cardiol.* 1987; 60(12):23G

59. Cunnane, S.C. 1995. Metabolism and function of alpha-linolenic acid in humans. In: *Flaxseed in Human Nutrition.* Ed. S.C. Cunnane and L.U. Thompson, AOCS Press, Champaign, IL. pg 99-127

60. Horrobin, D.F. 1990. Interactions between n-3 and n-6 essential fatty acids (EFAs). In: *Int. Symp. New Aspects Diet. Lipids: Benefits, Hazards, Use.* pg 11

61. Nelson, G.J. and Chamberlain, J.G. 1995. The effect of dietary alpha-linolenic acid on blood lipids and lipoproteins in humans. In: *Flaxseed in Human Nutrition,* ed. S.C. Cunnane and L.U. Thompson. Champaign, IL: AOCS Press, pg 187-206

62. Allman, M.A., et al. 1995. Supplementation with flaxseed oil versus sunflower seed oil in healthy young men consuming a low fat diet: Effects on platelet composition and function. *Europ J. Clin. Nutr.* 49(3):169

63. Mantzioris, J. E., et al. 1995. Differences exist in the relationships between dietary linoleic and a-linolenic acids and their respective long-chain metabolites. *Amer. J. Clin. Nutr.* 61:320

64. Boudreau, M.D., et al. 1991. Lack of dose response by dietary n-3 fatty acids at a constant ratio of n-3 and n-6 fatty acids in suppressing eicosanoid biosynthesis from arachidonic acid. *Am. J. Clin. Nutr.* 54:111

65. Horrobin, D.F. 1990. Interactions between n-3 and n-6 essential fatty acids (EFAs). In: *Int. Symp. New Aspects Diet. Lipids: Benefits, Hazards, Use.* pg11

66. Budowskik, P. and Crawford, M.A. 1985. Alpha-linolenic acid as a regulator of the metabolism of arachidonic acid: dietary implications of the ratio, n-6:n-3 fatty acids. *Proc. Nutr. Soc.* 44:221

67. Whitney, E.N., et al. 1991. *Understanding Normal and Clinical Nutrition,* 3rd Ed. St. Paul, MN: West Publishing Co. pg 123

68. Albers, C. M., et al. 1998. Fish consumption and risk of sudden cardiac death. *JAMA* 279(1):23

69. Ibid

70. Cunnane, S.C. 1995. Metabolism and function of alpha-linolenic acid in humans. In: *Flaxseed in Human Nutrition.* Ed. S.C. Cunnane and L.U. Thompson. Champaign, IL: AOCS Press, pg 99-127

71. Leaf, A. and Weber, P.C. 1988. Cardiovascular effects of n-3 fatty acids, *N. Engl. J. of Medicine* 318: 549

72. Whitney, E.N., et al. 1991. *Understanding Normal and Clinical Nutrition,* 3rd Ed. St. Paul, MN: West Publishing Co. pg 111

73. Peat, R. *Ray Peat's Newsletter* 1997 Issue. pg 4

74. Peat, R. *Ray Peat's Newsletter* Membrane Issue. pg 5

75. Sorisky, A. and Robbins, D.C. 1989. Fish oils and diabetes: The net effect. *Diabetes Care* 12(4):302

76. Marwick, C. 1989. What to do about dietary saturated fats? *JAMA* 262(4):453

77. Ibid

78. Budowskik P. and Crawford, M.A. 1985. Alpha-linolenic acid as a regulator of the metabolism of arachidonic acid: dietary implications of the ratio, n-6:n-3 fatty acids. *Proc. Nutr. Soc.* 44:221

79. Marwick, C. 1989. What to do about dietary saturated fats? *JAMA* 262(4):453

Chapter 5—The Facts on Flax

1. Albers, C. M., et al. 1998. Fish consumption and risk of sudden cardiac death. *JAMA* 279(1):23

2. Nestel, P.J., et al. 1997. Arterial compliance in obese subjects is improved with dietary plant n-3 fatty acid from flaxseed oil despite increased LDL oxidizability. *Arteriscler. Thromb. Vasc. Biol.* 17:6

3. Vijay Kumar, K. and Das, U.N. 1994. Lipid peroxides and essential fatty acids in patients with doronary heart disease. *J. Nutr. Med.* 4(1):33

4. Thompson, L.U., et al. 1996. Flaxseed and its lignan and oil components reduce mammary tumour growth at a late stage of carcinogenesis. *Carcinogenesis* 17 (6):1373

5. Fukui, H., et al. 1994. Physicochemical perturbation of a-linolenic acid related to cell proliferation. *Bull. Chem. Soc. Jpn.* 67:2213

6. deBravo, M.G., et al. 1994. Effects of dietary gamma and alpha linolenic acid on a human lung carcinoma grown in nude mice. *Med. Sci. Res.* 22:667

7. Devi, M.A. and Das, N.P. 1994 Antiproliferative effect of polyunsaturated fatty acids and interleukin-2 on normal and abnormal human lymphocytes. *Experientia* 50:489

8. Cantrill, R.C., et al., 1993 Concentration-dependent effect of iron on gamma-linolenic acid toxicity in ZR-75-1 human breast tumor cells in culture. *Canc. Lett.* 72:99

9. Das, U.N. 1995. Tumoricidal action of gamma-linolenic acid with particular reference to the therapy of human glioma. *Med. Sci. Res.* 23:507

10. Ramanathan, R., et al. 1994. Effects of Gamma-linolenic acid, flavonoids, and vitamins on cytotoxicity and lipid peroxidation. *Free Rad. Biol. Med.* 16:43

11. Das, U.N. 1992. Anti-cancer effects of cis-unsaturated fatty acids both in vitro and invivo. In : *Lipid-Soluble Antioxidants: Biochemistry and Clinical Applications.* Ong. A.S.H. and Packer, L., eds. Basel/Switzerland: Birkhauser Verlag, pg 482

12. Kumar, G.S. and Das, U.N. 1995. Free radical-dependent suppression of growth of mouse myeloma cells by alpha linolenic acid and eicosapentaenoic acids in vitro. *Cancer Lett.* 92:27

13. Ells, G.W., et al. 1996. Vitamin E blocks the cytotoxic effect of gamma-linolenic acid when administered as late as time of onset of cell death - insight into the mechanism of fatty acid induced cytotoxicity. *Cancer Lett.* 98:207

14. Ramanathan, R., et al. 1994. Effects of gamma-linolenic acid, flavonoids, and vitamins on cytotoxicity and lipid peroxidation. *Free Rad. Biol. Med.* 16:43

15. Levander, O.A. and Ager, A.L. 1995. Antimalarial effects of flaxseed and flaxseed oil. In: *Flaxseed in Human Nutrition.* ed. S.C. Cunnane and L.U. Thompson. Champaign, IL: AOCS Press, pg 237-243

16. Fukui, H., et al. 1994. Physicochemical perturbation of a-linolenic acid related to cell proliferation. *Bull. Chem. Soc. Jpn.* 67:2213

17. Rose, D.P., et al. 1995. Effects of linoleic and gamma-linolenic acid on the growth and metastasis of a human breast cancer cell line in nude mice and on its growth and invasive capacity in vitro. *Nutr. Cancer.* 24:33

18. DeVries, D.E.E. and Van Noorden, C.J.F., 1992. Effects of dietary fatty acid composition on tumor growth and metastasis. *Anticancer Res.* 12:1513

19. Levander, O.A. and Ager, A.L. 1995. Antimalarial effects of flaxseed and flaxseed oil. In: *Flaxseed in Human Nutrition.* ed. S.C. Cunnane and L.U. Thompson. Champaign, IL: AOCS Press, pg 237-243

20. Thompson, L., et al. 1994. Inhibitory effect of polyunsaturated fatty acids on the growth of *Helicobacter pylori*: a possible explanatin of the effect of diet on peptic ulceration. *Gut* 35:1557

21. Madhavi, N., et al. 1994. Supression of human T-cell growth in vitro by cis-unsaturated fatty acids: Relationship to free radicals and lipid peroxidation. *Prostagland. Leukotri. Ess. Fatty Acids* 51:33

22. DeMarco, D.M. et al. 1994. Effects of fatty acids on proliferation and activation of human synovial compartment lymphocytes. *J. Leukocyte Biol.* 56:612

23. Madhavi, N., et al. 1994. Supression of human T-cell growth in vitro by cis-unsaturated faty acids: relationship to free radicals and lipid peroxidation. *Prostagland. Leukotri. Ess. Fatty Acids* 51:33

24. DeMarco, D.M. et al. 1994. Effects of fatty acids on proliferation and activation of human synovial compartment lymphocytes. *J. Leukocyte Biol.* 56:612

25. Kelley, D.S., et al. 1991. Dietary alpha-linolenic acid and immuno-competence in humans. *Amer. J. Clin. Nutr.* 53:40

26. Ingram, A.J., et al. 1995. Effects of flaxseed and flax oil diets in a rat-5/6 renal ablation model. *Amer. J. Kidney Dis.* 25(2):320

27. Kelley, D.S. 1995. Immunomodulatory effects of flaxseed and other oils rich in alpha-linolenic acid. In: *Flaxseed in Human Nutrition.* ed. S.C. Cunnane and L.U. Thompson. Champaign, IL: AOCS Press, pg 147-163

28. Raloff, J. 1989. Fish oil slows some developing cancers. *Science News* 135(25):390

29. Peat, R. *Ray Peat's Newsletter* 1997 Issue, pg 3

30. Mascioli, E.A. et al. 1987. *Lipids* 22(6):421. Cited by Ray Peat, *Ray Peat's Newsletter* 1997 Issue, pg 3

31. C.J. Meade and J. Martin, 1978. *Adv. Lipid Res.* 127. Cited by Ray Peat, *Ray Peat's Newsletter* 1997 Issue, pg 3

32. Yetiv, J.Z. 1988. *Clinical applications of fish oils.* JAMA 260(5):665

33. Whitney, E.N., et al. 1991. *Understanding Normal and Clinical Nutrition,* 3rd Ed. St. Paul, MN: West Publishing, pg 257

34. Haung, Y-S., et al. 1996. In vivo and in vitro metabolism of linoleic and gamma-linolenic acids. In: *Gamma-linolenic Acid: Metabolism and Its Roles in Nutriton and Medicine.* Huang, Y-S. and Mills, D.E. eds. Champaign, IL: AOCS Press, pg 84-105

35. Phinney, S. 1994. Potential risk of prolonged gamma-linolenic acid use. *Ann. Intern. Med.* 120:692

36. Barre, D.E., et al. 1993. The effect of borage oil supplementation on human platelet aggregation, thromboxane B2, prostaglandin E1 and E2 formation. *Nutr. Res.* 13:739

37. Barre, D.E. and Holub, B.J. 1992. The effects of borage oil consumption on human plasma lipid levels and the phosphatidylcholine and cholesterol ester composition of high density lipoprotein. *Nutr. Res.* 12:1181

38. Johnson, P.V. 1995. Flaxseed oil and cancer: alpha-linolenic acid and carcinogenesis. In: *Flaxseed in Human Nutrition.* ed. S.C. Cunnane and L.U. Thompson. Champaign, IL: AOCS Press, pg 207-218

39. Cunnane, S.C., et al. 1994. Nutritional attributes of traditional flaxseed in healthy young adults. *Amer. J. Clin. Nutr.* 61:62

40. Aldercreutz, H. and Mazur, W. 1997. Phytoestrogens and Western diseases. *Ann. Med.* 29:95

41. Ingram , D., et al. 1997. Case-control study of phytoestrogens and breast cancer. *Lancet* 350(9083):990

42. Rickard, S.E. 1997. Healtheffects of flaxseed mucilage, lignans. *INFORM* 8(8):860

43. Knight, D.C. and Eden, J.A. 1996. A review of the clinical effects of phytoestrogens. *Obstet. Gynecol.* 87:897

44. Classen, N. et al. 1995. The effect of different n-6/n-3 essential fatty acid ratios on calcium balance and bone in rats. *Prosta. Leukot. Essent. Fatty Acids.* 53(1):13

45. Cunnane, S.C., et al. 1993. High a-linolenic acid flaxseed: Some nutritional properties in humans. *Brit. J. Nutr.* 69:443

46. Bricklin, M. 1993. The facts on flax: Could this be the new, super cholesterol fighter? *Prevention* 45(8):37

Chapter 6—The Polyunsaturated Cow

1. Cunnane, S.C. 1996. The Canadian Society for Nutritional Sciences 1995 Young Scientist Award Lecture: Recent studies on the synthesis, beta-oxidation, and deficiency of linoleate and alpha-linolenate: are essential fatty acids more aptly named indispensable or conditionally dispensable fatty acids? *Can. J. Physiol. Pharmacol.* 74:629

2. Crayer, D.L. and Brown, J.B.J. 1943. *Biol Chem.* 151:427

3. Prior, I.A., et al. 1981. Cholesterol, coconuts, and diet on Polynesian atolls: a natural experiment: the Pukapuka and Tokelau island studies. *Am. J. Clin. Nutr.* 34(8):1552

4. Kummerow, F.A. 1975. Lipids in atherosclerosis. *J. Food Sci.* 40:12

5. Reichlmayr-Lais, A.M., et al. 1994. Fatty acid composition of brain and heart of rats fed various dietary oils. *Nutr. Res.* 14:829

6. Chapkin, R.S. and Carmichael, S.L. 1990. Effects of dietary n-3 and n-6 polyunsaturated fatty acids on macrophage phosphoipid classes and subclasses. *Lipids* 25:827

7. Cherian, G. and Sim, J.S. 1995. Dietary alpha-linoleic acid alters the fatty acid composition of lipid classes in swine tissues. *J. Agric. Food Chem.* 43(11):2911

8. Oomah, B.D. and Mazza, G. 1995. Functinal properties, uses of flaxseed protein. *INFORM.* 6(11):1246

9. Cherian, G. and Sim, J.S. 1995. Dietary alpha-linoleic acid alters the fatty acid composition of lipid classes in swine tissues. *J. Agric. Food Chem.* 43(11):2911

10. Budowski, P., and Crawford, M.A. 1985. Alpha-linolenic acid as a regulator of the metabolism of arachidonic acid: dietary implications of the ratio, n-6:n-3 fatty acids. *Proceedings of the Nutrition Society* 44:221

11. Gutteridge, J.M.C. and Halliwell, B. 1994. *Antioxidants in Nutrition, Health, and Disease.* Oxford: Oxford University Press, pg 79

12. Renee, D.R.M., et al. 1993. Lipid Peroxidation of phospholipid liposomes is influened by their fatty acid composition. *Am. J. Clin. Nutr.* 57(5):8185

13. Gutteridge, J.M.C. and Halliwell, B. 1994. *Antioxidants in Nutrition, Health, and Disease.* Oxford: Oxford University Press, pg 113

14. Ziboh, V.A. and Miller, C.C. 1990. Essential fatty acids and polyunsaturated fatty acids significance in cutaneous biology. *Ann. Rev. Nutr.* 10:433

15. Brod, J., et al. 1988. Evolution of lipid composition in skin treated with black currant seed oil. *Int. J. Cosmetic Sci.* 10:149

16. *Free Radical Biology and Medicine* Vol. 22, Is. 7, 1997. Vitamin E and melanoma. As reported in *Life Extension* pg 30 Nov. 1997

17. Passwater, R.A. 1985. *The Antioxidants.* New Canaan, CT: Keats Publishing, pg 10-11

18. Burk, K., et al. 1992. The effects of topical and oral l-selenomethionine on pigmentation and skin cancer incidence by ultraviolet irradiation. *Nutrition and Cancer* 17:123

19. Delver, E and Pence, B. 1993. Effects of dietary selenium level on uv-induced skin cancer and epidermal zntioxidant status. *FASEB Journal* 7:A290

20. Epstein, J.H. 1977. Effets of beta-carotene on ultraviolet induced cancer formation in the Harless mouse skin. *Photochem Photobiol* 25:211

21. *Life Extension.* December 1997, pg 5-8

22. Thibodeau, G.A., and Patton, K.T. 1992. *The Human Body in Health and Disease.* St. Louis: Mosby-Year Book, pg 355-366

23. Kappus, H. 1991. *Free Radicals and Food Additives.* Aruoma, O.I. and Halliwell, B. eds, London: Taylor and Francis, pg 69

24. Bateson-Koch, C., 1994, *Allergies: Disease in Disguise.* Burnaby, BC: Alive Books pg 39-41

25. Madhavi, N., et al. 1994 Supression of human T-cell growth in vitro by cis-unsaturated fatty acids: relationship to free radicals and lipid peroxidation. *Prostagland. Leukotri. Ess. Fatty Acids* 51:33

26. DeMarco, D.M., et al. 1994. Effects of fatty acids on proliferation and activation of human synovial compartment lymphocytes. *J. Leukocyte Biol.* 56:612

27. Jeffery, N.M., et al. 1996. The ratio of n-6 to n-3 polyunsaturated fatty acids in the rat diet alters serum lipid levels and lymphocyte function. *Lipids* 31(7):737

28. Inui, K., et al. 1996. The effect of alpha-linolenic acid-rich emulsion on fatty acid metabolism and leukotriene generation of the colon in a rat model with inflammatory bowel disease. *Ann. Nutr. Metab.* 40(3):175

29. Clark, W.F., et al. 1995. Flaxseed: A potential treatment for lupus nephritis. *Kidney Inter.* 48:475

30. Parbtani, A. and Klark, W.F. 1995. Flaxseed and its components in renal disease. In: *Flaxseed in Human Nutrition.* ed. S.C. Cunnane and L.U. Thompson. Champaign, IL: AOCS Press, pg 245-260

31. Ingram, A.J., et al. 1995. Effects of flaxseed and flax oil diets in a rat-5/6 renal ablation model. *Amer. J. Kidney Dis.* 25(2):320

32. Kelley, D.S. 1995. Immunomodulatory effects of flaxseed and other oils rich in alpha-linolenic acid. In: *Flaxseed in Human Nutrition.* ed. S.C. Cunnane and L.U. Thompson. Champaign, IL: AOCS Press, pg 147-163

33. Caughey, G.E., et al. 1996. The effect on human tumour necrosis factor alpha and interleukin 1-beta production of diets enriched in n-3 fatty acids from vegetable oil or fish oil. *Amer. J. Clin. Nutr.* 63(1):116

34. Jeffery, N.M., et al. 1996. The ratio of n-6 to n-3 polyunsaturated fatty acids in the rat diet alters serum lipid levels and lymphocyte function. *Lipids* 31(7):737

35. Inui, K., et al. 1996. The effect of alpha-linolenic acid-rich emulsion on fatty acid metabolism and leukotriene generation of the colon in a rat model with inflammatory bowel disease. *Ann. Nutr. Metab.* 40(3):175
36. Jeffery, N.M., et al. 1996. The ratio of n-6 to n-3 polyunsaturated fatty acids in the rat diet alters serum lipid levels and lymphocyte function. *Lipids* 31(7):737
37. Clark, W.F., et al. 1995. Flaxseed: A potential treatment for lupus nephritis. *Kidney Inter.* 48:475
38. Parbtani, A. and Klark, W.F. 1995. Flaxseed and its components in renal disease. In: *Flaxseed in Human Nutrition.* ed. S.C. Cunnane and L.U. Thompson. Champaign, IL: AOCS Press, pg 245-260
39. Wright, S. and Bolton, C. 1989. Breast milk fatty acids in mothers of children with atopic eczema. *British J. Nutr.* 62:693
40. Innis, S.M. 1993. Essential fatty acid requirements in human nutrition. *Can. J. Phys. Pharma.* 71:699
41. Saarinen, U.M., et al. 1979. Prolonged breat feeding as prophylaxis for atopic disease. *Lancet* 11:163
42. Midwinter, R.E., et al. 1982. Infant feeding and atopou. *Lancet* 1:339

Chapter 7—The Cholesterol Controversy

1. McGee, C.T. 1993. *Heart Frauds: The Misapplication of High Technology in Heart Disease.* Coeur d'Alene, ID: MediPress, pg 67
2. Liebman, B. 1999. Solving the diet-and-disease puzzle. *Nutriton Action Health Letter* 26(4):6
3. Rosenberg, H. *The Doctor's Book on Vitamin Therapy.* New York: Putnam, pg 308
4. Krumholz, H.M. 1994. Lack of association between cholesterol and coronary heart disease and morbidity and all-cause mortality in persons older than 70 years. *JAMA* 272:1335
5. Addis, P.B. and Warner, G.J. 1991. *Free Radicals and Food Additives.* Aruoma, O.I. and Halliwell, B. eds. London: Taylor and Francis, pg 79
6. Gutteridge, J.M.C. and Halliwell, B. 1994. *Antioxidants in Nutrition, Health, and Disease.* Oxford: Oxford University Press, pg 126
7. Ibid. pg 23
8. McCully, K.S. 1997. *The Homocysteine Revolution.* New Canaan, CT: Keats Publishing, pg 38
9. Napier, K.1995. Partial absolution. *Harvard Health Letter.* 20(10):1
10. *Life Extension* November 1997. HDL not protective, pg 31
11. White, P. D.1971. *Prog Cardiovascular Dis.* 14:249
12. *Statistical Abstracts of the United States*, United States Department of Commerce. Cited by McGee, C. T. 1993. *Heart Frauds: The Misapplication of High Technology in Heart Disease.* Coeur D'alene, ID: MediPress. pg 69-71
13. Addis, P.B. and Warner, G.J. 1991. *Free Radicals and Food Additives.* Aruoma, O.I. and Halliwell, B. eds. London: Taylor and Francis, pg 87
14. Ignatovsky, M.A. 1908. Influence de la nourriture animale sur l'organisme des lapins. *Archives of Experimental Medicine and Pathological Anatomy* 20:1
15. Ignatovsky, M.A. 1909. Uber die wirkung des tierischen eiweisses auf die aorta und die parenchymatosen organe der kaninschen. *Virchow's Archive for Pathological Anatomy, Physiology and Clinical Medicine,* 198:248
16. Anitschkow, N. and Chalatow, S. 1913. Uber experimentelle cholesterinsteatose und ihre bedeutung fur die entstehung einiger pathologische prozesse, *Centralblatt fur Allgemeine Pathologie und Pathologische Anatomie* 24:1
17. Hausman, P. 1981. *Jack Sprat's Legacy—The Science and Politics of Fat and Cholesterol*, New York: Richard Mauk Publishers, pg 53-61
18. Gutteridge, J.M.C. and Halliwell, B. 1994. *Antioxidants in Nutrition, Health, and Disease.* Oxford: Oxford University Press. pg 23
19. McGee, C. T. 1993. *Heart Frauds: The Misapplication of High Technology in Heart Disease.* Coeur d'Alene, ID: MediPress, pg 72
20. Fallon, S.1996. Why butter is good for you, *Consumers' Research,* 79(3):10
21. Nichols, A.B. 1976. *JAMA* 236:1948
22. Davis, G.P. and Park, E.1984. *The Heart: The Living Pump.* New York: Torstar Books
23. Wilson, E.N. 1969. *Among the Shoshones.* Salt Lake City, UT: Bookcraft
24. Prior, I.A. et al. 1981. Cholesterol, coconuts, and diet on Polynesian atolls: a natural experiment: the Paukapuka and Tokelau island studies. *American Journal of Clinical Nutrition* 34 (8):1552
25. *Medical World News* June 7, 1982
26. Moore, Thomas, 1989. *Heart Failure.* New York: Touchstone
27. McCully, K.S. 1997. *The Homocysteine Revolution.* New Canaan, CT: Keats Publishing. pg 48
28. McGee, C. T. 1993. *Heart Frauds: The Misapplication of High Technology in Heart Disease.* Coeur d'Alene, ID: MediPress, pg 81-82
29. McCully, Kilmer S. 1990. Atherosclerosis, serum cholesterol and the homocysteine theory: a study of 194 consecutive atutpsies. *American Journal of the Medical Sciences* 299:217
30. Naito, H.K. and Hoff, H.F. 1983 Jeffrey Bland, ed., *Medical Applications of Clinical Nutrition.* New Canaan, CT: Keats Publishing. Chapter 7
31. Fallon, S. and Enig, M.G. 1996. Diet and heart disease: not what you think, *Consumers' Research,* 79(7):15
32. Gutteridge, J.M.C. and Halliwell, B. 1994. *Antioxidants in Nutrition, Health, and Disease.* Oxford: Oxford University Press, pg 128
33. Mann, G. 1977. Diet-heart: end of an era, *New England Journal Of Medicine* 297:664
34. Mann, G. 1978. *American Heart Journal* 96:569
35. Fallon, S. and Enig, M.G. 1996. Diet and heart disease: not what you think, *Consumers' Research,* 79(7):15
36. Moore, T.J. 1989. The cholesterol myth. *Atlantic Monthly,* September.
37. Fallon, S. and Enig, M.G. 1996. Diet and heart disease: not what you think, *Consumers' Research,* 79(7):15
38. Brisson, G.J. 1981. *Lipids in Human Nutrition,* Englewood NJ: Jack K. Burgess
39. Ravaskov, U. 1992. *British Medical Journal* 305:15
40. Addis, P.B. and Warner, G.J. 1991. *Free Radicals and Food Additives.* Aruoma, O.I. and Halliwell, B. eds, Taylor and Francis London pg81
41. Heimlich, Jane. 1990. *What Your Doctor Won't Tell You.* New York: Harper Perennial
42. McGee, C. T. 1993. *Heart Frauds: The Misapplication of High Technology in Heart Disease.* Coeur d'Alene, ID: MediPress, pg 202
43. Ibid. pg 97
44. *The New York State Medical Journal.* 1958. 59:2343
45. Yudkin, J. 1972. *Sweet and Dangerous.* New York: Bantam
46. Ornish, D. 1990. *Dr. Dean Ornish's Program for Reversing Heart Disease.* New York: Random House. Chapter 3
47. Ibid. Chapter 1
48. Blankenhorn, D.H., et al. 1987. Beneficial effects of combined colestipol-niacin therapy on coronary atherosclerosis and coronary venous bypass grafts. *JAMA* 257:3223
49. Brown, B.G., et al. 1989. Niacin or lovastatin, combined with colestipol, regress coronary atherosclerosis and prevent clinical events in men with elevated apolipoprotein B. *Circulation* 80(4):II-266
50. Ornish, D. 1990. *Dr. Dean Ornish's Program for Reversing Heart Disease.* New York: Random House. Chapter 3
51. Ibid. Chapter 1
52. Addis, P.B. and Warner, G.J. 1991. *Free Radicals and Food Additives.* Aruoma, O.I. and Halliwell, B. eds. London: Taylor and Francis, pg 78
53. Hully, Stephen, et al. 1992. Childhood cholesterol screening: Contraindicated. *JAMA* 267:100
54. Fallon, S. and Enig, M.G. 1996. Diet and heart disease: not what you think, *Consumers' Research,* 79(7):15
55. Willis, R. A., et al. 1990. Lovastatin decreases coenzyme Q levels in rats. *Proceedings of the National Academy of Sciences* USA 87:8928
56. Cleave, T.L. 1985. *Lancet* May 11, pg 1085
57. Biss, L., et al.1971. *New England Journal of Medicine* 284:694
58. Walker, A.R.P., et al. 1978. *British Medical Journal* 1:1336
59. Leaf, A. 1975. *Youth in Old Age.* New York: McGraw Hill
60. Benet, Sula, 1976. *How to Live to Be 100.* New York: Dial Press
61. Drury, R.A. 1976. *Tropical and Geographic Medicine* 24:385
62. Smith, et al. 1976. *Tropical Medicine and Hygiene* 25:(4):637
63. Gsel, D., et al. 1962. *American Journal of Clinical Nutrition* 10:471

64. Cohen, J.C., et al. 1962. *Lancet* 2:1399

65. Biss, K, et al. 1971. *New England Journal of Medicine* 284:694

66. Marmot, M.G. 1975. Epidemiologic studies of coronary heart disease and stroke in Japanese men. *American Journal of Epidemiology* 102:511

67. Davis, G.P. and Park, E. 1984. *The Heart: The Living Pump*. New York: Torstar Books, pg 81

68. *The Colorado Springs Gazette*. Heart disease the leading cause of death worldwide, study finds. May 3, 1997

69. Malhotra. 1967. *American Journal of Clinical Nutrition* 20:462-75

70. Fallon, S. 1996. Why butter is good for you. *Consumers' Research* 79(3):10

71. Whitney, E.N. 1991. *Understanding Normal and Clinical Nutrition*, 3rd Ed. St. Paul, Mn: West Publishing, pg 881

72. Gutteridge, J.M.C. and Halliwell, B. 1994. *Antioxidants in Nutrition, Health, and Disease*. Oxford: Oxford University Press, pg 129

73. Cathcart, M.K., et al. 1985. *Journal of Leukocyte Biology* 38:341

74. MacDougall, D.B., et al. 1965. The effects of certain C27 steroids on organ cultures of rabbit aortas, *British Journal of Experimental Pathology* 46:549

75. Passwater, R. 1992. *The New Superantioxidant—Plus*. New Canaan CT: Keats Publishing, pg 22

76. Imai, H., et al. 1976. Angiotoxicity and atherosclerosis due to contaminants of USP-grade cholesterol, *Archives of Pathology and Laboratory Medicine* 100:565

77. Steinberg, D., et al.1989. Beyond Cholesterol. *N. Engl. J. of Medicine* 320:915

78. Addis, P.B. and Warner, G.J. 1991. *Free Radicals and Food Additives*. Aruoma, O.I. and Halliwell, B. eds. London: Taylor and Francis, pg 112

79. Steinberg, D., et al. 1989. Beyond cholesterol: modifications of low-density lipoprotein that increase its atherogenicity. *N. Engl. J. of Medicine* 320:915

80. Addis, P.B. and Warner, G.J. 1991. *Free Radicals and Food Additives*. Aruoma, O.I. and Halliwell, B. eds. London: Taylor and Francis, pg 78

81. McGee, C. T.1993. *Heart Frauds: The Misapplication of High Technology in Heart Disease*, MediPress, Coeur d'Alene, ID, pg 130-131

82. Addis, P.B. and Park, S.W. 1989. *Food Toxicology. A Perspective on the Relative Risks* Taylor, S.L. and Scanlan, R.A. eds. New York: Marcel Dekker. pg 297-330

83. McGee, C. T. 1993. *Heart Frauds: The Misapplication of High Technology in Heart Disease*. Coeur d'Alene, ID: MediPress, pg 155-156

84. McCully, K.S. 1997. *The Homocysteine Revolution*. New Canaan, CT: Keats Publishing, pg 51

85. Sampsidis, N. 1983. *Homogenized!* Glenwood Landing, NY: Sunflower Publishing. pg 5

86. Fallon, S. and Enig, M.G. 1996. Diet and heart disease: not what you think, *Consumers' Research*, 79(7):15

87. Harman, D. 1969. Prolongation of life; role of free radical reactions in aging. *J. Am. Geriatrics Soc.* 17:721

88. *American Journal of Clinical Nutrition* 1967. 20: 462-75

89. Ornish, D., 1990. *Dr. Dean Ornish's Program for Reversing Heart Disease*. New York: Random House. Chapter 3

90. Ibid. Chapter 1

91. Thampan, P.K.1994. *Facts and Fallacies About Coconut Oil*. Jakarta: Asian and Pacific Coconut Community, pg 17

92. Rose, G.A. 1965. *British Medical Journal* 1:1531

93. *Atherosclerosis, Thrombosis and Vascular Biology*. Nov 1997 as reported in *Energy Times* March 1998, Nutritional news, pg 12

94. *Lancet*. 1997. From what will we die in 2020? 349:1263

95. Fernandex, N.A. 1975. Nutrition in Puerto Rico. *Cancer Res.* 35:3272

96. Martinex, I., et al.1975. Cancer incidence in the United States and Puerto Rico. *Cancer Res.* 35:3265

97. Moore, T.J. 1989. The cholesterol myth. *Atlantic Monthly* September, pg 37

98. Ibid

99. Ibid

100. *The Colorado Springs Gazette* February 7, 1999. High cholesterol can be very bad, but not enough isn't good either

101. Suarez, E. 1999. *Psychosomatic Medicine* May/June as reported in *The Colorado Springs Gazette*, June 1, 1999

102. Sampsidis, N. 1983. *Homogenized!* Glenwood Landing, NY: Sunflower Publishing, pg.3

Chapter 8—Saturated Fat

1. Budowski, P. and Crawford, M.A. 1985. Alpha-linolenic acid as a regulator of the metabolism of arachidonic acid: dietary implications of the ratio, n-6:n-3 fatty acids. *Proceedings of the Nutrition Society* 44:221

2. Simon, H. 1990. The scales of evidence: eating fish cuts heart attacks, but fish oils may not, *American Health* 9(6):91

3. Yamori, Y., et al. 1987. Pathogenesis and dietary prevention of cerebrovascular diseases in animal models and epidemiological evidence for the applicability in man. In: Yamori Y, Lenfant C eds. *Prevention of Cardiovascular Diseases: An Approach to Active Long Life*. Amsterdam, the Netherlands: Elsevier Science Puiblishers, pg 163-177

4. Ikeda, K., et al. 1987. Effect of milk protein and fat intake on blood pressure and incidence of cerebrovascular disease in stroke-prone spontaneously hypertensive rats (SHRSP). *J. Nutr. Sc.i Vitaminol.* 33:31

5. Kimura, N. 1985. Changing patterns of coronary heart disease, stroke, and nutrient intake in Japan. *Prev. Med.* 12:222

6. Omura, T., et al. 1987. Geographical distribution of cerebrovascular disease mortality and food intakes in Japan. *Soc Sci Med.* 24:401

7. McGee, D., et al. 1985. The relationship of dietary fat and cholesterol to mortality in 10 years. *Int. J. Epidemiol.* 14:97

8. Gillman, M. W., et al. 1997. Inverse association of dietary fat with development of ischemic stroke in men. *JAMA* 278(24):2145

9. Thampan, P.K. 1994. *Facts and Fallacies About Coconut Oil*. Jakarta: Asian and Pacific Coconut Community, pg 8

10. Kiyasu G.Y., et al. 1952. The portal transport of absorbed fatty acids. *Journal of Biological Chemistry* 199:415-19

11. Thampan, P.K. 1994. *Facts and Fallacies About Coconut Oil*. Jakarta: Asian and Pacific Coconut Community, pg 9

12. Ibid. pg 15

13. Geliebter, A. 1980. Overfeeding with a diet containing medium chain triglyceride impedes accumulation of body fat. *Clinical Research* 28:595A

14. Bray, G.A., et al. 1980. Weight gain of rats fed medium-chain triglycerides is less than rats fed long-chain triglycerides. *Int. J. Obes.* 4:27-32

15. Geliebter, A., et al. 1983. Overfeeding with medium-chain triglycerides diet results in diminished depositionof fat. *Am. J. Clin. Nutr.* 37:1-4

16. Thampan, P.K. 1994. *Facts and Fallacies About Coconut Oil*. Jakarta: Asian and Pacific Coconut Community, pg 1-2

17. Baba, N. 1982. Enhanced thermogenesis and diminished deposition of fat in response to overfeeding with diet containing medium chain triglyceride. *Am. J. of Clin. Nutr.* 35:678-82

18. Murray, M. T. 1996. *American Jouranal of Natural Medicine* 3(3):7

19. Hill, J.O., et al. 1989. Thermogenesis in man during overfeeding with medium chain triglycerides. *Metabolism* 38:641-8

20. Seaton, T.B., et al. 1986. Thermic effect of medium-chain and long-chain triglycerides in man. *Am. J. of Clin. Nutr.* 44:630-4

21. Peat, R. *Ray Peat's Newsletter* 1997 Issue, pg 2-3

22. *Encyclopedia Briticanica Book of the Year*, 1946. Cited by Ray Peat, *Ray Peat's Newsletter*, 1997 Issue, pg 4

23. Hegsted, D.M., et al. 1965. Qualitative effects of dietary fat on serum cholesterol in man. *Am. J. of Clin. Nutrition* 17:281

24. Hashim, S.A., et al. 1959. Effect of mixed fat formula feeding on serum cholesterol level in man. *Am. J. of Clin. Nutr.* 1:30

25. Bray, G.A., et al. 1980. Weight gain of rats fed medium-chain triglycerides is less than rats fed long-chain triglycerides. *Int. J. Obes.* 4:27-32.

26. Geliebter, A. 1983. Overfeeding with medium-chain triglycerides diet results in diminished deposition of fat. *Am. J. of Clin. Nutr.* 37:104

27. Baba, N. 1982. Enhanced thermogenesis and diminished deposition of fat in response to ovefeeding with a diet containing medium chain triglycerides. *Am. J. of Clin. Nutr.* 35:678

28. Greenberger, N.J. and Skillman, T.G. 1969. Medium-chain triglycerides: physiologic considerations and clinical implications. *N. Engl. J. Med.* 280:1045-58

29. Fino, J.H. 1973. Effect of dietary triglyceride chain length on energy utilized and obesity in rats fed high fat diets. *Fed. Proc.* 32:993

30. Sindhu Rani, J.A., et al, 1993. Effect of coconut oil and coconut kernel on serum and tissue lipid profile. *Ind. Coco. J.* XXIV(7):2

32. Thampan, P.K. 1994. *Facts and Fallacies About Coconut Oil.* Jakarta: Asian and Pacific Coconut Community. pg 31

33. Ibid. pg 31

34. Hornung, B., et al. 1994. Lauric acid inhibits the maturation of vesicular stomatitis virus. *Journal of General Virology* 75:353

35. Wan, J.M. and Grimble, R.F. 1987. Effect of dietary linoleate content on the metabolic response of rats to Escherichia coli endotoxin. *Clinical Science* 72(3):383-5

36. Ibid

37. Thampan, P.K. 1994. *Facts and Fallacies About Coconut Oil.* Jakarta: Asian and Pacific Coconut Community, pg 4-5

38. Wickremasinghe, R.L.1994. Coconut oil, not the villain. *Cocoinfo International* 1(2):6

39. Brod, J., et al. 1988. Evolution of lipid composition in skin treated with black currant seed oil. *Int. J. Cosmetic Sci.* 10:149

40. Prior, I.A. 1981. Cholesterol, coconuts, and diet on Polynesian atolls: a natural experiment: the Pukapuka and Tokelau island studies. *Am. J. of Clin. Nutr.* 34 (8): 1552-61

41. Stanhope, J.M., et al. 1981.The Tokelau Island migrant study. Serum lipid concentrations in two environments. *J. Chron. Dis.* 34:45

42. Ibid

43. Prior, I.A.1981. Cholesterol, coconuts, and diet on Polynesian atolls: a natural experiment: the Pukapuka and Tokelau island studies. *Am. J. of Clin. Nutr.* 34 (8): 1552-61

44. Blonz, Edward R. Scientists revising villain status of coconut oil. *Oakland Tribune* Jan 23, 1991

45. Heimlich, J. 1990. *What Your Doctor Won't Tell You.* New York: Harper Perennial

46. Spencer, P. L. 1995. Fat faddists. *Consumers' Research* 78(5):43

Chapter 9—Nutrition and Physical Degeneration

1. Brennan, R.O. 1975. *Nutrigenetics.* New York: M. Evans and Co, Inc. pg 43ff

2. McGee, C. T. 1993. *Heart Frauds: The Misapplicatin of High Technology in Heart Disease.* Coeur d'Alene, ID: MediPress, pg 182

3. Trowell, H. C. *Executive Health,* Nov. 1977

4. Price, Weston, 1945. *Nutrition and Physical Degeneraton.* New Canaan, CT: Keats Pub.

5. Schaefer, O. 1971.When the Eskimo comes to town. *Nutrition Today,* Nov/Dec, pg 8-16

6. Prior, I.A.M. 1971. The price of civilization. *Nutriton Today,* July/Aug, pg 2-11

7. Fife, B. 1997. *The Healing Crisis.* Colorado Springs: HealthWise, pg 31-35

8. Fallon, S. 1996. Why butter is good for you. *Consumers' Research* 79(3):10

Chapter 10—The Antioxidant Connection

1. Brandt, J. *The Grape Cure.* Yonkers, NY: Ehret Literature Publishing CO.

2. Ibid. pg 109-110

3. Rosquist, L. 1993. *Dr. Lamar Rosquist and Pycnogenol.* audiotape

4. Halvorson, G. A. 1994. *Pycnogenols—Nature's Superstar Antioxidant.* audiotape

5. Passwater, R. A. 1985. *The Antioxidants.* New Canaan, CT: Keats Publishing

6. Ibid

7. Ibid

8. Gaziano, J. M. 1990. *Circulation* 82:111

9. *Life Extension* December 1997. Following the best science, pg 5-8.

10. Ibid. pg 6

11. Gaby, A.G.1983. *American Journal of Holistic Medicine* 5:107

12. Passwater, R. A. 1985. *The Antioxidants.* New Canaan, CT: Keats Publishing

13. Stampfer, M. J., et al. 1993. Vitamin E consumption and the risk of coronary disease in women. *N. Eng. J. Med.* 328:1444

14. Gazis, A., et al. 1997. *British Medical Journal.* 324(7098):1845

15. Passwater, R. 1992. *The New Superantioxidant—Plus.* New Canaan, CT: Keats Publishing, pg 22

16. Gey, K. Fred, et al. 1991. *American Journal of Clinical Nutrition* 53:326S

17. Passwater, R. A. 1985. *The Antioxidants.* New Canaan, CT: Keats Publishing

18. Stampfer, M.J., et al. 1993. Vitamin E consumption and the risk of coronary disease in women. *N. Eng. J. Med.* 328:1444

19. Rimm, E.B., et al. 1993. Vitamin E consumption and the risk of coronary heart disease in men. *N. Eng. J. Med.*328:1450

20. Lieberman, S. and Bruning, N. 1990. *The Real Vitamin & Mineral Book.* Garden City Park, NY: Avery Publishing Group. Chapter 8

21. Ethridge, E. Brain food, *Energy Times,* October 1997, pg 65

22. Harman, D., et al. 1976. Free radical theory of aging: effect of dietary fat on central nervous system function. *Journal of the American Geriatrics Society* 24 (7):301

23. Whitney, E. N., et al.1991. *Understanding Normal and Clinical Nutrition,* 3rd Ed. St Paul , MN: West Publishing Company. Chapter 9

24. Shamberger, R.J. 1976. *Federation proceedings* 35:578 abstract #2016

26. Ibid. pg 10

27. Lieberman, S. and Bruning, N. 1990. *The Real Vitamin & Mineral Book.* Garden City Park, NY: Avery Publishing Group, pg 170

28. Ibid. pg 171

29. Bland, J. 1984. *Bioflavonoids: The Feiends and Helpers of Vitamin C in Many Hard-To-Treat Ailments.* New Canaan, CT: Keats Publishing. pg 8

30. Ibid. pg 7

31. Passwater, R. 1992. *The New Superantioxidant—Plus.* New Canaan, CT: Keats Publishing. pg 8-9

32. St. Leger, A.S., 1979. Eighteen country study of mortality due to ischemic heart disease. *Lancet* 1017, May 12

33. Fay-Morgan, A. 1957. Protective effect of wine in laboratory animals fed a cholesterol-enriched diet. *Amer. J. Physiol.* 189:290

34. *Life Extension* Dec. 1997. pg 7

35. Yu, C.L. and Swaminathan, B. 1987. Mutagenicity of proanthocyanidins *Food Chem. Toxicol.* 25 (2):135-9

36. Lauffer, R.B. 1991. *Iron and Your Heart.* New York: St. Martin's Press. Chapter 2

37. Salonen, J.T., et al. 1991. *American Journal of Clinical Nutrition* 53(5):1222

38. Esterbauer, H., et al. 1989. In:Vitamin E: biochemisty and Health Implications. Diplock, A. et al. eds, *Ann N.Y. Acad. Sci* pg 254-67

39. Passwater, R. 1992. *The New Superantioxidant—Plus.* New Canaan, CT: Keats Publishing, pg 23

Chapter 11— Iron and Your Health

1. Hill, H.A.O.1981. *Philosophical Transactions of the Royal Society of London, Series B* 294:119

2. Gutteridge, J.M.C. and Halliwell, B. 1994. *Antioxidants in Nutrition, Health, and Disease.* Oxford: Oxford University Press, pg 113

3. Jiun, Y.S. and Hsien, L. 1994. Lipid peroxidation in workers exposed to lead. *Archives of Environmental Health* 49(4):256

4. Halliwell, B. and Gutteridge, J.M.C.1986. *Archives of Biochemistry and Biophysicis,* 246:501

5. McLaren, G.D., et al, 1983. *CRC Critical Reviews in Clinical Laboratory Science,* 19:205

6. Gutteridge, J.M.C. and Halliwell, B. 1994. *Antioxidants in Nutrition, Health, and Disease.* Oxford: Oxford University Press, pg 36

7. McGee, C. T. 1993. *Heart Frauds: The Misapplicatin of High Technology in Heart Disease.* Coeur d'Alene, ID: MediPress, pg 146

8. Lauffer, R.B. 1991. *Iron and Your Heart.* New York: St. Martin's Press

9. Ibid

10. Bothwell, T, H., et al. 1979. *Iron Metabolism in Man.* Oxford: Blackwell Scientific Publications

11. Lauffer, R.B. 1991. *Iron and Your Heart.* New York: St. Martin's Press. Chapter 2

12. Ibid. pg 20

13. Cook, J.D., et al. 1976. Evaluation of the Iron Status of a Population. *Blood* 48:449

14. Casale, G., et al. 1981. Serum Ferritin and Ageing. *Age and Ageing* 10:119

15. Leggett, B.A., et al. 1990. Factors Affecting the Concentrations of Feritin in Serum in a healthy Australian population. *Clinical Chemistry* 36:1350

16. Lauffer, R.B. 1991. *Iron and Your Heart*. New York: St. Martin's Press. Chapter 2

17. Gutteridge, J.M.C. and Halliwell, B. 1994. *Antioxidants in Nutrition, Health, and Disease*. Oxford: Oxford University Press. pg 75

18. Cross, C.E., et al. 1987. Oxygen radicals and human disease, *Ann. Int. Med.* 107:526

19. Lauffer, R.B. 1991. *Iron and Your Heart*. New York: St. Martin's Press Chapter 2

20. Ibid. Chapters 10 and 11

21. McCord, J.M. 1996. Effects of positive iron status at a cellular level. *Nutrition Reviews* 54(3):85, 1996

22. Halliwell, B. 1987 *FASEB Journal* 1:456

23. Gutteridge, J.M.C. and Halliwell, B. 1994. *Antioxidants in Nutrition, Health, and Disease*. Oxford: Oxford University Press, pg 115

24. Brody, J.E. 1989. Countering the myth that women have little to fear from heart disease. *New York Times*, February 2, 1989 pg B7

25. Braunwald, E. ed. 1988. *Heart Disease: A Textbook of Cardiovascular Medicine*. Philadelphia: W.B. Saunders. Chapter 36

26. Gordon, T., et al. 1976. Menopause and risk of cardiovascular disease: The Framingham Study. *Ann. Intern, Med.* 85:447

27. Sullivan K.L. 1989. The Iron Paradigm of Ischemic Heart Disease. *American Heart Journal* 117:1177

28. Fraser, G.E. 1988. Determinants of ischemic heart disease in Seventh-Day Adventists: A review. *Am. J. Clin. Nutr.* 48:833

29. Sullivan, J.L., et al. 1983. Vegetarianism, ischemic heart disease, and iron, *Am. J. Clin.Nutr.* 37: 882

30. Lauffer, R.B. 1991. *Iron and Your Heart*. New York: St. Martin's Press

31. Gutteridge, J.M.C. and Halliwell, B. 1994. *Antioxidants in Nutrition, Health, and Disease*. Oxford: Oxford University Press, pg 32

32. Cohen, L. A. 1987. Diet and Cancer. *Scientific American* 257:42

33. Irving, D. and Drasar, B.S. 1973. Fibre and Cancer of the Colon. *British Journal of Cancer* 28:462

34. Chapman, R.W., et al. 1983. Hepatic iron uptake in alcoholic liver disease. *Gastroenterology* 84:143

35. Friedman, I.M., et al.1988. Elevated serum iron concentration in adolescent alcohol users. *American Journal of Diseases of Children* 142:156

36. Harman, D. 1986. Free radical theory of aging: role of free radicals in the origination and evolution of life, aging, and disease processes, In: *Free Radicals, Aging and Degenerative Diseases*. New York: Alan R. Liss, pg 3-50

37. Cross, C.E., et al. 1987. Oxygen radicals and human disease. *Ann. Intern. Med.* 107:526

38. Katz, M.L. and Robison, W.G. 1986. Nutritional influences on autoxidation, lopofuscin accumulation, and aging, In: *Free Radicals, Aging, and Degenerative Diseases*. New York: Alan R. Liss, pg 221-262

39. Marzabadi, et al. 1988. Effect of ferric iron and desferrioxamine on lipofuscin accumulation in cultured rat heart myocytes. *Mech. Ageing Devel.* 46:145

Chapter 12—The Homocysteine Revolution

1. Newburgh, L.H. and Clarkson, S. 1923. The production of atherosclerosis in rabbits by feeding diets rich in meat. *Archives of Internal Medicine* 31:653

2. Newburgh, L.H. and Marsh, P.L. 1925. Renal injuries by amino acids. *Archives of Internal Medicine*, 36:682

3. Rinehart, J.F. and Greenberg, L.D. 1956. Vitamin B-6 deficiency in the Rhesus monkey with particular reference to the occurrence of atherosclerosis, dental caries and hepatic cirrhosis. *Am. J. of Clin.Nutrition*, 4:318

4. Mushett, C.W. and Emerson, G. 1956. Atherosclerosis in pyridoxine-deficient monkeys and dogs. *Federation Proceedings* 15:526

5. McCully, K. S. 1997. *The Homocysteine Revolution*. New Canaan, CT: Keats Publishing, pg 33

6. Mann, G.V. 1968. Blood changes in experimental primates fed purified diets: pyridoxine and riboflavin deficiency. *Vitamins and Hormones* 26:465

7. Case Records of the Massachusetts General Hospital, Case 19471, 1933. Marked cerebral symptoms following a limp of three months' duration. *N. Eng. J. Med.* 209:1063

8. McCully, K. S. 1997. *The Homocysteine Revolution*. New Canaan, CT: Keats Publishing, pg 87

9. McCully, K.S. and Ragsdale, B.D. 1970. Production of atherosclerosis by homocysteinemia. *American Journal of Pathology* 61:1

10. McCully, K. S. 1997. *The Homocysteine Revolution*. New Canaan, CT: Keats Publishing. pg 80

11. Ibid. pg 115

12. Donahue, S., et al. 1974. Atherosclerosis due to homocysteinemia. Failure to reproduce the model in weaning rabbits. *Americna Journal of Pathology* 77:167

13. Mitchell, T. The resurrection of Kilmer McCully. *Life Extension* 21, Nov. 1997

14. Kuzuya, F. and Yoshimine, N. 1978. Homocysteine theory of atherosclerosis, *Domyakukoka (Journal of Japan Atherosclerosis Society)* 6:135

15.Brattstrom, L.E. et al.1984. Moderate homocysteinemia—a possible risk factor for arteriosclerotic cerebrovascular disease. *Stroke* 15:1012

16. Wilcken, David E. and Wilcken, B. 1976. The pathogenesis of coronary artery disease. A possible role for methionine metabolism. *Journal of Clinical Investigation* 57:1079

17. Boushey, C.J., et al. 1995. A quantitative assessment of plasma homocysteine as a risk factor for vascular disase. *JAMA* 274:1049

18. Stampfer, M.J., et al. 1992. A prospective study of plasma homocysteine and risk of myocardial infarction in U.S. physicians. *JAMA* 268:877

19. Selhub, J., et al. 1995. Association between plasma homocysteine concentrations and extracranial carotid artery stenosis. *N. Engl. J. of Med.* 332: 286

20. McCully, K. S. 1997. *The Homocysteine Revolution*. New Canaan, CT: Keats Publishing, pg 22

21. Clarke, R., et al. 1991. Hyperhomocysteinemia as an independent risk factor for vascular disease. *N. Engl. J. of Med.* 324:1149

22. Ubbink, J.D., et al. 1991. The prevalence of homocysteinemia and hypercholesterolemia in angiographically defined coronary heart disease. *Klinische Wochenschrift* 69:527

23. McCully, K. S. 1997. *The Homocysteine Revolution*. New Canaan, CT: Keats Publishing, pg 48

24. *Nutrition Reviews* . 1967.Vitamin status of cardiac patients. 25:116

25. Selhub, J., et al. 1993. Vitamin status and intake and primary determinants of homocysteinemia in an elderly population. *JAMA* 270:2693

26. Robinson, K., et al.1995. Hyperhomocysteinemia and low pyridoxal phosphate. Common and independent reversible risk factors for coronary artery disease. *Circulation* 92:2825

Chapter 13—Meat, Eggs, and Dairy

1. Ornish, D. 1990. *Dr. Dean Ornish's Program for Reversing Heart Disease*. New York: Random House. Chapter 10

2. Allen, L.H. 1982. Calcium bioavailability and absorption: A review. *Am. J. Clin. Nutr.* 35:783

3. Morter, M.T., Jr. 1990. *Your Health Your Choice*. Hollywood, FL: Lifetime Books

4. Murry, F. 1995.*The Big Family Guide to All the Minerals*. New Canaan, CT: Keats Publishing. pg 147-171

5. Crawford, T., et al. 1967. *Lancet* 1:229

6. DeCarli, C., et al. 1986. Serum magnesium levels in symptomatic atrial fibrillation and their relation on rhythm control by intravenous digoxin. *American Journal of Cardiology* 57:956

7. Reinhart, R., et al. 1985. Hypomagnesemia in patients entering the ICU. *Critical Care Medicine* 13(6):506

8. Altura, B.M.1980. *Medical Tribune* Aug. 20, pg 3

9. Parsons, R.S., et al. 1959. *Medical Proceedings* 5:487

10. Peticone, F., et al. 1988 Protective magnesium treatment in ischemic dilated cardiomyopathy, *Journal of the American College of Nutrition* 7:403

11. Brodsky, M.S. 1992. Magnesium, myocardial infarction and arrhythmias. *Journal of the American College of Nutrition* 11(5)607/ Abstract 36

12. Shechter, M., et al. 1992. Rationale of magnesium supplementation in acute myocardial infarction: A review of the literature. *Archives of Internal Mediciane* 152:2189

13. Brodsky, M.S.1992. Magnesium, myocardial infarction and arrhythmias. *Journal of the American College of Nutrition* 11(5)607/ Abstract 36

14. Murry, F. 1995. *The Big Family Guide to All the Minerals*. New Canaan, CT: Keats Publishing, pg 160

15. McCully, K.S. 1997. *The Homocysteine Revolution*. New Canaan, CT: Keats Publishing, pg 154

16. Malmos, H. The relation of Nutrition to Health, *Acta Med. Scand.* 1950

17. Spencer, P.L. 1995. Fat faddists. *Consumers' Research* 78(5):43

18. Ibid

19. Fallon, S. 1996. Why cholesterol is good for you. *Consumers' Research* 79(3):13

20. Oster, K.A. 1973. St. Vincent Park City Hospitals Medical Bulletin March 1973. Cited by Sampsidis, N. 1983. *Homogenized!* Glenwood Landing , NY: Sunflower Publishing

21. Sampsidis, N. 1983. *Homogenized!* Glenwood Landing, NY: Sunflower Publishing, pg 22

22. Sander, B.D., et al. 1989. *Journal of Food Protection*. 52:109

23. Park, S.W. and Addis, P.B. 1987. *Journal of Food Science*, 52:1500

24. Addis, P.B. and Park, S.W. 1989. *Food Toxicology. A Perspective on the Relative Risks* Taylor, S.L. and Scanlan, R.A. eds.New York: Marcel Dekker, pg 297-330

25. Mitchell, T. The resurrection of Kilmer McCully. *Life Extension* 21, Nov. 1997

Chapter 14—How to Stop Premature Aging and Degenerative Disease

1. Kaunitz, H. 1983. *Coconuts Today* 1(2):27

2. Chan, J.K., et al. 1993. Effect of dietary a-linolenic acid and its ratio to linoleic acid on platelet and plasma fatty acids and thrombogenesis. *Lipids* 28:811

3. Wolff, S.P. and Dean, R.T.1987. *Biochemical Journal* 245:243

4. Nygard, O., et al. 1995. Total plasma homocysteine and cardiovascular risk profile. The Hordaland homocysteine study. *JAMA* 274:1526

5. Harman, D. 1971. Free radical theory of aging: Effect of the amount and degree of unsaturation of dietary fat on mortality rate. *J. Geront.* 26:451

6. Lieberman, S. and Bruning, N. 1990. *The Real Vitamin and Mineral Book*. Garden City Park, NY: Avery Publishing Group, pg 146

7. Leon, A. 1987. Leisure-time physical activity levels and risk of coronary heart disease and death, *JAMA* 258:2388

8. Ginsburg, G.S. et al. 1996. Effects of a single bout of ultraendurance exercise on lipid levels and susceptibility of lipids to peroxidation in triathletes. *JAMA* 276(3):221

SUGGESTED READING

Cholesterol and Your Health—the Great American Rip-Off! Chris Mudd, 1990: American Lite Company.

The Cholesterol Conspiracy. Russell Smith, 1991: Warren H. Green, Inc.

The Cholesterol Hoax. Sheldon Zerden, 1997: Bridger House Publications, Inc.

Dr. Kennith H. Cooper's Antioxidant Revolution. Kennith H. Cooper, 1997: Thomas Nelson Pub.

Free Radicals, Aging and Degenerative Diseases. D. Harman, 1986: Alan R. Liss.

Heart Frauds: The Misapplication of High Technology in Heart Disease. Charles T. McGee, 1993: MediPress.

Heart Failure: A Critical Inquiry Into the Revolution in Heart Care. Thomas J. Moore, 1989: Random House.

The Homocysteine Revolution. Kilmer S. McCully, 1997: Keats Publishing.

Iron and Your Heart. Randall B. Lauffer, 1991: St. Martin's Press.

Nutrition and Physical Degeneraton. Weston Price, 1945: Keats Publishing.

Racketeering in Medicine: The Suppression of Alternatives. James Carter, 1992: Hampton Roads Pub.

Sunlight Could Save Your Life. Zane R. Kime,1980: World Health Publications

INDEX

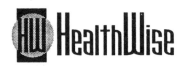

Additional Resources
to Help You Improve
Your Health

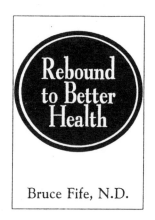

Rebound
to Better
Health

Bruce Fife, N.D.

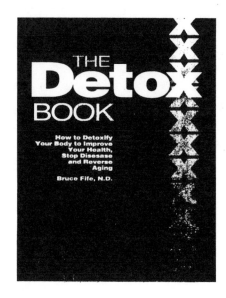

REBOUND TO BETTER HEALTH

by Bruce Fife, ND

Rebound exercise is known as *the most efficient, most effective form of exercise ever devised by man.* With a simple rebounder (mini-tramp) you have a device that is equal to *all* the fancy machines and equipment found in a gymnasium or health spa. This little trampoline will do it all for you, and in most cases, more effectively too. You can gain all the benefits of running without suffering from injuries caused by pounding on a hard surface. Studies by NASA scientists have shown that rebounding is 68% *more* effective than jogging, and yet requires *less* effort! You can also develop both upper and lower body strength just as effectively as weight lifting—without the strain or threat of pulled or torn muscles. Rebounding has been shown to out perform swimming as an all round exercise. Even the elderly and crippled can rebound to better health. And you can do it all in the privacy of your own home.

Rebound exercise is the only form of exercise that is capable of building physical strength, as well as help reverse degenerative health conditions. Rebounding enhances the immune system in a way that is unlike any other form of exercise. Many people suffering from a variety of degenerative conditions have achieved better health using this unique form of exercise. No other exercise can compare, because they all lack an essential element found only in rebounding.

On this audio tape you will learn about the miraculous benefits of rebound exercise and why it's used by professional athletes to build strength and improve coordination. You will learn about a lady crippled by arthritis and confined permanently to a wheelchair who was able to regain the strength and mobility in her legs and become active again. You will see how it helped reverse the effects of heart disease in an elderly couple and gave them back their lives. You will also learn how it's been used as an effective tool against osteoporosis. You will discover *why* it is called the most efficient, most effective, and most beneficial form of exercise ever devised by man and, best of all, you will learn what it can do for you.

THE DETOX BOOK
How to Detoxify Your Body to Improve Your Health, Stop Disease, and Reverse Aging

by Bruce Fife, ND

We live in a toxic world. Environmental pollution and disease-causing germs assault us continually day after day. Our food is nutrient deficient and our water supply dangerously contaminated. People today are exposed to chemicals in far greater concentrations than were previous generations. Thousands of tons of man-made chemicals and industrial pollutants are poured into our environment and our food supply daily.

With such a massive attack on our health we should all be sick from toxic overload. And we are! In no other time in the history of the world has degenerative disease been as prominent as it is today. Diseases that were rare or unheard of a century ago are now raging upon us like a plague. Millions are dying from diseases that were virtually unknown in the past.

Nature, however, has provided us with the solution. Our bodies are amazingly resilient. If the disease-causing toxins are removed, the body will heal itself. This book outlines the steps you need to take to thoroughly detoxify and cleanse your body from these disease-causing agents. You will also learn how to reduce your toxic exposure and how to strengthen your immune system.

Through detoxification you will free yourself from the chains of pain, reverse degenerative conditions, gain more energy, feel and look younger, improve your memory, and be happier. Virtually all the diseases of modern society, including many infectious illnesses, can be avoided or even cured by sensible systematic detoxification.

Although we live in a toxic world we can take control of our health. This book will show you how.

Look for these informative resources at you local book or health food store. For a free catalog write to HealthWise Publications, P.O. Box 25203, Colorado Springs, CO 80936